T0248685

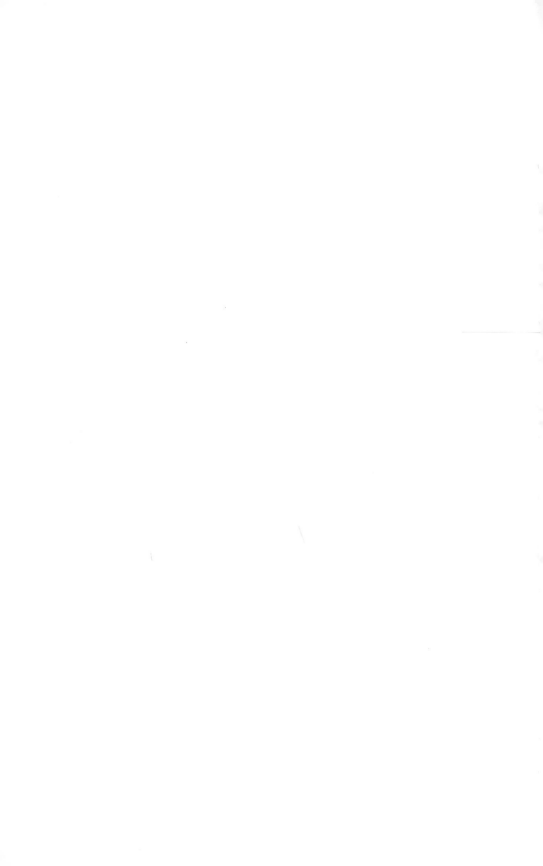

Psychiatric Disorders: New Insights

Psychiatric Disorders: New Insights

Edited by **Harvey Wilson**

New Jersey

Published by Foster Academics,
61 Van Reypen Street,
Jersey City, NJ 07306, USA
www.fosteracademics.com

Psychiatric Disorders: New Insights
Edited by Harvey Wilson

International Standard Book Number: 978-1-63242-336-8 (Hardback)

Printed in the United States of America.

Contents

Preface

Various studies have approached the subject by analyzing it with a single perspective, but the present book provides diverse methodologies and techniques to address this field. This book contains theories and applications needed for understanding the subject from different perspectives. The aim is to keep the readers informed about the progresses in the field; therefore, the contributions were carefully examined to compile novel researches by specialists from across the globe.

Psychiatric disorders are regarded as one of the most significant, serious and agonizing illnesses because of their universality, prevalence and burden inflicted on today's women and men. This deterioration of emotional, cognitive, or behavioral working is in few cases very disturbing. Apart from knowing the physical organic factors, like endocrinal illnesses, infections or head injuries, the aetiology of these disorders has stayed a question. However, current developments in neuroscience and psychiatry have been successful in uncovering following pathophysiology and encompassing related bio-psycho-social factors. The book contains current trends and advancements in psychiatry from across the globe, illustrated in the form of diverse and descriptive research chapters. The book covers addiction psychiatry, associated not only with socio-cultural but also biological changes. Towards the end, the book talks about Biological Neuropsychiatry, elucidating topics like clinical neuropsychiatric conditions, basic neuroscience and latest molecular biology. Undoubtedly, this book will serve as a valuable source for future growth and collaboration in the world of psychiatry.

Indeed, the job of the editor is the most crucial and challenging in compiling all chapters into a single book. In the end, I would extend my sincere thanks to the chapter authors for their profound work. I am also thankful for the support provided by my family and colleagues during the compilation of this book.

Editor

Part 1

Addiction Psychiatry

Drug Use Disorders and Recovery

Arthur J. Lurigio
Department of Psychology
Department of Criminal Justice
Loyola University Chicago
USA

1. Introduction

Drug abuse and dependence disorders are chronic but treatable brain diseases, involving compulsive drug-seeking and -using behaviors that persist despite immediate or potentially harmful consequences for users and their families and communities. Drug abuse and dependence are serious threats to public health and safety, costing hundreds of billions of dollars in yearly healthcare expenditures, crime, poor work productivity, and job loss (Hoffman & Fromeke, 2007). For example, illegal drug use in the United States cost nearly 200 billion dollars in 2002; approximately two-thirds of the costs (129 billion) were economic losses attributable to people's inability to work because of drug-precipitated illness, premature death, or incarceration. The treatment of the healthcare problems of drug addicts cost 16 billion dollars, while drug-related criminal justice and welfare costs totaled 36 billion dollars in 2002 (Office of National Drug Control Policy, 2004). Addiction also can result in intangible costs, such as homelessness, academic failure, and troubled relationships, and is one of the most pervasive and intransigent mental health disorders in the world, affecting the thoughts, feelings, and behaviors of millions of people annually (World Health Organization, 2004).

2. Drug effects and classification

Drugs are psychoactive substances that change moods and behaviors by altering brain chemistry and function (Hyman & Malenka, 2001). Drugs of abuse include medically prescribed (e.g., barbiturates and pain relievers), legal (e.g., alcohol and nicotine), and illegal (e.g., marijuana and heroin) substances. Some drugs, such as alcohol, have been used since ancient times, whereas others, such as methamphetamine and designer drugs (e.g., Ecstasy), are relatively new. People consume drugs to feel good (some drugs produce euphoria, confidence, and relaxation), to keep from feeling bad (some drugs combat anxiety, depression, and hopelessness), to accelerate performance (some drugs sharpen attention and enhance physical strength and athletic prowess), and to experience altered sensory perceptions (some drugs cause visual, auditory, or tactile hallucinations) (National Institute on Drug Abuse [NIDA], 2007).

Drugs of abuse can be classified into five groups according to effects. The first class consists of stimulants, which increase alertness and decrease fatigue; examples include amphetamines, Benzedrine, caffeine, Dexedrine, ephedrine, and nicotine. The second class consists of depressants, which reduce tension, alleviate nervousness, and induce sedation. Among these drugs are Nembutal, Seconal, Tunial, Veronal, Valium, and Xanax. The third class, hallucinogens, changes sensory perceptions; examples include cannabis, Lysergic Acid Diethylamide (LSD), Mescaline, Phencyclidine (PCP), and psilocybin. The fourth class consists of opiates, which induce sleep, euphoria, and relaxation as well as relieve pain and anxiety; opiates include codeine, heroin, opium, OxyContin, Percodan, and morphine. The fifth class consists of performance enhancers; they increase athletic strength and speed and stimulate the growth and recovery of skeletal muscles. Anadrol, Depo-Testosterone, Dianabol, and Winstrol are some examples of such performance enhancers (Abadinsky, 2007).

Drug abusers typically prefer one class of drugs over others. However, when they have difficulty obtaining their drug of choice, they often turn to other drugs in the same class that produce similar effects. Psychoactive drugs in the same class can be compared on the basis of their potency and efficacy. The potency of a drug is the amount that must be ingested to produce a desired effect whereas efficacy is a drug's ability to produce a desired effect regardless of dosage. Both the strength and the potency of a substance can determine an abuser's drug of choice as well as the drug's potential for abuse and dependence (see below) (NIDA, 2007).

3. The addictive process

Drug use can escalate to substance use disorders: abuse or dependence. The progression to uncontrolled use depends on several risk factors. For example, biological factors play a role in addiction; in other words, genetics can predispose a person to addictive behavior—a predisposition that is shared among close biological relatives. Scientists estimate that genes account for nearly half of a person's vulnerability to a substance use disorder (NIDA, 2007). Age of first use and psychiatric history are also important factors for explaining drug use problems. Younger users are more likely to become addicted because developing adolescent brains are more susceptible to a drug's ability to change brain chemistry and functions. Likewise, people with mental illness are also more likely to abuse or become dependent on drugs. In addition, a person's exposure to a parent's or a peer's use of drugs can increase his or her risk of addiction. The mode of drug ingestion can also raise the potential for abuse and dependence: a drug that is inhaled or injected is more addictive than one that is ingested orally. Inhalation and injection send the drug to the brain faster and produce more intense highs and lows. Drug-seeking behavior intensifies in response to the cycle of peaks and valleys that the user experiences (Hoffman & Fromeke, 2007).

Psychoactive drugs are thought to become addictive through their activation of the brain's mesocorticolimbic dopamine pathway, extending from the brain's ventral tegmental area to the nucleus accumbens to the frontal cortex. Drugs of abuse stimulate this pleasure circuit by increasing the amount of dopamine in the brain two- to ten-fold, creating an extremely pleasurable experience for users that compels them to repeat the incident. Drugs of abuse either mimic the effects of dopamine on neurotransmitters (i.e., they act as agonists) or block the re-absorption of dopamine so that it can continue to activate neurons (i.e., they act as antagonists). Eventually, the brain shuts down its own production of dopamine, causing the user to ingest the drug merely to stave off feelings of listlessness, depression, and other withdrawal symptoms. Drugs of abuse also affect the brain's frontal regions, impairing judgment and leading addicts to crave drugs even as the rewards of use steadily diminish. Hence, relapses—a return to drug use after a period of abstinence—are common among people with substance use disorders and can be triggered by stress, mood changes, and cues that remind the abuser of the substance (Karch, 2007; NIDA, 2007).

4. Substance use disorders

Substance abuse and dependence disorders are diagnosed according to criteria in the American Psychiatric Association's Diagnostic and Statistical Manual IV-TR (American Psychiatric Association, 2007). A substance abuse disorder is diagnosed when drug use in the previous 12 months has led to significant distress and impairment in functioning and meets at least one of several diagnostic criteria—namely, failure to fulfill obligations at work, school, or home; recurring use of substances in dangerous situations (e.g., driving while intoxicated); recurring substance use-related criminal justice involvement; and continued substance use that leads to interpersonal conflicts.

A drug-dependence disorder—more serious than a drug-abuse disorder—is diagnosed when drug use in the previous 12 months has reached the level of abuse and meets at least three of seven criteria that include tolerance (i.e., increasing amounts of the drug must be taken to achieve desired effects), physical withdrawal (i.e., symptoms that accompany the cessation of drug use, such as tremors, chills, drug craving, restlessness, bone and muscle pain, sweating, and vomiting), and persistent failure to reduce drug consumption.

5. Prevalence of drug use and substance use disorders

The National Survey on Drug Use and Health assesses the prevalence of substance use and substance use disorders in the United States. In 2005, an estimated 20 million Americans age 12 or older (or 8 percent of the total population in this age group) reported having used an illicit substance in the previous month; marijuana was the most commonly used drug (15 million), followed by cocaine (2 million), hallucinogens (1 million), methamphetamine (580,000), and heroin (166,000). Meanwhile, an estimated 22 million people age 12 or older were classified with a substance abuse or dependence problem (9 percent of the population). Among them, more than 3 million were classified with abuse of or dependence on both alcohol and illicit drugs; more than 3.5 million had abused or were dependent on illicit drugs but not alcohol; and more than 15 million had abused or were dependent on alcohol but not illicit drugs (Substance Abuse and Mental Health Services Administration, 2007).

In 2005, the order of lifetime illicit drug use among members of the general population paralleled past-month illicit drug use in 2005. Nearly half (46 percent) of people age 12 or older reported the lifetime use of any illicit substance. The most popular drug was marijuana (40 percent), followed by powder or crack cocaine (17 percent), hallucinogens (14 percent), methamphetamine (4 percent), and heroin (2 percent).

6. A public health approach to addiction

The most widely used definition of *health* is found in the World Health Organization's (WHO) 1948 charter: "Health is a state of complete physical, mental, and social well-being and not merely the absence of disease or infirmity." This definition was expanded by the WHO in its 1986 *Ottawa Charter for Health Promotion* in order to underscore the notion that health is "a resource for everyday life, not the objective of living. Health is a positive concept emphasizing social and personal resources as well as physical capacities" (WHO, 1986, p. 11). By this definition, drug addiction is a serious public health problem that adversely affects all of these domains. As I have discussed in this chapter, drug abuse and dependence are formidable threats to public health and safety, costing hundreds of billions of dollars in yearly healthcare expenditures, crime, poor work productivity, and job loss (Hoffman & Fromeke, 2007; United Nations Office on Drugs and Crime, 2006). Treating addiction as a crime rather than a health problem compounds its negative impact on individuals and communities in terms of public health and safety. Not only do most addicted ex-offenders emerge from behind bars with untreated substance use disorders, but they are likely to have been exposed to a variety of contagious diseases in prison, to have learned criminogenic behaviors that discourage contributive citizenship, and to have lost connections with family and friends whose support is critical for their healthy reintegration into society.

7. Importance of treatment

Prevention and education programs for nonusers and treatment programs for users are widely recognized as the most effective means of decreasing the demand for drugs. However, throughout the long history of the drug war, approximately two-thirds of government expenditures have been on supply reduction efforts. Numerous experts acknowledge that supply-side interventions have done little to curtail drug use or the violence that accompanies the sale and distribution of illegal drugs in the United States (MacCoun & Reuter, 2001). Moreover as I noted above, prohibition and strict penalties for drug possession and sales have spawned many unanticipated problems. Nonetheless, few government officials are willing to shift the emphasis of the war on drugs away from punitive measures and toward treatment and rehabilitation programs for people with substance use disorders. Most politicians are particularly reluctant to decry punitive drug policies out of fear of being labeled as "soft on crime" and losing the support of their constituents (Kleinman, 1992; Nadelmann, 1989).

Offenders with drug use problems are a diverse group, and the relationship between drugs and crime is complicated (Bureau of Justice Statistics, 1991). Offenders become addicted to drugs and commit crimes as a result of various events in their lives (Lurigio & Swartz, 1999). Whatever the road to addiction and criminality, drug control policies must fully incorporate what research has consistently shown: drug addiction is a chronic relapsing brain disease with biological, psychological, social, and behavioral concomitants. Therefore, programs for drug-abusing offenders should be comprehensive and include a wide range of treatment and adjunctive social services (Gerstein & Harwood, 1990).

One of the most successful examples of drug treatment as an alternative to incarceration has been Arizona's Proposition 200, the Drug Medicalization, Prevention and Control Act of 1996. This initiative prohibits incarceration for first- and second-time non-violent drug offenders, mandating probation and drug treatment instead of prison. A 1999 evaluation of the initiative by the Arizona Supreme Court found that it saved taxpayers 2.6 million dollars annually. Furthermore, nearly 75% of the drug offenders who had been sentenced to probation and drug treatment as a result of Proposition 200 remained drug-free during their participation in the program and paid their own money to offset the cost of treatment (Arizona Supreme Court, 1999).

A similar initiative in California has also significantly reduced incarceration rates and criminal justice expenditures. California's Proposition 36, the Substance Abuse and Crime Prevention Act (SACPA), allows first- and second-time non-violent drug offenders to enter substance abuse treatment programs as opposed to being incarcerated. Although the impact of SACPA varied by county based on the characteristics of drug treatment programs (in-patient vs. outpatient, duration of treatment), results showed that after 5 years, SACPA reduced the prison population of those convicted of drug possession by 27%. This resulted in an estimated savings of $350 million in prison costs alone (Ehlers & Ziedenberg, 2006). The costs associated with arrests and convictions were also significantly lower among drug offenders who completed treatment, compared to those who never entered treatment and those who entered but did not complete treatment (Longshore, Hawken, Urada, & Anglin, 2006). California saved more than $2.50 for every dollar spent on drug treatment; for those who completed treatment, the savings increased to $4 saved for every dollar spent (UCLA, 2007).

Studies of substance abuse treatment for drug offenders have repeatedly demonstrated the success of these programs in reducing drug use and its attendant problems, as well as in significantly decreasing the costs associated with crime and the criminal justice system. Drug treatment programs have proven effective as an alternative to incarceration and as a prison-based, post-release, or work-release intervention for addicted offenders. Hence, drug treatment is suitable for a wide range of offenders, and it is a cost-effective intervention at various points in the criminal justice process.

Considerable research shows the crime-reducing benefits and cost effectiveness of treatment relative to other antidrug measures (e.g., interdiction) and supports a greater investment in drug treatment (Anglin & Hser, 1990). Nonetheless, the treatment infrastructure in the criminal justice system has eroded over the past several years, a disheartening development that bodes ill for future efforts to control crime and reduce illegal drug use (Lipton, 1995). For example, despite record numbers of people incarcerated for drug crimes, the proportion of drug offenders who received drug treatment in prison declined throughout the 1990s and remained at a low level during the early 2000s (Belenko, Patapis, & French, 2005; Inciardi, 1996).

The economic benefits of drug treatment accrue mostly from reductions in incarceration, criminal victimization, medical treatment, and lost wages (Hoffman & Fromeke, 2007). A recent study in California found that the state saved $7,500 in aggregate reductions in crime and incarceration for every addicted person treated (Ettner, Huang, Evans, Ash, Hardy, Jourabchi, & Hser, 2007). A similar study found that every dollar spent on drug treatment resulted in an average savings of seven dollars, stemming from decreased crime and its corollaries (e.g., increased employment and major reductions in healthcare expenditures) (McCarthy, 2007). In an extensive review of hundreds of studies of drug treatment programs, Belenko, Patapis, and French (2005) found that drug treatment reduces drug use and crime, incarceration, and victimization as well as health care expenses and other medical costs. Belenko et al. (2005) concluded that "it is clear from research on the economic impacts of substance abuse addictions on health, crime, social stability, and community well-being that the costs to society of *not* (authors' italics) treating persons with substance abuse problems would be quite substantial" (p. 58).

8. Types of drug treatment: A brief overview

As I mentioned previously in this chapter, addiction is a recurring disease that often requires repeated episodes of treatment. The ultimate goal of treatment is sustained abstinence. During the process of recovery, treatment is designed to improve overall functioning while minimizing the social and medical consequences of substance abuse and dependence disorders. The recovery process begins with treatment and progresses as addicts gain insights into their uncontrolled use of alcohol and drugs and start to manage their thoughts, feelings, and behaviors (Center for Health and Justice, 2006).

The course of treatment for drug-dependent persons follows a general therapeutic process and lies on a continuum of care (NIDA, 2006b). Drug treatment encompasses a broad range of services, including detoxification, educational and vocational training, urine testing, counseling, HIV education and prevention, life and interpersonal skills training, psychiatric care, pharmacotherapy, psychotherapy, relapse prevention strategies, and self-help groups (see section on drug treatment principles below) (Anglin & Hser, 1990; Hoffman & Fromeke, 2007; Peters, 1993). Depending on the nature and severity of the addiction and an individual's progress toward recovery, treatment can occur at various levels and in diverse settings: inpatient, intensive outpatient, outpatient, or sobriety maintenance (Center for Health and Justice, 2006). NIDA (2006b) classifies treatment into two broad categories: pharmacological and behavioral.

The use of medication in recovery typically begins during detoxification. Persons who are physically dependent on alcohol and drugs are placed on medications to safely alleviate the painful symptoms and control the adverse physical consequences of withdrawal. Medication is used in the treatment and relapse prevention process to "help re-establish normal brain function and to prevent relapse and diminish [drug] cravings" (NIDA, 2006b, p. 3). For example, buprenorphine and methadone effectively treat opiate addiction by blocking withdrawal symptoms and reducing drug cravings. The passage of the Drug Addiction Treatment Act in 2000, permits physicians to prescribe these medications in medical settings; previously, such medications could be dispensed only in specialized drug treatment clinics. Promising new medications for drug addiction are pending FDA approval, including Baclofen (for cocaine addiction), Nalemfene (for opiate addiction), Topitamate (for alcohol, opiate, and cocaine addiction), and Disulfiram (for cocaine addiction [although for many years used for alcohol addiction]) (Hoffman & Fromeke, 2007).

Behavioral therapy consists of interventions designed to change addicts' attitudes and behaviors as well as help them acquire the skills and competencies they need to avoid relapses. Several behavioral approaches have proved successful in treating addicts — used by themselves or in combination with medications. The most common are cognitive behavioral therapy (helps addicts avoid relapse triggers), multidimensional family therapy (focuses on adolescents and their peers and family members), motivational enhancement therapy (capitalizes on addicts' readiness to change their behaviors and begin treatment), and motivational incentive therapy (employs positive reinforcement and contingency management techniques to promote abstinence) (NIDA, 2006b).

9. Drug treatment studies

Abundant research demonstrates that drug treatment reduces illegal drug use, crime, and recidivism in the general and correctional population (Anglin & Hser, 1990; Anglin et al., 1996; Gerstein & Harwood, 1990; Office of Technology Assessment, 1990). Since the 1960s, numerous studies at the local, state, and federal levels have shown that drug treatment works (Lurigio, 2000). The best research on drug treatment consists of large-scale, federally funded studies that involve large samples of participants and employ longitudinal designs and a comprehensive range of outcome measures. These studies have provided the most compelling evidence that addiction is a treatable disease and have identified the principles of drug treatment that characterize the most useful and effective programs (see below).

10. Large-scale studies of drug treatment

Three large-scale, multisite investigations, funded by NIDA, strongly support the conclusion that drug treatment works: the Drug Abuse Reporting Program (DARP), the Treatment Outcome Prospective Study (TOPS), and the Drug Abuse Treatment Outcome Study (DATOS). These evaluations of community-based treatment have contributed greatly to our knowledge about the benefits of drug treatment and significantly influenced drug treatment policies, programs, and research (Gerstein & Harwood, 1990; McLellan, Metzger; Alterman, Cornish, & Urschel, 1992; Simpson, Chatham, & Brown, 1995). As Lillie-Blanton (1998) stated, "these studies are generally considered by the research community to be the major evaluations of drug abuse treatment effectiveness, and much of what is known about 'typical' drug abuse treatment outcomes comes from these studies" (p. 3).

10.1 Drug abuse reporting program
DARP involved more than 44,000 persons admitted to drug treatment between 1969 and 1973. Participants were in 52 federally funded treatment programs that administered four types of treatment modalities: methadone maintenance, therapeutic communities, outpatient drug-free treatment, and detoxification. Conducted by researchers at Texas Christian University, data were collected through client interviews with treated clients and persons who applied for treatment but never returned for services (intake-only clients). Information was also collected from clients' progress reports and other program records. Follow-up intervals occurred from 3 to 12 years after treatment. "The DARP findings have been widely used to support continued public funding of drug-abuse treatments and to influence federal drug policy in the United States" (DARP, 2007, p.3)

DARP found that clients' daily use of opiates declined from 100 percent prior to treatment to 36 percent in the first year after treatment and to 24 percent 3 years after treatment. In the DARP study, addicts who were in treatment for more than 90 days were significantly less likely to use drugs in the year after treatment than those who were in treatment for fewer than 90 days (Simpson & Sells, 1982). Outpatient drug-free treatment, methadone maintenance, and therapeutic communities were equally effective at producing positive outcomes; clients in detoxification programs or those who dropped out of treatment within 3 months showed no positive outcomes. Moreover, among drug treatment clients in general, arrest rates declined 74 percent and employment rates increased 24 percent after treatment. Twelve years after treatment, daily heroin use remained 74 percent lower (Simpson, 1993; Simpson & Sells, 1982, 1990).

Approximately three-fourths of the opiate addicts studied in DARP reported at least one relapse to daily use after they had experienced a period of sobriety. The highest percentage of addicts (85%) who quit using drugs, did so while in treatment. The most common reasons reported for staying sober referred primarily to the adverse consequences of addiction. For example, 83 percent of the treatment participants indicated that they quit because they were "tired of the hustle," 56 percent, because they were "afraid of going to jail," and 54 percent, because they had to "meet family responsibilities" (Simpson & Sells, 1990).

10.2 Treatment outcome prospective study

TOPS involved 11,000 people admitted from 1979 through 1981 to 41 drug treatment programs in 10 cities. Three types of programs were examined—outpatient drug free, residential, and methadone maintenance—and clients were followed 1, 2, and 3 to 5 years after treatment. TOPS found that drug treatment reduced drug use for as many as 5 years after a single treatment episode; different treatment modalities appeared to be equally effective in helping drug users recover. Declines in drug use were most dramatic among heroin and cocaine users (Hubbard et al., 1989)

TOPS also produced solid evidence that drug treatment reduces drug users' criminal activities. Three to 5 years after treatment, the proportion of clients engaged in pretreatment predatory crimes decreased by one-third to one-half among the three treatment modalities. Moreover, TOPS demonstrated that drug treatment is cost-effective and cost-beneficial; data showed that the costs of treatment were recouped largely during treatment and that additional cost savings accrued with reductions in post-treatment drug use. Criminal justice savings were significant. Researchers reported a 30 percent decline in costs to victims of drug-related crimes and a 24 percent decline in costs to the criminal justice system (Harwood, Collins, Hubbard, Marsden, & Rachal, 1988). TOPS' principal investigators, Hubbard et al. (1989), concluded that "publicly funded drug abuse treatment is essential to our national effort to reduce the demand for drugs and its related social and economic costs" (p. 12)

10.3 Drug abuse treatment outcome study

DATOS, the third NIDA-funded comprehensive evaluation of drug abuse treatment (Leshner, 1997), followed a sample of 10,000 clients in 96 programs located in 11 large- and medium-sized cities in the United States for 36 months, from 1991 through 1993. DATOS participants were selected from four treatment programs: outpatient drug-free, outpatient methadone maintenance, short-term inpatient, and long-term residential. According to Leshner (1997), DATOS was "the first national study of treatment outcomes since the AIDS epidemic began, the first to examine outcomes for community-based cocaine abuse treatment, the first since the transition to NIDA block grants in 1981, and the first to include public and private short-term inpatient hospitals as a treatment modality" (p. 211) (also see Hubbard, Craddock, Flynn, Anderson, & Etheridge, 1997).

DATOS found that a larger percentage of drug-free outpatients than similar TOPS participants were involved in the criminal justice system and that clients with psychiatric disorders were more likely to be poly-drug users (Flynn, Craddock, Luckey, Hubbard, & Dunteman, 1996). Drug treatment significantly reduced drug use from pretreatment baseline levels to 12-month post-treatment levels for persons addicted to heroin, cocaine, and other types of drugs (Hubbard, et al., 1997; Simpson, Brown, & Joe 1997). DATOS also found that ancillary services for addicts had declined, but drug treatment programs were delivering core services (i.e., assessment, treatment, and aftercare) more effectively than they had in the DARP and TOPS studies (Etheridge, Hubbard, Anderson, Craddock, & Flynn, 1997).

In a five-year study of cocaine addicts, DATOS researchers reported that treatment reduced cocaine use from 100 percent at intake to 25 percent 5 years after discharge from treatment. Illegal activity declined from 40 percent in year 1 post-treatment to 25 percent in year 5 post-treatment. In general, the study found that clients with more serious drug and psychosocial problems at intake had poorer outcomes in treatment. However, more exposure to treatment was related to more positive long-term outcomes (Simpson, Brown, & Joe, 1997).

11. National treatment improvement evaluation study

Another federally funded, national evaluation of drug treatment was the National Treatment Improvement Evaluation Study (NTIES). Funded by the Center for Substance Abuse Treatment and conducted by the National Opinion Research Center and the Research Triangle Institute, NTIES used a highly rigorous methodology and extensive outcome measures. The purpose of the project was to investigate the impact of drug treatment on more than 4,000 clients in publicly supported drug treatment programs across the country.

NTIES found that drug treatment had numerous favorable effects on clients, including reductions in drug use. For example, one year after treatment, clients' use of heroin dropped from 73 to 38 percent while cocaine use dropped from 40 to 18 percent. The study also found post-treatment reductions in arrests rates, self-reported criminal activities, drug selling, and illegal earnings. Among treatment participants, homelessness, unemployment, and welfare dependency declined while overall physical and mental health problems became less severe. Moreover, participants engaged in safer sex practices after drug treatment than before; specifically, the percentage of participants who reported having sex for money declined 56 percent, and the number who had sex with an intravenous drug user declined 51 percent (Substance Abuse and Mental Health Services Administration [SAMHSA], 2007).

12. Services research outcome study

The Services Research Outcome Study (SROS), conducted by the Substance Abuse and Mental Health Services Administration (SAMHSA), was the first nationally representative study of drug treatment in the United States. SROS involved 1,800 participants in inpatient, outpatient, and residential care who were discharged in 1990 from a random sample of 100 facilities in rural, suburban, and urban areas nationwide. Five years after treatment, participants were interviewed; the results showed consistent reductions in drug use — namely, 45 percent in cocaine use, 28 percent in marijuana use, 17 percent in crack cocaine use, and 14 percent in alcohol and heroin use. The study also reported 23 to 38 percent reductions in criminal activity, such as burglary, the selling of drugs, and prostitution. Finally, after completing drug treatment, participants were less likely to be involved in physically abusive relationships or to attempt suicide and were more likely to live in secure housing (SAMHSA, 1998).

13. Principles of effective drug treatment

Several basic principles underlie and characterize successful drug treatment practices. These principles have largely been derived from studies of whether and how drug treatment works to change addicts' behaviors; many of these studies were discussed earlier in this chapter (Anglin et al., 1996, 1998; Prendergast, Anglin, & Wellisch, 1995; Taxman & Spinner,

1997). With funding and guidance from NIDA, researchers explored the implementation of drug treatment programs and their effects on a variety of populations. Their aggregate findings led to the identification of core program elements that assist addicts in achieving sobriety and improving their lives in many areas of functioning (NIDA, 2006a; 2006b). The following is a synthesis and distillation of NIDA's principles of effective drug-treatment programs.

13.1 Drug assessment and treatment matching

The first principle is that no single drug treatment regimen is useful for all addicts (NIDA, 2006a). To develop successful treatment approaches, tailored to each client's addiction and service needs, clinical evaluations must be conducted to assess the specific nature and extent of clients' substance use disorders. The fundamental clinical question is what type of treatment or intervention is most appropriate for what type of client, in which type of setting, and for what length of time (NIDA, 2006a.

A crucial first step in the formulation of an individualized treatment plan is the use of comprehensive and standardized assessment protocols that collect accurate information about a client's current and previous drug use; criminal history; medical conditions; drug and psychiatric treatment experiences; education and employment records; cognitive, psychological, and interpersonal adjustment; and social support networks (Anglin et al., 1996). Before treatment begins, a client's readiness and motivation for change must also be thoroughly evaluated (NIDA, 1999).

At intake, clients should be tested for communicable diseases (e.g., HIV/AIDS, tuberculosis, and Hepatitis B and C), which are significantly more prevalent among people who use drugs (NIDA, 2006a). If they test positive, clients should be counseled on treatment options and the importance of avoiding behaviors that can spread infections to others. If they test negative, clients should be counseled on ways to prevent infection through safer sex and drug-use practices (so-called harm reduction strategies) as they strive for recovery.

Following assessment, clients' problems and needs should be matched to treatment settings and strategies (NIDA, 2006a). Addicts who openly acknowledge their drug problems and commit fully to the recovery process can benefit greatly from drug treatment and adjunctive social and medical services (Simpson, 1998b). Repeated, unfavorable consequences from substance abuse can lead addicts to realize that professional interventions are necessary to achieve sobriety (Hoffman & Fromeke, 2007). Thus, addicts with extensive drug use and criminal histories are often amenable to treatment (Anglin et al., 1996).

Clients in the early stages of drug use can also be excellent candidates for drug treatment programs (Center for Substance Abuse Treatment, 1994). With the implementation of proper assessment and treatment-matching techniques, most persons with substance use disorders can be helped by treatment at any juncture in their addiction careers. The old adage that drug abusers must "hit rock bottom" before they can begin recovery is supported by neither research nor clinical experience (Hoffman & Fromeke, 2007).

13.2 Availability and length of participation

The second principle is that effective treatment takes time and must be highly accessible and readily available to take advantage of addicts' readiness for change (NIDA, 2006a). People with substance use disorders can lose their interest and willingness to enter treatment when they languish on waiting lists for services. Drug users must break through their denial and hesitancy and become motivated in the early stages of the recovery process, paving the way for long-term care (Anglin et al., 1996). Motivational interviewing techniques can be quite effective in encouraging engagement in the initial phases of treatment (NIDA, 2006a).

Treatment takes time. Addiction is an intractable disease and cannot be overcome with brief interventions. Hence, the goal of treatment should be the management of addiction, not its cure. Many studies show that the length of stay in treatment is positively related to outcomes (De Leon, 1991; Simpson, 1979, 1998a; Simpson, Joe, Lehman, & Sells, 1986). However, clients frequently leave drug treatment prematurely; therefore, different strategies must be used to engage and retain addicts in services long enough for them to gain therapeutic benefit from their participation. The threshold for achieving significant improvement in treatment is generally reached in three months, and several episodes of treatment, aftercare, and relapse are expected before abstinence is attained (Gendreau, 1996; Wexler, Falkin, Lipton, & Rosenblum, 1992).

Fletcher, Tims, and Brown (1997) observed that the "association between treatment duration and outcomes is strong enough to warrant research simply to improve retention." Furthermore, they stated that "time itself is a surrogate measure that might represent, for example, motivation, willingness to adhere to treatment, a process of behavioral change, or the ability of the practitioner to engage the patient" (p. 223). Therefore, favorable treatment outcomes depend not only on time spent in treatment but also on what happens during treatment to change clients' behaviors (Anglin et al., 1996). Recovery is a nonlinear process. Addicts learn to eschew old patterns of thinking (e.g., criminogenic attitudes and beliefs) and behaving and to replace them with new problem-solving skills for reducing cravings, avoiding relapse triggers (i.e., places, persons, and paraphernalia that remind the addict of drug use), and re-establishing healthy interpersonal relationships. Recovery involves steady progress toward a responsible, abstinent, and productive life (NIDA, 2006a).

13.3 Treatment structure and coercion

The third principle is that treatment should be both highly structured and adaptable, involving medical detoxification for persons with a substance dependence disorder and a contingency management component for all clients. Detoxification safely alleviates the acute physical symptoms of withdrawal and is a necessary (but not sufficient) precursor to successful drug treatment. Under a physician's care, detoxification is conducted in a hospital or residential setting and lasts from three to five days (Hoffman & Fromeke, 2007; NIDA, 2006a). After a client becomes stabilized through detoxification, progressive incentives can be incorporated into treatment. Different types of contingency contracts include positive and negative reinforcements to encourage addicts to remain drug free and engaged in the therapeutic process (Onken, Blain, & Boren, 1997). Voucher-based incentives can be combined with non-monetary rewards, such as verbal recognition, reward ceremonies, and certificates of completion (NIDA, 2006a).

Graduated sanctions should be leveled against participants who do not adhere to program regulations, and rewards should be given to those who do. To be most effective, positive and negative sanctions must be clearly specified, explicitly tied to behaviors, and swiftly administered (NIDA, 2006a). They should also be progressive and commensurate with the severity of clients' rule breaking or their degree of improvement. Clients should be monitored throughout treatment to overcome their struggles to identify and avoid the triggers for relapse. The continued use of drugs should be tracked through urinalysis or other objective drug tests (NIDA, 2006a).

Treatment success depends on the adaptability of services in meeting addicts' changing life circumstances (McLellan, Arndt, Metzger, Woody, & O'Brien, 1993). Interventions are most effective when they are responsive to addicts' evolving needs at different points in the recovery process (Anglin et al., 1996). Treatment and service plans should be continually renewed and modified throughout recovery. They must always be sensitive and responsive to differences in clients' age, gender, race, ethnicity, and sexual orientation. Practitioners should be skilled at combining several modalities, including medication, individual and group psychotherapy, family interventions, childcare assistance, and legal services.

Medications, such as methadone, LAAM, Naltrexone, and bupropion, can be essential aspects of care, especially when administered with psychotherapy and other supportive interventions (NIDA, 2006a). In addition, "self help can complement and extend the effects of professional treatment" (NIDA, 2006a, p. 20). Self-help interventions include 12-step programs (e.g., Alcoholics Anonymous, Narcotics Anonymous, and Cocaine Anonymous) (NIDA, 2006a).

Drug treatment programs must be flexible in their responses to relapses—expected, not exceptional, setbacks on the pathway to sobriety. Relapses can occur even after prolonged periods of abstinence, although addicts are most vulnerable to relapse in the first three to six months after treatment (Hoffman & Fromeke, 2007; NIDA, 2006a). Occasional drug use by participants, which minimally disrupts the recovery process, should be handled immediately through placement in detoxification, exposure to graduated sanctions, or return to a higher level of care. As a rule, one or two minor relapses should not result in participants being summarily dropped from drug treatment programs as the termination of treatment after relapse is ill-advised, unjustified, and unethical from a medical standpoint (Hoffman & Fromeke, 2007).

Addicts who are coerced into drug treatment by legal mandates are just as successful in recovery as those who enter treatment programs voluntarily, and legally coerced participants typically remain in treatment programs longer (Anglin et al., 1990). Whenever possible, legal mandates should be used to order offenders to participate in drug treatment programs and to hold them accountable for their progress in recovery (NIDA, 2006a). Coercion involves entering and complying with drug treatment or facing legal consequences. Participation is mandatory and noncompliance can result in sanctions, such as incarceration, the loss of child custody rights, or more stringent conditions of community supervision. Coerced treatment can be mandated at various stages of the criminal justice process and imposed with varying degrees of restrictiveness. Judges can offer a defendant the choice between treatment and incarceration. Probation officers can recommend and enforce treatment as a court-ordered condition of probation. Prison administrators can place inmates involuntarily into drug treatment programs (Lurigio, 2002).

A willingness to enter treatment is not a prerequisite for success (Hoffman & Fromeke, 2007). Legal coercion compels addicts make decisions that they might not be able to make on their own. Coercion is leverage that keeps addicted offenders in treatment long enough to benefit from the positive effects of a supportive therapeutic experience and become intrinsically motivated to remain and succeed in care. In short, coerced treatment provides services for addicts that would otherwise have been unavailable to them (Lurigio, 2002).

13.4 Evidence-based treatment

The fourth principle is that drug treatment must be evidence-based (science-validated) and implemented in accordance with proven models of recovery (Hoffman & Fromeke, 2007).

Evidence-based practices are never grounded in a drug treatment agency's traditions or the experiences or preferences of its staff; instead, they are supported by independent research that demonstrates their effectiveness in achieving outcomes that are broadly endorsed by experts and practitioners in the addiction field (Lurigio, 2006). As Brady states in Hoffman and Fromeke (2007, p. 135), "Evidence-based treatment is treatment that has been proven to work through rigorous scientific studies. Evidence-based treatment is particularly important in the addictions field because many myths and personal biases have infiltrated the treatment area and are often accepted without question."

The most compelling evidence of a program's effectiveness emerges from research that includes representative samples of participants, random assignment to treatment and control groups, and baseline and follow-up measures of client performance that are valid (accurate) and reliable (consistent). Moreover, the most useful results of studies — for the purpose of establishing evidence-based practices — are based on evaluations of programs that are manualized and implemented by trained, credentialed, and experienced staff persons. Practitioners must implement treatment protocols carefully and consistently, and participate regularly in professional development activities (Lurigio, 2006). Evidence-based drug treatment services include: relapse prevention therapy, supportive-expressive psychotherapy, individualized drug counseling, motivational enhancement therapy, multidimensional family therapy for adolescents, and the matrix model (NIDA 2006b).

13.5 Network of services

The fifth principle is that people with substance use problems should receive services that address their other difficulties (NIDA, 2006a). Drug abusers tend to suffer from a variety of psychological, medical, and social problems as well as deficits in education, employment, and housing (Swartz & Lurigio, 1999). Many of these problems persist throughout the recovery process (McLellan, et al., 1981). Drug treatment practitioners should collaborate with other service providers (e.g., psychiatrists and psychologists, vocational training experts, and housing advocates) in addressing the multifaceted problems of drug addicts, especially those with comorbid psychiatric disorders who need integrated substance use and psychiatric treatment services. Addicts must be treated comprehensively; their various problems should be addressed simultaneously, not sequentially (Waller & Weiner, 1989).

13.6 Continuity of care

The sixth principle is that residential (short- or long-term) treatment must be followed by a continuum of care, namely, intensive outpatient treatment, aftercare, and relapse prevention services. Seamless interventions are instrumental in achieving sobriety (NIDA, 2006a; Russell, 1994). As mentioned throughout this chapter, drug abuse and dependence disorders are chronic, and several cycles of treatment and aftercare services — often "with a cumulative impact" — are required to minimize relapses and sustain recovery (NIDA, 1999, p. 16). If drug abusers remain in intensive treatment for at least 90 days and receive continuous care after treatment, they are more likely to attain sobriety, get a job, and stop committing crimes (NIDA, 2006b).

Continuity of care is particularly crucial to the recovery of drug-involved offenders leaving correctional settings (NIDA, 1999; Peters, 1993). Offenders who complete structured drug treatment programs in jails or prisons should be assisted in their transition to community-based services by engaging in prerelease planning and programming activities. Without aftercare services (i.e., continuity of care), the gains that offenders make in prison or jail treatment programs are frequently diminished or lost altogether (Lipton, 1995; NIDA, 2006a).

Prison inmates who participated in a drug treatment program with follow-up services in work release centers demonstrated significantly lower drug use and recidivism rates than those who participated in institutional treatment only (Inciardi, 1998). Similarly, offenders participating in both prison- and community-based treatment programs were less likely to commit subsequent crimes than offenders who participated in drug treatment without follow-up care (Wexler, 1996; Wexler, De Leon, Thomas, Kressel, & Peters, 1999).

Numerous obstacles can impede the delivery of aftercare services, including the fragmented nature of the criminal justice system, the lack of coordination between criminal justice practitioners and treatment providers, and the absence of incentives and sanctions for offenders to remain drug free after unsupervised release from jails and prisons. The paucity of community treatment programs and treatment providers' inexperience with offenders are also impediments to recovery (Field, 1998). Relapse prevention services for offenders should be more thoroughly studied and understood (Vigdal, 1995) as suggested by the following under-investigated and unresolved issues:

- Reasons why offenders are especially vulnerable to relapse, including stressors related to release from correctional facilities and psychosocial factors related to crime and drug use;
- The evolving recovery process at its various stages;
- The destabilized and stabilized relapse-prone individual;
- Methods to overcome recovery plateaus;
- Basic components of relapse prevention therapy (e.g., self-knowledge and identification of warning signs, coping skills and management of warning signs, and involvement of family members and others in the relapse prevention plan; and
- The timing of relapse prevention efforts, particularly in advance of release from jail and prison.

13.7 Service coordination

The seventh principle is that drug treatment programs for offenders work best when criminal justice professionals (e.g., probation, parole, and detention officers) and service providers communicate with one another and coordinate their efforts (NIDA, 2006a). Cross-training can help both groups understand the competencies and limitations of the other and work more effectively as a case management team. As stated in NIDA (2006a), "The coordination of drug abuse treatment with correctional planning can encourage participation in drug abuse treatment and can help treatment providers incorporate correctional requirements as treatment goals." (p. 3)

Treatment Alternatives for Safe Communities (TASC) was the culmination of a federal effort to establish and promote coordination between criminal justice agencies and treatment providers at the local level. Seeded in 1972 with funding from the Law Enforcement and Assistance Administration, TASC's first pilot program was implemented in Wilmington, Delaware. By 2007, more than 220 TASC programs were operating in 30 states. TASC identifies, assesses, and refers offenders at the pretrial and post-adjudication levels to treatment and adjunctive services. TASC monitors clients' treatment progress through case management, urine testing, and other techniques, and reports violations of the conditions of release to the court.

Case managers establish linkages between treatment providers and correctional staff in order to develop coordinated strategies that hold offenders accountable and protect community safety (Anglin et al., 1996; Inciardi & McBride, 1991; Swartz, 1993; Weinman, 1990). The critical elements of TASC operations include "a process to coordinate justice, treatment, and other systems; procedures for providing information and cross-training to justice, treatment, and other systems; policies and procedures for regular staff training; clearly defined client eligibility criteria; and performance of client-centered case management" (National TASC, 2007).

13.8 Program evaluation

The eighth principle is that drug treatment programs should be routinely examined by outside evaluators to determine whether services are being implemented as planned (treatment fidelity) and to measure the overall impact of services (treatment effectiveness). Process evaluations should provide program staff members with real-time information that can be used to improve service delivery and preserve treatment integrity. Outcome evaluations should be based on internally valid research designs that incorporate random assignment and control groups; such designs yield data that permit confident conclusions about program effectiveness. Researchers should also consider client selection criteria and attrition (i.e., program dropouts) when interpreting results.

Evaluations of program impact must include a variety of outcome measures, such as number and type of drugs used; frequency of drug use; treatment retention; desistence from criminal activities; length of time to relapse and rearrest; vocational skills; employment; social, psychological, and family functioning; reliance on social service agencies; physical and emotional health; HIV risk behaviors; and mortality rates (Anglin & Hser, 1990; Swartz, 1993; Vigdal, 1995). Finally, researchers should test different treatment modalities to ascertain which approaches work best with which groups of clients; they should also employ longitudinal and nested research designs to understand more precisely the effectiveness of interventions as well as the trajectories of participants' addiction and criminal careers (Leukefeld & Tims, 1992).

14. Conclusions

The use of illicit substances is common in the United States. The casual use of drugs can escalate to misuse, abuse, and dependence, resulting in distress and impairment in functioning as well as hardship for users' families and the larger community. The criteria for rendering a clinical diagnosis of drug abuse and dependence are enumerated in the 4th Edition of the Diagnostic and Statistical Manual of the American Psychiatric Association (DSM-IV-TR). These criteria help diagnosticians in evaluating the nature and severity of substance use disorders. Although substance use disorders produce serious harm for those affiliated with such problems, they are considered treatable conditions. Many studies have demonstrated the effectiveness of drug treatment in leading to recovery. Substance use changes brain chemistry and functioning; therefore addiction is a chronic disease that requires a life-long commitment to achieve long-term sobriety.

Since the War on Drugs was declared 40 years ago, people arrested for drug crimes have been the fastest-growing subpopulations at every step in the criminal justice process from arrest to post-incarcerative release from prison. The criminal justice system often provides the first and only opportunity for criminally involved drugs users to obtain substance abuse treatment and other recovery services. NIDA has discussed several principles of effective care for drug-involved members of the general and correctional populations, including assessment, treatment matching, relapse prevention, the use of medications and adjunctive services, and the evaluation of services to identify evidence-based practices.

15. References

Abadinsky, H. (2007). *Drug use and abuse: A comprehensive introduction.* Pacific Grove, CA: Wadsworth Publishing.

American Psychiatric Association. (2007). *Diagnostic and statistical manual of mental disorders IV-TR.* Washington, DC; Author.

Anglin, M.D., Brecht, M.L. & Maddahian, E. (1990). Pretreatment characteristics and treatment performance of legally coerced versus voluntary methadone maintenance admissions *Criminology, 27,* 537-557.

Anglin, M.D., & Hser Y. (1990). Treatment of drug abuse. In M. Tonry & J.Q. Wilson (Eds.), *Drugs and crime* (pp.393-460). Chicago: University of Chicago Press.

Anglin, M.D., Longshore, D., Turner, S. McBride, D., Inciardi, J.A., & Prendergast, M.L. (1996). *Studies of the functioning and effectiveness of Treatment Alternatives to Street Crime (TASC) programs.* Los Angeles: University of California, Los Angeles Drug Abuse Research Center.

Anglin, M D., Prendergast, M .L., & Farabee. D (1998). *The effect of coerced drug treatment for drug-abusing offenders.* Paper presented at the Office of National Drug Control Policy's Conference of Scholars and Policy Makers, Washington, DC.

Arizona Supreme Court (1999). Proposition 200 working, saving money. Phoenix, AZ: Author

Belenko, S., Patapis, N., & French, M.T. (2005). *Economic Benefits of Drug Treatment: A critical review of evidence for policy makers.* Philadelphia, PA: Treatment Research Institute, University of Pennsylvania.

Bureau of Justice Statistics. (1991). *Drugs and crime data. Fact sheet: Drug data summary.* Washington, D.C.: Author.

Center for Health and Justice. (2006). *Understanding treatment and recovery.* Chicago, IL: Treatment Alternatives for Safe Communities.

Center for Substance Abuse Treatment. (1994). *Screening and assessment for alcohol and other drug abuse among adults in the criminal justice system* (DHHS Publication Number SMA 94-2076). Rockville, MD: Author.

De Leon, G. (1991) Retention in drug-free therapeutic communities In R W Pickens, C. G. Leukefeld, & C. R. Shuster (Eds.), *Improving drug abuse treatment* (pp 21-38) Rockville, MD: National Institute on Drug Abuse.

Drug Abuse Reporting Program. (2007). *DATOS background.* Washington, DC: Author. http://www.datos.org/background.html. Retrieved on December 16, 2007.

Ehlers, S. & Zeidenberg, J. (2006). *Proposition 36: Five years later.* Washington, DC: Justice Policy Institute.

Etheridge, R.M., Hubbard, R. L., Anderson, J., Craddock, S.G., & Flynn, P.M. (1997). Treatment structure and program services in the Drug Abuse Treatment Outcome Study. *Psychology of Addictive Behaviors, 11,* 244-260.

Ettner, S.L., Huang, D., Evans, E., Ash, D.R., Hardy, M., Jourabchi, M., & Hser, Y. (2006). *Health Services Research, 41,* 192-213.

Field, G. (1998). *Continuity of offender treatment: Institution to the community* Paper presented at the Office of National Drug Control Policy's Conference of Scholars and Policy Makers, Washington, DC.

Fletcher, B.W., Tims, F.M., & Brown, B.S. (1997). The Drug Abuse Treatment Outcome Study (DATOS): Treatment evaluation research in the United States *Psychology of Addictive Behaviors, 11,* 216-229.

Flynn, P.M., Craddock, S. G. Luckey, J. W., Hubbard, R.L., Dunteman, G.H. (1996). Comorbidity of antisocial personality and mood disorders among psychoactive substance-dependent treatment clients. *Journal of Personality Disorders, 10,* 56-67.

Gendreau, P. (1996). The principles of effective intervention with offenders. In A T. Harland (Ed.), *Choosing correctional options that work* (pp 121-146) Thousand Oaks, CA: Sage

General Accounting Office. (1995). Drug courts: Information on a new Washington, DC: GAO.

Gerstein, D., & Harwood, H.J. (Eds.). (1990) *Treating drug problems: A study of the evolution, effectiveness, and financing of public and private drug treatment systems.* Washington, DC: National Academy Press.

Hardwood, H.J., Collins, J.J., Hubbard, R.L., Marsden, M.E., & Rachal, J.V. (1988). The costs of crime and benefits of drug abuse treatment: A cost benefit analysis using TOPS data. In C.G. Leukefeld & F.M. Tims (Eds.), Compulsory treatment of drug abuse: Research and clinical practice (NIDA Research Monograph 86, NIH Publication Number 94-3713) (pp. 209-235). Washington, DC: Government Printing Office.

Hoffman, J., & Froemke, S. (2007). *Addiction: New knowledge, new treatments, new hope.* New York: Rodale.

Hubbard, R.L., Craddock, S.G., Flynn, P.M., Anderson, J., & Etheridge, R.M. (1997). Overview of 1-year follow-up outcomes in the Drug Abuse Treatment Outcome Study (DATOS). *Psychology of Addictive Behaviors, 11,* 261-278.

Hubbard, R.L., Marsden, M.E., Rachal, J.V., Hardwood, H.J., Cavanaugh, E.R., & Ginzburg, H.M. (1989). *Drug Abuse treatment: A national study of effectiveness.* Chapel Hill: University of North Carolina Press.

Hyman S.E. & Malenka R.C. (2001). Addiction and the brain: the neurobiology of compulsion and its persistence. *Nature Reviews: Neuroscience, 2,* 695–703.

Inciardi, J. A. (1996). *A corrections-based continuum of effective drug abuse treatment.* Washington, DC: National Institute of Justice.

Inciardi, J. A., & McBride, D. C. (1991). Treatment alternatives to street crime History, experiences, and issues. *Rockville, MD: National Institute on Drug Abuse.*

Karch, S. (Ed.). (2007). *Drug abuse handbook.* Boca Raton, FL: CRC Press.

Kleiman, M. A. R. (1992). *Against excess: drug policy for results.* New York: Basic Books.

Leshner, A. I. (1997) Drug abuse and addiction treatment research. The next generation. *Archives of General Psychiatry, 54,* 730-735.

Leukefeld, C.G., & Tims, F M. (1992). *Drug abuse treatment in prisons and jails.* Rockville, MD: National Institute on Drug Abuse.

Lillie-Blanton, M. (1998). *Studies show treatment is effective, but benefits may be overstated.* Washington, DC: General Accounting Office.

Lipton, D.S. (1995). *The effectiveness of treatment for drug abusers under criminal justice supervision.* Washington, DC: National Institute of Justice.

Longshore, D., Hawken, A., Urada, D., & Anglin, M.D. (2006). *Evaluation of the Substance Abuse and Crime Prevention Act: SACPA cost-analysis report. Los Angeles: UCLA.*

Lurigio, A. J. (2002). Coerced drug treatment for offenders: Does it work? *GLATTC Research Update, 4,* 1-2.

Lurigio, A.J. (2000). Drug treatment availability and effectives: Studies of the general and criminal justice populations. *Criminal Justice and Behavior, 27,* 495-528.

Lurigio, A.J. (2000). Drug treatment availability and effectives: Studies of the general and criminal justice populations. *Criminal Justice and Behavior, 27,* 495-528.

Lurigio, A. J., & Swartz, J. A. (1999). The nexus between drugs and crime: Theory, research, and practice. *Federal Probation, 63,* 67-72.

MacCoun, R. J., & Reuter, P. (2001). *Drug war heresies.* New York: Cambridge University Press.

McCarthy, D. (2007). *Substance abuse treatment benefits and costs: Knowledge assets policy brief.* Greenburo, NC: Substance Abuse Policy Research Program.

McLellan, A.R., Arndt, I.O., Metzger, D. S., Woody, G.E., & O'Brien, C.P. (1993). The effects of psychosocial services in substance abuse treatment. *Journal of the American Medical Association, 269,* 1953-1996.

McLellan, A.T., Luborsky, L., Woody, G.E., O'Brien, C.P., & Kron, R. (1981). Are the "addiction-related" problems of substances abuses really related? *The Journal of Nervous and Mental Disease, 173,* 94-102.

McLellan, A. T., Metzger, D., Alterman, A.I., Cornish, J., & Urschel, H. (1992). How effective is substance abuse treatment-Compared to what? In C. P. O'Brien & J. Jaffe (Eds.), *Advances in understanding the addictive states* (pp. 231-252). New York: Raven Press.

Nadelmann, E. (1989). Drug prohibition in the United States: Costs, consequences, and alternatives. *Science, 245,* 939-947.

National Institute on Drug Abuse (2007). *Drugs, brains, and behavior.* Washington, DC: National Institutes of Health: U.S. Department of Health and Human Services.

National Institute on Drug Abuse. (2006a). *Principles of drug abuse treatment for criminal justice populations: A research based guide.* Washington, DC: Author.

National Institute on Drug Abuse. (2006b). *Treatment approaches for drug addiction.* Washington, DC: Author.

National TASC. (2007). *National TASC: Treatment Accountability for Safer Communities.* www.nationaltasc.org.

Office of National Drug Control Policy. (2004). *National drug control strategy: Update.* Washington, DC: White House.

Office of Technology Assessment. (1990). *The effectiveness of drug abuse treatment: Implications for controlling AIDS/HIV infection.* Washington, DC: Government Printing Office.

Onken, L.S., Blain, J.0., & Boren, J. J. (Eds.) (1997). *Beyond the therapeutic alliance: Keeping the drug-dependent individual in treatment* (NIDA Research Monograph 165, NIH Publication Number 97-4142). Washington, DC: Government Printing Office.

Peters, R.H. (1993). Drug treatment in jails and detention settings. In J.A. Inciardi (Ed.), *Drug treatment and criminal justice* (pp. 44-80) Newbury Park, CA: Sage.

Prendergast, M., Anglin, M D , & Wellisch, J. (1995). Treatment for drug-abusing offenders under community supervision. *Federal Probation, 59,* 66-75.

Simpson, D.D. (1993). Drug treatment evaluation in the United States. *Psychology of Addictive Behaviors, 7*, 120-128.

Simpson, D. D (1998a). *Ingredients of effective treatment* Fort Worth, IX: Institute of Behavioral Research, Texas Christian University.

Simpson, D. D. (1998b). *Patient engagement and duration of treatment.* Paper presented at the Office of National Drug Control Policy's Conference of Scholars and Policy Makers, Washington, DC.

Simpson, D. D. (1979). The relation of time spent in drug abuse treatment to post-treatment outcome *American Journal of Psychiatry, 36*, 1449-1453.

Simpson D. D., Brown B. S., Joe, G. W. (1997) Treatment retention and follow-up outcomes in the Drug Abuse Treatment Outcome Study (DATOS). *Psychology of Addictive Behaviors 11*:294-307.

Simpson, D.D. Chatham, L.R., & Brown, B.S. (1995) The role of evaluation research in drug abuse policy. *Current Directions in Psychological Science, 4*, 123-126.

Simpson, D. D., Joe, G.W., Lehman W. E. K., & Sells, S B. (1986). Addiction careers: Etiology, treatment, and 12-year follow-up procedures. *Journal of Drug Issues, 16*, 107-121.

Simpson, D.D., & Sells, S.B. (Eds.). (1982). Effectiveness of treatment for drug abuse: An overview of the DARP research program. *Advances in Alcohol and Substance Abuse, 2*, 7-29.

Simpson, D. D., & Sells, S. B. (Eds.). (1990), *Opioid addiction and treatment: A twelve year follow-up.* Malabar, FL: Robert E. Krieger Publishing Co.

Substance Abuse and Mental Health Services Administration. (2007). *Results of the 2005 national survey on drug use and health: National findings.* Washington, DC: Department of Health and Human Services.

Swartz. J. A. (1993) TASC—the next 20 years: Extending, refining, and assessing the model. In J A. Inciardi (Ed.), *Drug treatment and criminal justice* (pp. 127-148). Newbury Park, CA: Sage.

Swartz, J A., & Lurigio, A. J (1999). Psychiatric illness and comorbidity among adult male detainees in drug treatment. *Psychiatric Services, 50,* 1628-1630.

Taxman, F., & Spinner, D. (1997). *Fail Addiction Services (JAS) Demonstration Project in Montgomery County, MD. Jail and community-based substance abuse treatment program model.* College Park: University of Maryland. College Park.

United Nations Office on Drugs and Crime. (2006). *World drug report: Volume I analysis.* Vienna, Austria: United Nations.

University of California, Los Angeles Integrated Substance Abuse Programs (2007). *Evaluation of the substance abuse and crime prevention act: Final report.* Prepared for the California Department of Alcohol and Drug Programs (ADP), California Health and Human Services Agency.

Vigdal, G L. (1995). Planning for alcohol and other drug abuse treatment for adults in the criminal justice system. Rockville, MD: Department of Health and Human Services.

Waller, M., & Weiner, H. (1989). The dually diagnosed patient in an inpatient chemical dependency treatment program *Alcoholism Treatment Quarterly, 5,*197-218.

Weinman, B. (1990). Treatment Alternatives to Street Crime (TAW) In J. A. Inciardi (Ed.), *Handbook of drug control in the United States* (pp 139-150).Westport CT: Greenwood.

Wexler, H. K. (1996). *The Amity Prison TC evaluation: Inmate profiles and reincarceration outcomes.* Presentation for the California Department of Corrections, Sacramento, CA.

Wexler, H K, De Leon, G. Thomas, G., Kiessel, D., & Peters, 3. (1999) .The Amity Prison T'C evaluation: Reincarceration outcomes. *Criminal Justice and Behavior, 26,* 147-.167.

Wexler, H. K., Falkin, G P., Lipton, D. S & Rosenblum, A. B. (1992). Outcome evaluation of a prison therapeutic community for substance abuse treatment In C. G Leukefeld & F. M Tims *(Eds.), Drug abuse treatment in prisons and jails* (NIDA Research Monograph 118, DIMS Publication Number ADM 92-1884, pp. 54-72). Washington, DC: National Institute on Drug Abuse.

World Health Organization. (2004). *Neuroscience of psychoactive substance use and dependence.* Geneva, Switzerland:Author.

World Health Organization. (1986). *Ottawa charter for health promotion.* Presented at the first international conference on health promotion. Ottawa, Canada. (November 21, 1986).

http://www.intechweb.org/booksprocess/authorguidelines/chapter/36007

The Epidemiology and Treatment of Prescription Drug Disorders in the United States

Scott P. Novak,[1] Sara L. Calvin,[1] Cristie Glasheen[1] and Mark J. Edlund[2]
[1]RTI International, Department of Behavioral Epidemiology;
[2]University of Arkansas School of Medicine, Department of Psychiatry
USA

1. Introduction

The drug problem in the United States is a complex mosaic involving different types of drugs, consumption practices, and biological and psychological responses to their effects. Over the past two decades, the fields of psychiatry and neurology have witnessed dramatic scientific breakthroughs in understanding the actions of drugs that can be used to regulate the nervous system (Nestler, Hyman, & Malenka, 2009). This has led to a dramatic increase in use of these medications for treating a wide range of physical and mental disorders (Dasgupta et al., 2006). An unintended consequence of this increased level of availability is that a large proportion of these drugs are being consumed in excess of the dosage recommended by the manufacturer or prescriber, used to self-treat illnesses instead of seeking professional medical care, and/or combined with other drugs increase the desired effects. As a result, the numbers of unintentional poisonings and emergency room visits have nearly doubled. For instance, the latest figures from the Drug Abuse Warning Network (DAWN) indicate that in 2008, that nearly half of the 2 million emergency room visits to U.S. hospitals involved prescription medications. Approximately two-thirds of those visits that involved prescription medications were for prescription pharmaceuticals only and no co-occurring illicit drug or alcohol abuse (SAMHSA, 2006). In addition to the tremendous economic costs associated with overdoses involving prescription medications, the adverse social and mental/physical health effects, though difficult to directly quantify, are considerable.

The goal of this chapter is to present an overview of the current state of knowledge about the nonmedical use of prescription medications. Because of the sheer volume of the literature, this chapter cannot cover the entire breadth of this complex phenomenon. Therefore, the discussion is limited to those exhibiting features of dependence on prescription medications, as this is the most harmful pattern of use. Within the context of dependence, the goal is to present a concise review of the epidemiological data on the prevalence of dependence on prescription medications within various population sub-groups (e.g. youth, those with co-occurring illicit substance use disorders, and previous history of psychiatric illness). In addition, a brief summary is provided on the pharmacological properties that are likely to confer selective use of the particular drug class for nonmedical use. Information on the prevalence of seeking treatment for a substance use disorder involving prescription drugs, unmet need for treatment, and types of evidence-based treatment available for each drug class is also presented. Surveillance data also indicate that nonmedical use occurs in a wide range of medication classes (e.g., anabolic steroids, over-the-counter cough medicines, antihistamines) (Compton & Volkow, 2006; Kuehn, 2007; Lankenau, Sanders, Bloom, & Hathazi, 2008). However, this chapter focuses on the three classes of medications where the epidemiological and physiological literatures indicate that the likelihood of transitioning beyond experimentation to dependence is greatest—pain relievers, stimulants, and sedatives/tranquilizers (Blanco et al., 2007). Unless otherwise noted, the source of the surveillance data is the 2005-2009 National Survey on Drug Use and Health (NSDUH). It is a cross-sectional survey of non-institutionalized youth (age 12-17) and adults (age 18+) in the United States that is conducted on an annual basis and arguably contains the richest source of data covering topics related to the nonmedical use of prescription medications (Colliver, Kroutil, Dai, & Gfroerer, 2006).

2. Taxonomy of nonmedical prescription drug use

The term *nonmedical use of prescription drugs* has been criticized in the literature because studies typically define it use as a single item. However, NMPD is a multidimensional construct that encompasses a wide range of motivations to use prescription medications (Boyd & McCabe, 2008). Unlike heroin or other illicit drugs, prescription medications can be used to treat legitimate medical conditions. With the exception of cocaine, most illicit drugs are defined by the Drug Enforcement Agency in the United States as having no medical therapeutic value and therefore are considered illegal to possess or dispense (Table 1).

An important side note deserves mentioning. Marijuana and cocaine have some level of medically accepted therapeutic value and are available in certain States only under extremely unique circumstances. For instance, marijuana is currently treated by the US federal government as having no medically accepted therapeutic value and is therefore considered illegal (See Table 2). A small number of States (e.g., California, Colorado) consider marijuana an acceptable treatment, such as for patients with glaucoma. In those states, it is available from a licensed prescriber and may be obtained from a specialized pharmacy licensed to dispense limited quantities to patients. Cocaine is used as a topical anesthetic for conditions of the eye and nose, including nasal cauterization. However, prescriptions for cocaine and marijuana are highly regulated.

Substances: Categories and Names	Examples of *Commercial* and Street Names	DEA Schedule*/ How Administered**	Intoxication Effects/ Potential Health Consequences
Depressants			
barbiturates	*Amytal, Nembutal, Seconal, Phenobarbital;* barbs, reds, red birds, phennies, tooies, yellows, yellow jackets	II, III, V/injected, swallowed	Reduced pain and anxiety; feeling of well-being; lowered inhibitions; slowed pulse and breathing; lowered blood pressure; poor

Substances: Categories and Names	Examples of *Commercial* and Street Names	DEA Schedule* / How Administered**	Intoxication Effects / Potential Health Consequences
benzodiazepines (other than flunitrazepam)	*Ativan, Halcion, Librium, Valium, Xanax;* candy, downers, sleeping pills, tranks	IV/swallowed	concentration/confusion, fatigue; impaired coordination, memory, judgment; respiratory depression and arrest, addiction
flunitrazepam****	*Rohypnol;* forget-me pill, Mexican Valium, R2, Roche, roofies, roofinol, rope, rophies	IV/swallowed, snorted	*For barbiturates* – sedation, drowsiness/depression, unusual excitement, fever, irritability, poor judgment, slurred speech, dizziness *For benzodiazepines* – sedation, drowsiness/dizziness *For flunitrazepam* – visual and gastrointestinal disturbances, urinary retention, memory loss for the time under the drug's effects
Opioids and Morphine Derivatives			
codeine	*Empirin with Codeine, Fiorinal with Codeine, Robitussin A-C, Tylenol with Codeine;* Captain Cody, Cody, schoolboy; (with glutethimide doors & hours, loads, pancakes and syrup	II, III, IV/injected, swallowed	Pain relief, euphoria, drowsiness/respiratory depression and arrest, nausea, confusion, constipation, sedation, unconsciousness, coma, tolerance, addiction *For codeine* – less analgesia, sedation, and respiratory depression than morphine
fentanyl	*Actiq, Duragesic, Sublimaze;* Apache, China girl, China white, dance fever, friend, goodfella, jackpot, murder 8, TNT, Tango and Cash	II/injected, smoked, snorted	
morphine	*Roxanol, Duramorph;* M, Miss Emma, monkey, white stuff	II/injected, swallowed, smoked	
opium	laudanum, paregoric; big O, black stuff, block, gum, hop	II, III, V/swallowed, smoked	

Substances: Categories and Names	Examples of *Commercial* and Street Names	DEA Schedule*/ How Administered**	Intoxication Effects/ Potential Health Consequences
other opioid pain relievers (oxycodone, meperidine, hydromorphone, hydrocodone, propoxypene)	*Tylox, OxyContin, Percodan, Percocet*; oxy 90s, oxycotton, oxycet, hillbilly heroin, percs *Demerol, meperidine hydrochloride*; demmies, pain killer *Dilaudid*; juice, dillies *Vicodin, Lortab, Lorcet, Darvon, Darvocet*	II, III, IV/swallowed, injected, suppositories, chewed, crushed, snorted	
Stimulants			
amphetamines	*Biphetamine, Dexedrine*; bennies, black beauties, crosses, hearts, LA turnaround, speed, truck drivers, uppers	II/injected, swallowed, smoked, snorted	Increased heart rate, blood pressure, metabolism; feelings of exhilaration, energy, increased mental alertness/rapid or irregular heart beat; reduced appetite, weight loss, heart failure *For amphetamines* – rapid breathing; hallucinations/tremor, loss of coordination; irritability, anxiousness, restlessness, delirium, panic, paranoia, impulsive behavior, aggressiveness, tolerance, addiction *For cocaine* – aggression, violence, psychotic behavior/memory loss, cardiac and neurological damage; impaired memory and learning, tolerance, addiction *For methylphenidate* – increase or decrease in blood pressure, psychotic episodes/ digestive problems, loss of appetite, weight loss
cocaine	*Cocaine hydrochloride*; blow, bump, c, candy, Charlie, coke, crack, flake, rock, snow, toot	II/injected, smoked, snorted	
methamphetamine	*Desoxyn*; chalk, crank, crystal, fire, glass, go fast, ice, meth, speed	II/injected, swallowed, smoked, snorted	
methylphenidate	*Ritalin*; JIF, MPH, R-ball, Skippy, the smart drug, vitamin R	II/injected, swallowed, snorted	

Schedule I and II drugs have high potential for abuse. They require greater storage security and have a quota on manufacturing, among other restrictions. Schedule I drugs are available for research only and have no approved medical use; Schedule II drugs are available only by prescription (unrefillable) and require a form for ordering. Schedule III and IV drugs are available by prescription, may have five refills in 6 months, and may be ordered orally. Most Schedule V drugs are available over the counter.
**Taking drugs by injections can increase the risk of infection through needle contamination with staphylococci, HIV, hepatitis, and other organisms.*
***Associated with sexual assaults.*
†Not available by prescription in the U.S.*

Table 1. Selected Prescription Drugs with Potential for Abuse

Substance Category	Definition	Example Drugs
Schedule I	• Most restrictive level • Includes drugs or other substances with a high potential for abuse • No currently accepted medical use in the United States • Low level of safety • Not approved for use, distribution, manufacture, or importation	Heroin Marijuana Phencyclidine (PCP) Lysergic acid dithylamide (LSD)

Schedule II	• Drugs have high abuse potential
	• Have currently accepted medical use in treatment, with severe restrictions
		Cocaine
		Methamphetamine
		Amphetamines
		    Dextroamphetamine
		    Adderall®
		Morphine
		Oxycodone
		    OxyContin®
		Methylphenidate
		    Ritalin®

Schedule III	• Drugs have abuse potential less than that of Schedule I or II drugs
	• Have currently accepted medical uses in treatment
		Hydrocodone
		    Vicodin®
		Butalbital
		    Fiorinal®

Schedule IV	• Drugs have lower abuse potential than those of Schedule III drugs
	• Have currently accepted medical uses in treatment
		Alprazolam
		    Xanax®
		Diazepam
		    Valium®
		Propoxyphene
		    Darvon®

Schedule V	• Drugs have low abuse potential • Have recognized medical uses • Some pharmaceuticals contain drugs with higher abuse potential but in much lower concentrations relative to other ingredients	Cough medicines with codeine Robitussin AC®

Table 2. Drug Enforcement Agency's Controlled Substances Act Definitions of Substances Subject to Food and Drug Administration Regulation

Notwithstanding marijuana and cocaine, many illicit drugs were originally developed for medicinal purposes, but were deemed to have little or no efficacy, or having such a high abuse liability that they were prohibited as a legal medical treatment (e.g., heroin, LSD).

Therefore, prescription medications are unique in that their use is motivated by factors other than euphoria. For instance, prescription pain relievers are often used to treat legitimate medical injuries, but many patients self-treat without a doctor's prescription when a dosage of the drug is readily available to them (e.g., using a spouses prescription).

Attempts to develop survey items to capture the concept of nonmedical use has been challenging because there is no universally accepted definition as to what constitutes nonmedical use prescription drug use (NMPD). The National Survey on Drug Use and Health (NSDUH) frames the question as whether the respondent "used a particular drug that was not prescribed for you or was used only for the experience or feeling it caused." It is sometimes argued that the NSDUH definition of NMPD is overly inclusive, as it could include drugs that are used for self-treatment of a medical condition, but were not specifically prescribed by a physician (Huang et al., 2006). In contrast, another annual cross-sectional surveillance study focused on youth, the Monitoring the Future (MTF) study defines nonmedical prescription drug use as 'use of prescription medications without a doctor telling you to take them' (Johnston, O'Malley, Bachman, & Schulenberg, 2009). Then, the survey follows with queries about motivations about the most important reason for use, such as: experimentation, pain relief, euphoria. Understanding motivations for use are important because nonmedical users who use only for therapeutic value and those using for other reasons, such as for euphoria, are likely to have different profiles of risk and protective factors for use, abuse liabilities, and prevention and treatment needs (Zachny and Lichtor, 1998; Boyd and McCabe).

In the United States, there is a tremendous gulf among legislative stakeholders in terms of a formal taxonomy for nonmedical prescription drug use and problematic levels of use. The Food and Drug Administration has urged manufactured to focus on "Physical Dependence" and "Tolerance" (Dasgupta, Henningfield, Ertischek, & Schnoll, 2011) in the assessment of abuse liability for prescription medications. The National Institutes of Health (NIH) is concerned both the physical and psychological aspects of addiction that are linked to extant diagnostic criteria, such as the American Psychiatric Association's Diagnostic and Statistical Manual (DSM) or the International Classification of Diseases (ICD) categories of abuse and dependence (Compton & Volkow, 2006). The United States Drug Enforcement Agency (DEA) takes a more scientific approach, focusing on the legal requirements (e.g., number and timing of refills, quantity dispensed under a single prescription, written versus ePrescribing) that is tied to a drug's particular abuse liability (Katz et al., 2007). The words "abuse" and "misuse" have often been used interchangeably, but may be used to define separate acts of nonmedical use. The term Abuse may refer to use that involves seeking a euphoric "high" and misuse typically refers to "intentional use that involves a legitimate prescription that is used in amounts not directed by the prescriber or to treat another medical condition." An additional piece of this complicated taxonomy is whether the drug was prescribed for the user or whether they obtained it illicitly (e.g., stole/obtained from friends/family, forged written prescription, feigned symptoms to a prescriber with liberal prescribing habits [pill mills] (Boyd & McCabe, 2008).

In 2003, the College on Problems on Drug Dependence, the largest professional society in the United States dedicated solely to the advancement of knowledge about drug abuse, published a position statement about prescription pain relievers (Zacny et al., 2003). The statement urged for a formal clarification of the term nonmedical use that is broad enough to include motivations for use for inclusion on national surveillance surveys, such as the NSDUH. However, the purpose of this chapter focuses on the epidemiology and treatment of levels of use that are problematic and in need of specialty substance abuse treatment. Therefore, clarification of the term nonmedical use is less important than resolution of the diagnostic criteria that can be used to assess problem use, such as the DSM or ICD classifications of abuse or dependence. There is some debate about the degree to which opioids differ in their abuse liability and phenotypic expression of abuse and/or dependence symptoms (Wu, Woody, Yang, & Blazer, 2011; Wu, Woody, Yang, Mannelli, & Blazer, 2011). However, DSM and ICD criteria are generally accepted measures that can be easily translated onto epidemiological surveys to estimate the population in need of substance abuse treatment services for prescription drug-related problems. There are many clinical tools that are used to diagnose problem use for different therapeutic classes, as well as biological challenge tests of physical dependence (Kosten, Bianchi, & Kosten, 1989). At one end of the continuum, there is concern that the "one-size fits all" approach to defining the concepts of abuse and dependence may not operate similarly across all substances even within a therapeutic class (e.g., extended release having lower abuse liability than immediate release oxycodone) (Dasgupta, et al., 2011). At the other end of the continuum, there is an argument that abuse and dependence are a continuum, which is derived from an underlying biopsychosocial propensity (Krueger et al., 2002). Regardless of the placement on the spectrum, the term *Addiction* refers to a chronic and relapsing pattern of use and is defined by essentially three characteristics: compulsive use, loss of control in limiting intake, and altering behavioral activities in support of drug consumption. Medical professionals typically employ more specific terminology aligned within clinical (e.g., DSM or ICD criteria) criteria when referencing disordered patterns of substance use, such as abuse and/or dependence.

For the remainder of this chapter, we present data on problem levels of prescription drug use using the DSM-IV/ICD classification scheme of abuse and/or dependence. This scheme is the most widely employed diagnostic tool for problem use on national surveillance data systems, and are used to frame the nation's perspective and conversation related to research, prevention, treatment, and public policy toward the nonmedical use of prescription drugs. Within this diagnostic taxonomy, hierarchical criteria are used to ensure that substance use disorders are classified by whether symptoms are directly tied to substance use or a separate psychiatric disorder or illness. For example, mood and anxiety disorders (APA, 2006) have exclusionary criteria because a common symptom of withdrawal (e.g., "dope sick") may involve symptomotology that overlaps with mood and anxiety disorders, such as "feeling downhearted and blue" or "nervousness". This task is complicated by the high rate of comorbidity between mental (i.e., mood, anxiety, and personality) and substance use disorders (McLellan, Lewis, O'Brien, & Kleber, 2000; NIDA, 1999; O'Brien et al., 2004).

Evaluating a substance use disorder has been established using criteria that can be implemented by a clinician, or a trained interviewer using a semi-structured instrument, such as the Structured Clinical Interview for DSM Axis II disorders (First, 2002). There are also many diagnostic tools that are fully structured and can be implemented in the context of a research interview. These include the Composite International Diagnostic Interview [CIDI] (Green et al., 2011; Haro et al., 2006; Kessler et al., 2004)and the Associated Disabilities Interview Schedule [AUDADIS] (Grant et al., 2003; Grant, Harford, Dawson, Chou, & Pickering, 1995). Ascertaining the count of the population in need of services is a challenge because of the resources needed to execute a full diagnostic exam on a sufficiently large enough sample that permits generalization to the population as a whole. However, such a task is critical for policymakers to help identify and prioritize placement of finite resources that are funded through public monies. As mentioned earlier, there are a small number of surveys that collect data annually on nonmedical use of prescription drugs, but only one implements a fully-structured diagnostic interview for substance use disorders annually for youth (age 12-17) and adults (ages 18 or older—the National Survey on Drug Use and Health (SAMHSA, 2008). Other annual surveys administer brief screening scales that can be used to assess probable case based on a small number of items. A drawback is that they lack the sensitivity and specificity to accurately assess the number in need of treatment (Aldworth et al., 2010; Novak, Colpe, Barker, & Gfroerer, 2010). Therefore, in-depth diagnostic scales provide the best approach to capturing the complex phenomena of substance abuse disorders, despite the length and expense in their implementation.

The Diagnostic and Statistical Manual of Mental Disorders (DSM-IV) distinguishes problematic substance use along two categorical rubrics (shown in Table 3):

- ABUSE: Captures a maladaptive pattern of use that causes significant impairment in social, mental, and physical life-world domains. An example is missing work or failing to attend to household obligations because of use. Continued use despite consistent interpersonal or social problems associated with use is another hallmark system.
- DEPENDENCE: Is defined by a maladaptive pattern of use with adverse clinical consequences. Dependence involves two physical aspects: (1) *Tolerance*—refers to the decrease in the physical or psychological effects of a constant dosage of a drug over time; and (2) *Withdrawal*—refers to a physiological state of adverse mental and physical symptoms (e.g., nausea, insomnia, muscle aches/pains, These symptoms will vary depending upon how long the medication was taken and the type of medication.

In the next section, we summarize the epidemiology of nonmedical prescription drug use, with an emphasis on disordered patterns of use as defined by DSM-IV criteria (APA, 2002). Surveillance data are drawn from the National Survey on Drug Use and Health (SAMHSA, 2009). The NSDUH is an annual, nationally representative survey of youth (age 12-17) and adults (age 18 or older) in the United States. The procedures and characteristics of the sample have been published extensively elsewhere (SAMHSA, 2008). Briefly, the sample includes approximately 65,000 respondents each year. The target population is the civilian, noninstitutionalized population of the United States (including civilians living on military bases) and residents of noninstitutional group quarters (e.g., college dormitories, group homes, civilians dwelling on military installations) and persons with no permanent residence (homeless people in shelters and residents of single rooms in hotels). The NSDUH collects information on a large range of illicit substances, including consumption patterns, treatment utilization, and diagnoses aligned with the Diagnostic and Statistical Manual of Mental Disorders (DSM-IV) criteria for abuse and/or dependence (APA, 2000) for alcohol and selected drugs. For this paper, Substance use treatment was coded if the respondent reported any therapy or treatment, including detoxification and treatment for any medical problems associated with their drug use. Unmet treatment need was defined as the presence of a past-year DSM-IV diagnosis for abuse and/or dependence on prescription medications, but the respondent did not report receiving substance abuse treatment. Due to the complex sampling design of the NSDUH, all descriptive and inferential analyses were conducted with SUDAAN release 10.0 (RTI, 2009).

Disorders	Definition
Substance Use Disorders	
Substance Dependence	A maladaptive pattern of substance use with adverse clinical consequences. The DSM-IV has widened the concept of dependence to include the association of substance use with uncontrolled use or with use in spite of adverse consequences.
Substance Abuse	A maladaptive pattern of substance use that causes clinically significant impairment, not meeting dependence criteria. This may include impairments in social, family, or occupational functioning, in the presence of a psychological or physical problem, or in satiations in which use of the substance is physically hazardous, such as driving while intoxicated.
Substance Induced Disorders	
Substance Intoxication	Reversible, substance-specific physiological and behavioral changes due to recent exposure to a psychoactive substance. Produced by all substances.
Substance Withdrawal	A substance-specific syndrome that develops following cessation of or reduction in dosage of a regularly used substance. Occurs with chronic use of all substances, except perhaps cannabis and hallucinogens.
Substance Induced Delirium (confusion, psychosis)	Occurs with overdose of many substances
Substance Induced Psychotic Disorder (psychosis)	May occur with phenylcyclidine (PCP) and hallucinogens, stimulants, cannabis, and alcohol.
Substance Induced Mood Disorder (depression, mania) **Anxiety**	Common with many substances, especially alcohol and stimulants. Disorder must be distinguished from primary psychiatric disorder that preceded drug use.
Substance Induced Sleep Disorder	A sleep disturbance attributable to acute or chronic substance use. Common with alcohol, sedatives, and stimulants.
Substance Induced Sexual Dysfunction	Alcohol, benzodiazepines, and opioids commonly reduce sexual responsiveness and performance.
Substance Induced Persisting Disorders	Substance-specific syndromes that persist long after drug use ceases (e.g., hallucinogen "flashbacks," memory impairments, or dementia).

* dsm-iv criteria (american psychiatric association, 1994)

Table 3. Classification of Substance Use and Substance Induced Disorders*

3. Patterns of prescription drug use and disordered use in the United States

Although trend data indicate that the prevalence of nonmedical use of prescription drugs has nearly doubled over the past two decades (Blanco, et al., 2007), the rate of nonmedical use remained fairly consistent over the past 5 years (Figure 1). Among youth (aged 12-17), the NSDUH showed that approximately 8 percent (8,000 per 100,000) used any class of prescription medication in the prior year. Among those that used, about 16% met the criteria for abuse or dependence (Figure 2). The rate of use far exceeds that of adults (aged 18 or older) where approximately 6% used any prescription medication non-medically and the

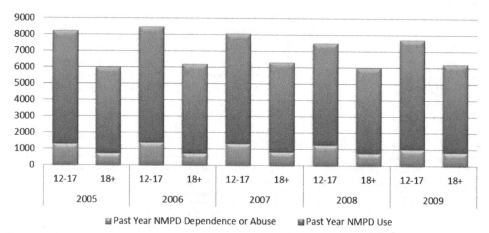

Fig. 1. Past Year Nonmedical Prescription Drug Use and Meeting Criteria for Dependence or Abuse of Nonmedical Prescription Drugs, by Age and Year: 2005-2009 NSDUH (per 100,000)

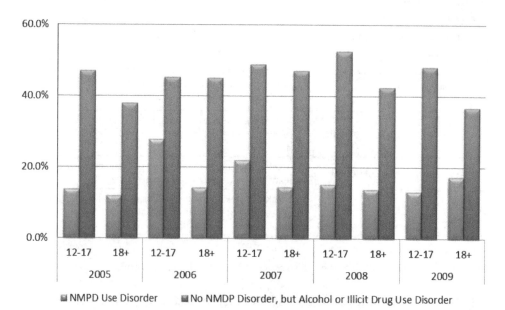

Fig. 2. Past Year Substance Use Disorder among Persons Receiving Drug Treatment in the Past Year, by Age and Year: 2005-2009 NSDUHs (In Percent)

rates of disordered use was about 16%, similar to adolescents. These data suggest that problematic levels of abuse are developing far earlier in lifecourse, especially compared to other drugs, such as heroin and cocaine where the median age of disordered use is in the mid 20s (SAMSHA, 2006). Additional data (Figure 2) indicate that adolescent females are progressing to abuse/dependence more rapidly than males. Among those that received any form of treatment for a substance use disorder in the United States (about 2.3 million in 2009), Figure 3 reveals that approximately 15% to 18% met the criteria for a prescription drug disorder. A concern about drug treatment is that care usually focuses on eliminating the most harmful substance in the client's drug-taking repertoire, so prescription drug disorders often go unrecognized and untreated compared to illicit drugs such as cocaine and heroin. When broken down by the amount of co-occurring disorders among those in treatment, Figure 4, shows that of those in drug treatment that have a prescription drug disorder, about 70% have a co-occurring drug and/or alcohol use disorder as well.

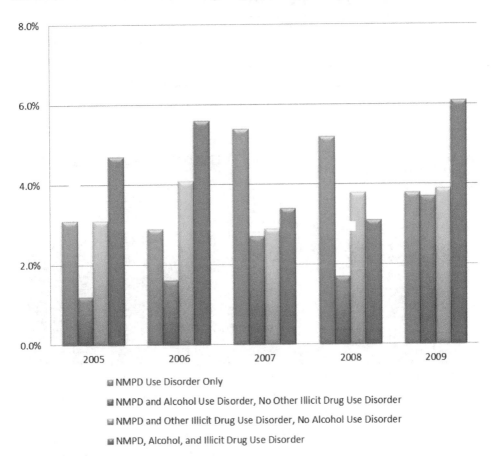

Fig. 3. Past Year Substance Use Disorders Among Persons Aged 18 or Older Receiving Past Year Drug Treatment, by Year: 2005-2009 NSDUHs

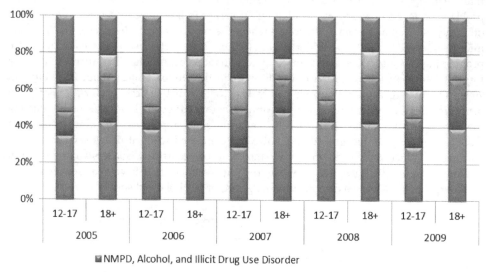

Fig. 4. Poly Drug Use Disorder among Persons with NMPD Use Disorder, by Age and Year: 2005-2009 NSDUHs

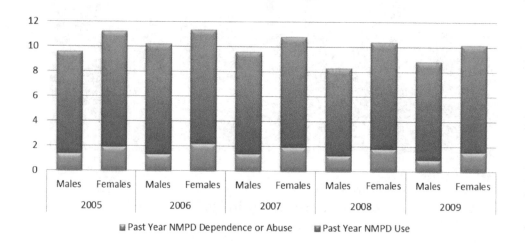

Fig. 5. Percent of Past Year Nonmedical Prescription Drug Use and Meeting Criteria for Dependence or Abuse of Nonmedical Prescription Drugs among 12-17 years olds, by Sex and year: 2005-2009 NSDUHs

4. Prescription pain relievers

Therapeutic Indications: Pain relievers as a therapeutic medication class are also referred to as analgesics. They are distinguished by the ways in which they act in the peripheral or central nervous system. Analgesics that are non-steroidal anti-inflammatory drugs (NSAIDS) are used to treat mild pain and act by reducing inflammation at the site of an injury or disease in the body. NSAIDS typically do not require a prescription in the United States and are available "over-the-counter" (OTC) at local pharmacies, drug stores, and even gas stations. Other types of (OTC) analgesics are not NSAIDS (e.g., acetaminophen), but act on the same physiological pathways to reduce the neuro-chemical sensation of pain.

Narcotic analgesics are used to treat moderate to severe pain, in many instances require a prescription from a prescriber that is licensed by the Drug Enforcement Agency (DEA). Perhaps the most widely used class of pain reliever in the United States is opioids, which can be subdivided into three types. First, naturally occurring (e.g., morphine or codeine) opioids are derived from the opium poppy plant. These drugs are typically altered into pro-drugs during the pharmaceutical manufacturing process, meaning that they are chemically converted to opioids as they are metabolized into the body. This manufacturing strategy is preferable to leaving the chemical structure unaltered (i.e., free base) because it increases the bioavailability of the drugs during metabolization and therefore maximizes their efficacy. Naturally occurring opioids are also used as chemical building blocks for semi-synthetic opiates (e.g., hydrocodone, oxycodone). Both naturally occurring and semi-synthetic opioids attach to specific opioid receptors in the brain (e.g., Mu, Kappa, Delta, and Epsilon). Heroin is a semi-synthetic opioid that is similar in chemical structure to morphine and was primarily developed as a legitimate treatment for pain in the 1800s. However, it was discovered to have high affinity to abuse because it quickly activates the brain's opioid neuro-receptors, thus producing a quick euphoric flush that is highly desirable by recreational abusers. Fully synthetic opioids (e.g., methadone, tramadol, dextropropoxyphene) are fully manufactured drugs and are not chemically related to opiates in structure, other than they selectively bind to the same neural receptors in the brain. There is controversy regarding the degree to which fully synthetic opioids have the same abuse liability as naturally occurring or semi-synthetic opioids (Aldworth, et al., 2010; Dasgupta, et al., 2011; Wu, Woody, Yang, Mannelli, et al., 2011). Overall, these drugs are known as exogenous opioids in that they are external stimuli, whereas endogenous opioids are produced internally (e.g., endorphins) in response to high levels of physical or emotional activity, and are secreted from the pituitary glands and attach to the opioid-like receptors in the brain.

Epidemiology of Nonmedical and Disordered Use: The United States has one of the highest levels per capital consumption of prescription opioids (United Nations, 2004). While the use of narcotic opioids is recognized as an important weapon in the physician's arsenal to combat mild to severe pain, studies have correlated high levels of exposure to nonmedical use and problematic levels to dependence (Dasgupta et al, 2006). Prescription pain relievers are the have the highest prevalence of nonmedical use, especially among youth aged 12-17 (Figure 6). Between 2005 to 2009, approximately 6.5% of youth (pop est. 6,000 per 100,000) used a prescription pain reliever non-medically in the prior year. About 1/6 of those who abused also used at levels consistent with DSM-IV abuse and/or dependence. Among adults aged 18 or older, the rates of nonmedical use were lower, approximately 4.5% (pop est. 4,500 per 100,000). The rates of disordered use were similar to youth, with about 16 percent reporting symptoms of abuse and/or dependence.

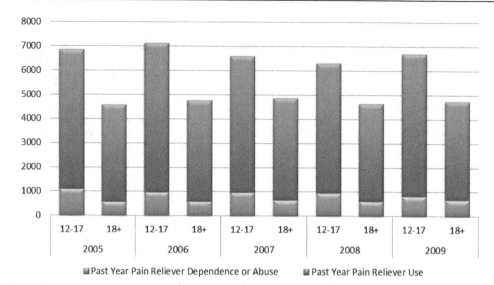

⬛Past Year Pain Reliever Dependence or Abuse   ⬛ Past Year Pain Reliever Use

Fig. 6. Past Year Pain Reliever Use and Meeting Criteria for Dependence or Abuse of Pain Relievers, by Age and Year: 2005-2009 NSDUHs (Per 100,000)

Treatment: Treatment for opioid pain medications tend toward the pharmacological spectrum, although some behavioral therapies do exist. The most common pharmacological treatment therapies for opioid pain medications include methadone, Buprenorphine, and Naltrexone or buprenorhpine/suboxone. Of the three, methadone is the oldest and most frequently used pharmacology (Amato et al., 2005), although limited evidence has shown that Buprenorphine may be slightly advantageous to methadone in terms of lessening withdrawal symptoms faster and overall completion of treatment (Gowing, Ali, & White, 2004). In contrast, a systematic review of Naltrexone indicates that the treatment may not be very effective on treatment retention or abuse relapse rates (Minozzi et al., 2006). Although pharmacotherapies are popular with clinicians, trials on behavioral therapies have shown to be effective in the treatment of opioid pain medication abuse. These therapies have been found to increase treatment adherence as well as increase social support variables known to increase positive outcomes (Amato et al., 2008). Specific behavioral therapies like motivational interventions among prescription drug abusers have been shown to reduce use by 25% in over half of users (Zahradnik et al., 2009).

5. Sedatives/tranquilizers

This class of therapeutic medications is primary used to treat used to treat anxiety and sleep disorders. They are also a major source of drug overdoses and adverse drug reactions (DAWN, 2008). The effects of most sedative medications are mediated through the GABA-chloride receptor complex, and there have been specific neural-receptors that have a high affinity to benzodiazepines. These effects are potentiated with co-ingestion with other depressants, such as alcohol. At extremely high levels of use, sedatives/hypnotics produce a loss of coordination, euphoria, dyskinesia, and even hallucinations. There are primarily two classes of medications. Barbiturates are among the oldest sedative/hypnotics and are sub-classified into their mechanism of duration (ultrashort acting, short acting, and long acting pharmacokinetics). The second major class is benzodiazepines. Unlike barbiturates, benzodiazepines are not useful for producing deep sedation and therefore are considered less powerful and of lower addictive potential. Because sedative/hypnotic drugs reduce neural excitability in the brain, neural adaption may occur after a period of weeks or months of prolonged use. Therefore, tapering rather than immediate withdrawal is recommended for patients who may develop physical tolerance after long-term exposure.

Epidemiology of Nonmedical and Disordered Use: The rate of nonmedical use and disordered use is far lower for sedative/hypnotics than prescription pain relievers. As shown in Figure 7, approximately 2% of youth and adults reported nonmedical use in the prior year. Use also appeared stable between 2005 to 2009. Among those reporting use in the past year, approximately 16% of youth and adults met the criteria for abuse and/or dependence.

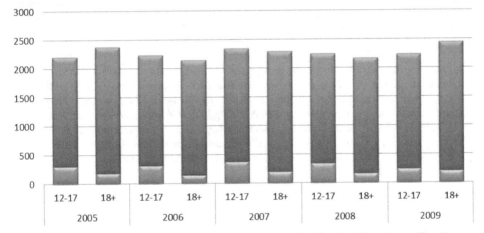

■ Past Year Sedative or Tranquilizer Dependence or Abuse   ■ Past Year Sedative or Tranquilizer Use

Fig. 7. Past Year Sedative and Tranquilizer Use and Meeting Criteria for Dependence or Abuse of Sedatives and Tranquilizers, by Age and Year: 2005-2009 NSDUHs (Per 100,000)

Treatment: Other than tapering, many types of treatment seem to be effective in treating benzodiazepine abuse. Minimal intervention, such as receiving physician advice or a form letter from a physician as well as treatment programs led by physicians or counselors are two effective treatments (Voshaar, Couvee, van Balkom, Mulder, & Zitman, 2006). Tailored behavioral interventions have also been found to be particularly effective in benzodiazepine abusers (Ten Wolde et al., 2008; Tyrer et al., 1996). Behavioral therapy programs augmented with pharmacotherapies, such as imipramine also help to reduce use among abusers. Other pharmacotherapies such as Carbamazepine have also significantly improved drug abstinence among benzodiazepine abusers (Voshaar, Couvee, et al., 2006; Voshaar et al., 2006; Voshaar et al., 2003). Behavioral interventions, such as cognitive behavioral therapy has also shown promise in reducing dependence (Denis, Fatseas, Lavie, & Auriacombe, 2006).

6. Psychostimulants

These drugs are typically used to treat attentional disorders (e.g., attention deficit disorder) and sleep disorders (e.g., narcolepsy). They are also compounds used in cold-medications because they are used to expand the nasal and esophageal airways and assist breathing (e.g., Ephedra). Ironically, low dosages of amphetamines actually produce a calming effect in those with attentional disorders. Drugs in this class are structurally related to a wide range of drugs that increase activation of the central nervous system. These include legitimate drugs such as caffeine and nicotine as illicit drugs such as crack cocaine. Prescription stimulants are typically referred to as amphetamines, and available in two chemical forms: l-amphetamine (e.g., Benzedrine) and d-amphetamine (aka dextroamphetamine). Amphetamines have a high resemblance to the dopamine (DA) transmitter in their chemical structure, therefore have a high affinity to DA receptors in binding. Methamphetamine is perhaps the most potent form of amphetamine in its effects on the central nervous system. Illicit forms of methamphetamine (e.g., crystallize methamphetamine or crystal meth) are manufactured using processes to increase the speed of uptake in the brain because amphetamine is first metabolized in the liver and has a slow uptake and a long half life (about 7-30 hours depending upon the formulation).

Epidemiology of Nonmedical and Disordered Use

The recent rise of diagnoses for attentional disorders in the United States (Birnbaum, 2004) has placed an increased volume of amphetamine stimulants used to treat ADHD/ADD within the public domain. An estimated 4% of youth aged 17 or younger have been projected to meet the diagnostic criteria for AHDH/ADD. Of importance is that much of the data indicate that youth and adults who use ADHD/ADD stimulants non-medically do so for its purported therapeutic value rather than euphoria or to "get high." (McCabe, et al., 2007; Novak et al., 2009). Epidemiological surveillance data from NSDUH (Figure 8) show

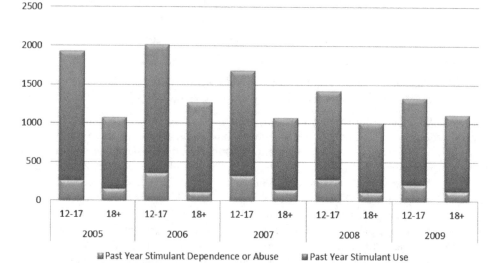

Fig. 8. Past Year Stimulant Use and Meeting Criteria for Dependence or Abuse of Stimulants, by Age and Year: 2005-2009 NSDUHs (Per 100,000)

that less than 2% of youth and 1% of adults reported nonmedical use, and of these, about 7% report levels consistent with abuse and/or dependence. Therefore, there may be a significant amount of nonmedical use of prescription psychostimulants, the level of problem use is far lower than prescription pain relievers and sedatives/hypnotics.

Treatment

Treatments for prescription stimulants and tranquilizers/sedatives are primarily limited to behavioral therapies (Rawson et al., 1995), though novel drug targets are being developed for cocaine and amphetamine use. Interventions such as cognitive behavioral therapy (CBT) and contingency management which have proven moderately effective for cocaine and methamphetamine use disorders in achieving drug abstinence can be applied to persons abusing or dependent upon prescription stimulants. Tapering can be used initially to begin treatment which will ease the symptoms of withdrawal, following by CBT and contingency management. An extensive review of the literature indicated that the behavioral therapies being applied to illicit stimulant abuse are currently the best options for treatment of prescription stimulant abuse (Vocci & Montoya, 2009). Currently, there is no Food and Drug Administration approved medication for the treatment of prescription stimulants.

7. Summary and future directions

Nonmedical prescription drug use had received a significant amount of policy and media attention in the past several years, with some using the term "epidemic" to describe the levels of use in the United States (Maxwell, 2011). In response, the Office of National Drug Control Policy (ONDCP), which is the policy arm of the President focused on substance abuse, issued a position statement in early 2011 (ONDCP, 2011). This policy release outlines the federal strategy for reducing nonmedical prescription drug abuse, and dictates various activities and a division of labor among federal agencies. The plan begins with patient and provider education programs across all federal health agencies. The content of which should focus on educating providers and patients on the safe and appropriate use of prescription medications, as well as the side effect profiles and the likelihood of abuse and diversion for nonmedical purposes. A more detailed understanding of the sequence of substance use initiation would help identify optimal points for prevention and treatment. For example, it is unknown how many persons develop a prescription drug disorder after long-term exposure to prescription medications used in the treatment of a legitimate medical condition. This pathway may be different in terms of etiology and treatment needs from a "garbage head" or poly-drug user who uses multiple illicit substances. For this latter type of user, prescription drugs are either substituted when illicit drugs are unavailable, used to self-treat withdrawal symptoms, or used concurrently to increase the feelings of euphoria. Research has shown differences in motivations to use based on therapeutic and euphoric reasons (McCabe, Cranford, Boyd, & Teter, 2007; McCabe, Teter, & Boyd, 2006; Novak, Kroutil, Williams, & Van Brunt, 2007; Novak, Reardon, & Buka, 2002), but additional knowledge is needed to articulate the pathways leading from initiation to regular use and dependence.

Tracking and enforcement are also primary goals outlined in the ONDCP Prescription Drug Control Strategy. While a large majority of the medications used for nonmedical purposes are obtained through friends and family, the highest volume consumers of prescription medications, who also meet the criteria for disordered use, obtain their medications through illicit channels such as doctor shopping, the internet, or theft (SAMHSA, 2009). There are a number of initiatives to reduce the availability of prescription medications for diversion, such as "Medication Take Back Days" sponsored by local law enforcement in various states. In addition, drugs with even modest abuse liability, such as Tramadol—a non-opioid prescription pain reliever, are being rescheduled by several States so that prescribing and refilling practices by doctors and patients is more restrictive.

In response to the public health threat that prescription drug abuse poses, federal and state initiatives in the United States have earmarked more than $500 million toward reducing the supply of NMPD through prescription monitoring programs, regulations for prescribing and dosing, and physician education programs (Fischer, Bibby, & Bouchard, 2010; Fishman, 2011; Manchikanti, 2007). These programs are implemented in more than 40 states, with some form of legislation pending in the rest. Several screening instruments have also been developed to help clinicians identify potential abuse liability for their patient. Unfortunately, these programs and assessments have been developed and implemented in the absence of a strong scientific understanding of characteristics of prescription drug abuse. Medical professionals need guidance about types of NMPD to identify those with the greatest potential for abuse of a particular medication. It is also unknown whether individuals are aware of these monitoring systems and programs and if they have significantly affected drug procuring behaviors.

This chapter began with an important statement about the complexities of the national drug problem involving prescription medications in the United States. This chapter presented descriptive epidemiological data on prescription drug disorders and their treatment. Unlike other drugs of abuse, the body of knowledge around prescription drug abuse is in its relative infancy. Many unresolved questions remain regarding the degree to which the risk factors for alcohol and tobacco and marijuana in adolescence are similar to prescription drug abuse. Resolution of this question would help frame primary prevention efforts toward either universal or specialized prevention programming in schools and in the community. Moreover, there are also many unknown questions about how the bio-pharmacological properties of prescription medications contribute toward abuse liability. Prescription drug manufacturers are developing abuse deterrent formulations (ADFs) of commonly abuse drugs. For example, several drugs in the FDA pipeline (Phase I to III) employ sequestered naltrexone, an opioid antagonist, to limit the nonmedical use of opioid-based pain medications. When the pill is crushed or tampered, the naltrexone becomes activated and counteracts the effects of the opioid concentrated in the medication. However, these methods are only effective against abuse by tampering (e.g., crushing, snorting, injecting), so additional methods are needed to curb routes of abuse that include oral ingestion as well. The health care delivery system for behavioral health is also under going tremendous transformation, which has wide-ranging implications for the prevention and treatment of prescription drug abuse. While the final proposed structure is likely to stay under significant and prolonged debate, experts agree that behavioral health, which is largely responsible for the delivery of substance abuse treatment services, will have greater integration into the primary and specialized health care systems. Taken together, it appears that a multi-pronged approach that involves effects at multiple systematic levels will be needed to reduce the epidemic of prescription drug abuse over the next several years.

8. Acknowledgements

The analyses for this paper were supported by a grant from the National Institute on Drug Abuse (R01DA030427, S. Novak, PI). The National Survey on Drug Use and Health was conducted by RTI International under a contract from the Substance Abuse and Mental Health Services Administration. The conclusions from this study are solely the authors. The authors would like to thank Richard Nowak, RPh. (CVS Pharmacy Group, USA) and David Brown, Ph.D. (Pfizer, Inc., USA) for their comments on early versions of this manuscript. The authors gratefully acknowledge the dedication of the NSDUH participants for their generosity and time.

9. References

Aldworth, J., Colpe, L. J., Gfroerer, J. C., Novak, S. P., Chromy, J. R., Barker, P. R., et al. (2010). The National Survey on Drug Use and Health Mental Health Surveillance Study: calibration analysis. *Int J Methods Psychiatr Res, 19 Suppl 1*, 61-87.

Amato, L., Davoli, M., Perucci, C. A., Ferri, M., Faggiano, F., & Mattick, R. P. (2005). An overview of systematic reviews of the effectiveness of opiate maintenance therapies: available evidence to inform clinical practice and research. *J Subst Abuse Treat, 28*(4), 321-329.

Amato, L., Minozzi, S., Davoli, M., Vecchi, S., Ferri, M. M., & Mayet, S. (2008). Psychosocial combined with agonist maintenance treatments versus agonist maintenance treatments alone for treatment of opioid dependence. *Cochrane Database Syst Rev*(4), CD004147.

APA. (2000). *Diagnostic and Statistical Manual of Mental Disorders* (4th ed.). Washington, DC: American Psychiatric Publishing, Inc.

Blanco, C., Alderson, D., Ogburn, E., Grant, B. F., Nunes, E. V., Hatzenbuehler, M. L., et al. (2007). Changes in the prevalence of non-medical prescription drug use and drug use disorders in the United States: 1991-1992 and 2001-2002. *Drug Alcohol Depend, 90*(2-3), 252-260.

Boyd, C. J., & McCabe, S. E. (2008). Coming to terms with the nonmedical use of prescription medications. *Subst Abuse Treat Prev Policy, 3*, 22.

Colliver, J. D., Kroutil, L. A., Dai, L., & Gfroerer, J. C. (2006). Misuse of prescription drugs: Data from the 2002, 2003, and 2004 National Surveys on Drug Use and Health (DHHS Publication No. SMA 06-4192, Analytic Series A-28). Rockville, MD: Substance Abuse and Mental Health Services Administration.

Compton, W. M., & Volkow, N. D. (2006). Abuse of prescription drugs and the risk of addiction. *Drug Alcohol Depend, 83 Suppl 1*, S4-7.

Dasgupta, N., Henningfield, J. E., Ertischek, M. D., & Schnoll, S. H. (2011). When drugs in the same controlled substance schedule differ in real-world abuse, should they be differentiated in labeling? *Drug Alcohol Depend.*

Dasgupta, N., Kramer, E. D., Zalman, M. A., Carino, S., Jr., Smith, M. Y., Haddox, J. D., et al. (2006). Association between non-medical and prescriptive usage of opioids. *Drug Alcohol Depend, 82*(2), 135-142.

Denis, C., Fatseas, M., Lavie, E., & Auriacombe, M. (2006). Pharmacological interventions for benzodiazepine mono-dependence management in outpatient settings. *Cochrane Database Syst Rev, 3*, CD005194.

Fischer, B., Bibby, M., & Bouchard, M. (2010). The global diversion of pharmaceutical drugsnon-medical use and diversion of psychotropic prescription drugs in North America: a review of sourcing routes and control measures. *Addiction, 105*(12), 2062-2070.

Fishman, S. M. (2011). Prescription drug monitoring programs serve a vital clinical need. *Pain Med, 12*(6), 845.

Gowing, L., Ali, R., & White, J. (2004). Buprenorphine for the management of opioid withdrawal. *Cochrane Database Syst Rev*(4), CD002025.

Grant, B. F., Dawson, D. A., Stinson, F. S., Chou, P. S., Kay, W., & Pickering, R. (2003). The Alcohol Use Disorder and Associated Disabilities Interview Schedule-IV (AUDADIS-IV): reliability of alcohol consumption, tobacco use, family history of depression and psychiatric diagnostic modules in a general population sample. *Drug Alcohol Depend, 71*(1), 7-16.

Grant, B. F., Harford, T. C., Dawson, D. A., Chou, P. S., & Pickering, R. P. (1995). The Alcohol Use Disorder and Associated Disabilities Interview schedule (AUDADIS): reliability of alcohol and drug modules in a general population sample. *Drug Alcohol Depend, 39*(1), 37-44.

Green, J. G., Avenevoli, S., Finkelman, M., Gruber, M. J., Kessler, R. C., Merikangas, K. R., et al. (2011). Validation of the diagnoses of panic disorder and phobic disorders in the US National Comorbidity Survey Replication Adolescent (NCS-A) supplement. *Int J Methods Psychiatr Res, 20*(2), 105-115.

Haro, J. M., Arbabzadeh-Bouchez, S., Brugha, T. S., de Girolamo, G., Guyer, M. E., Jin, R., et al. (2006). Concordance of the Composite International Diagnostic Interview Version 3.0 (CIDI 3.0) with standardized clinical assessments in the WHO World Mental Health surveys. *Int J Methods Psychiatr Res, 15*(4), 167-180.

Huang, B., Dawson, D. A., Stinson, F. S., Hasin, D. S., Ruan, W. J., Saha, T. D., et al. (2006). Prevalence, correlates, and comorbidity of nonmedical prescription drug use and drug use disorders in the United States: Results of the National Epidemiologic Survey on Alcohol and Related Conditions. *J Clin Psychiatry, 67*(7), 1062-1073.

Hubbard, R. L., Pantula, J., & Lessler, J. T. (1992). Effects of decomposition of complex concepts. In C. F. Turner & J. T. Lessler (Eds.), *Survey Measurement of Drug Use: Methodological Studies* (Vol. DHHS Publication no. (ADM) 92-1929). Washington, DC: Government Printing Office

Johnston, L. D., O'Malley, P. M., Bachman, J. G., & Schulenberg, J. E. (2009). *Monitoring the Future national results on adolescent drug use: Overview of key findings, 2008 (NIH Publication No. 09-7401). Bethesda, MD: National Institute on Drug Abuse, 73 pp. :* National Institute of Health (Number:)

Katz, N. P., Adams, E. H., Benneyan, J. C., Birnbaum, H. G., Budman, S. H., Buzzeo, R. W., et al. (2007). Foundations of opioid risk management. *Clin J Pain, 23*(2), 103-118.

Kessler, R. C., Abelson, J., Demler, O., Escobar, J. I., Gibbon, M., Guyer, M. E., et al. (2004). Clinical calibration of DSM-IV diagnoses in the World Mental Health (WMH) version of the World Health Organization (WHO) Composite International Diagnostic Interview (WMHCIDI). *Int J Methods Psychiatr Res, 13*(2), 122-139.

Kosten, T. A., Bianchi, M. S., & Kosten, T. R. (1989). Use predicts treatment outcome, not opiate dependence or withdrawal. *NIDA Res Monogr, 95*, 459-460.

Krueger, R. F., Hicks, B. M., Patrick, C. J., Carlson, S. R., Iacono, W. G., & McGue, M. (2002). Etiologic connections among substance dependence, antisocial behavior, and personality: modeling the externalizing spectrum. *J Abnorm Psychol, 111*(3), 411-424.

Kuehn, B. M. (2007). Many teens abusing medications. *JAMA, 297*(6), 578-580.

Lankenau, S. E., Sanders, B., Bloom, J. J., & Hathazi, D. (2008). Towards an Explanation of Subjective Ketamine Experiences among Young Injection Drug Users. *Addict Res Theory, 16*(3), 273-287.

Manchikanti, L. (2007). National drug control policy and prescription drug abuse: facts and fallacies. *Pain Physician, 10*(3), 399-424.

Maxwell, J. C. (2011). The prescription drug epidemic in the United States: a perfect storm. *Drug Alcohol Rev, 30*(3), 264-270.

McCabe, S. E., Cranford, J. A., Boyd, C. J., & Teter, C. J. (2007). Motives, diversion and routes of administration associated with nonmedical use of prescription opioids. *Addict Behav, 32*(3), 562-575.

McCabe, S. E., Teter, C. J., & Boyd, C. J. (2006). Medical use, illicit use, and diversion of abusable prescription drugs. *J Am Coll Health, 54*(5), 269-278.

McLellan, A. T., Lewis, D. C., O'Brien, C. P., & Kleber, H. D. (2000). Drug dependence, a chronic medical illness: implications for treatment, insurance, and outcomes evaluation. *Jama, 284*(13), 1689-1695.

Minozzi, S., Amato, L., Vecchi, S., Davoli, M., Kirchmayer, U., & Verster, A. (2006). Oral naltrexone maintenance treatment for opioid dependence. *Cochrane Database Syst Rev*(1), CD001333.

Nestler, E. J., Hyman, S. E., & Malenka, R. C. (2009). *Molecular Neuropharmacology: A foundation for clinical neuroscience* (Vol. II). New York: McGraw-Hill Companies

NIDA. (1999). *Principles of drug addiction treatment: a research based guide* (Vol. 2009). Rockville, MD: NIH.

Novak, S. P., Colpe, L. J., Barker, P. R., & Gfroerer, J. C. (2010). Development of a brief mental health impairment scale using a nationally representative sample in the USA. *Int J Methods Psychiatr Res, 19 Suppl 1*, 49-60.

Novak, S. P., Kroutil, L. A., Williams, R. L., & Van Brunt, D. L. (2007). The nonmedical use of prescription ADHD medications: results from a national Internet panel. *Subst Abuse Treat Prev Policy, 2*, 32.

Novak, S. P., Reardon, S. F., & Buka, S. L. (2002). How beliefs about substance use differ by socio-demographic characteristics, individual experiences, and neighborhood environments among urban adolescents. *J Drug Educ, 32*(4), 319-342.

O'Brien, C. P., Charney, D. S., Lewis, L., Cornish, J. W., Post, R. M., Woody, G. E., et al. (2004). Priority actions to improve the care of persons with co-occurring substance abuse and other mental disorders: a call to action. *Biol Psychiatry, 56*(10), 703-713.

ONDCP. (2011, June 21, 2011). Epidemic: Responding to America's Prescription Drug Abuse Crisis 5/11. Retrieved 5/11, 2011, from http://www.whitehousedrugpolicy.gov/publications/pdf/rx_abuse_plan.pdf

Rawson, R. A., Shoptaw, S. J., Obert, J. L., McCann, M. J., Hasson, A. L., Marinelli-Casey, P. J., et al. (1995). An intensive outpatient approach for cocaine abuse treatment. The Matrix model. *J Subst Abuse Treat, 12*(2), 117-127.

RTI. (2009). *SUDAAN User's Manual, Release 10.0.* Research Triangle Park, NC RTI International

SAMHSA. (2006). Drug Abuse Warning Network, 2005: National Estimates of Drug-Related Emergency Department Visits. *DAWN Series D-29, DHHS Publication No. (SMA)* 07-4256, Rockville, MD, 2007.

SAMHSA. (2008). *Results from the 2007 National Survey on Drug Use and Health: National Findings.*.

Ten Wolde, G. B., Dijkstra, A., van Empelen, P., van den Hout, W., Neven, A. K., & Zitman, F. (2008). Long-term effectiveness of computer-generated tailored patient education on benzodiazepines: a randomized controlled trial. *Addiction, 103*(4), 662-670.

Tyrer, P., Ferguson, B., Hallstrom, C., Michie, M., Tyrer, S., Cooper, S., et al. (1996). A controlled trial of dothiepin and placebo in treating benzodiazepine withdrawal symptoms. *Br J Psychiatry, 168*(4), 457-461.

Vocci, F. J., & Montoya, I. D. (2009). Psychological treatments for stimulant misuse, comparing and contrasting those for amphetamine dependence and those for cocaine dependence. *Curr Opin Psychiatry, 22*(3), 263-268.

Voshaar, R. C., Couvee, J. E., van Balkom, A. J., Mulder, P. G., & Zitman, F. G. (2006). Strategies for discontinuing long-term benzodiazepine use: meta-analysis. *Br J Psychiatry, 189*, 213-220.

Voshaar, R. C., Gorgels, W. J., Mol, A. J., van Balkom, A. J., Mulder, J., van de Lisdonk, E. H., et al. (2006). Predictors of long-term benzodiazepine abstinence in participants of a randomized controlled benzodiazepine withdrawal program. *Can J Psychiatry, 51*(7), 445-452.

Voshaar, R. C., Gorgels, W. J., Mol, A. J., van Balkom, A. J., van de Lisdonk, E. H., Breteler, M. H., et al. (2003). Tapering off long-term benzodiazepine use with or without group cognitive-behavioural therapy: three-condition, randomised controlled trial. *Br J Psychiatry, 182*, 498-504.

Wu, L. T., Woody, G. E., Yang, C., & Blazer, D. G. (2011). How do prescription opioid users differ from users of heroin or other drugs in psychopathology: Results from the National Epidemiologic Survey on Alcohol and Related Conditions. *J Addict Med, 5*(1), 28-35.

Wu, L. T., Woody, G. E., Yang, C., Mannelli, P., & Blazer, D. G. (2011). Differences in onset and abuse/dependence episodes between prescription opioids and heroin: results from the National Epidemiologic Survey on Alcohol and Related Conditions. *Subst Abuse Rehabil, 2011*(2), 77-88.

Zacny, J., Bigelow, G., Compton, P., Foley, K., Iguchi, M., & Sannerud, C. (2003). College on Problems of Drug Dependence taskforce on prescription opioid non-medical use and abuse: position statement. *Drug Alcohol Depend, 69*(3), 215-232.

Zahradnik, A., Otto, C., Crackau, B., Lohrmann, I., Bischof, G., John, U., et al. (2009). Randomized controlled trial of a brief intervention for problematic prescription drug use in non-treatment-seeking patients. *Addiction, 104*(1), 109-117.

3

Tobacco Addiction

Stephan Muehlig
Chemnitz University of Technology
Germany

1. Introduction

"Tobacco is the single most preventable cause of death in the world today. This year, tobacco will kill more than five million people – more than tuberculosis, HIV/AIDS and malaria combined. By 2030, the death toll will exceed eight million a year. Unless urgent action is taken tobacco could kill one billion people during this century. Tobacco is the only legal consumer product that can harm everyone exposed to it – and it kills up to half of those who use it as intended." (WHO Report on the global tobacco epidemic, 2008, p. 8)

Although nearly all smokers are aware of the outstanding healthy risks of cigarette smoking and the majority of them is willing to quit, only a small proportion of regular smokers is able to stop smoking successfully. Within 12 months after a stop smoking trial, only 2-6% of quitters remain abstinent. This high relapse rate can only be explained by mechanisms of addiction. The term *"tobabacco addiction"* refers to the definition of substance use disorders, which includes harmful substance use as well as physiological and psychological dependence. This chapter aims to summarize the current state of knowledge regarding to the phenomenon of tobacco addiction and tobacco use related disorder.

2. Classification, epidemiology, etiology, and treatment of tobacco addiction

2.1 Diagnostic classification

Tobacco addiction states a mental disorder with severe somatic and mental symptoms and consequences. The term *'addiction'* was, due to its terminological vagueness, discarded as an official name for a diagnostic category by the WHO in 1964, however it is still used today in everyday speech and as part of the technical language. Within the current clinical classification systems DSM-IV and ICD-10 the phenomene of addiction caused by psychotropic substances is classified in two different diagnostic categories: DSM-IV differenciates *'substance dependence'* (303.xx) and *'substance abuse'* (305.xx) whereas ICD-10 refers to *'dependence'* and *'harmful use'* (F1x.1). According to DSM, drug dependence is defined by seven diagnostic core criteria of which three must be met along with clinically important suffering in order to confirm the diagnosis. In contrast, abuse is determined by repeated, maladjusted substance use and psychosocial impairments (e.g., interpersonal problems, legal problems, high risk behaviour) over a period of at least 12 months (cf. Tab. 1).

There is a clinical and neurobiological distinction between somatic and mental addiction. *Somatic addiction* is primarily defined by development of tolerance and physiological withdrawal symptoms. That means, the organism "gets used" to the regular dose of the

DSM-IV-TR		DSM-V
Nicotine Abuse	**Nicotine Dependence**	**Tobacco Use Disorder**
at least one of the following *criteria* within the same 12 months period: (1) Severe problems regarding family, home, profession or school due to substance use (2) Substance use in dangerous situations (3)Legal problems due to substance use (4) Social and/or interpersonal problems due to substance use The symptoms have never fulfilled the criteria for substance addiction of the respective substance class.	*at least three* of the following *criteria* within the same 12 months period: (1) Development of tolerance (2) Withdrawal symptoms (3) Substance use longer or in larger quantities than intended (4) Permanent wish or failure to control substance use (5) Time-consuming procurement, use and recovery from substance (6) Important social, professional or recreational activities are given up or limited due to substance use (7) Continued substance use despite physical or psychic problems	*maladaptive pattern of substance use leading to clinically significant impairment or distress, as manifested by 2 (or more) of the following, occurring within a 12-month period:* 1. recurrent substance use resulting in a failure to fulfill major role obligations at work, school, or home 2. recurrent substance use in situations in which it is physically hazardous 3. continued substance use despite having persistent or recurrent social or interpersonal problems caused or exacerbated by the effects of the substance 4. tolerance, as defined by either of the following: a need for markedly increased amounts of the substance to achieve intoxication or desired effect b) markedly diminished effect with continued use of the same amount of the substance 5. withdrawal, as manifested by either of the following: a) the characteristic withdrawal syndrome for the substance; b) the same (or a closely related) substance is taken to relieve or avoid withdrawal symptoms 6. the substance is often taken in larger amounts or over a longer period than was intended 7. there is a persistent desire or unsuccessful efforts to cut down or control substance use 8. a great deal of time is spent in activities necessary to obtain the substance, use the substance, or recover from its effects 9. important social, occupational, or recreational activities are given up or reduced because of substance use 10. the substance use is continued despite knowledge of having a persistent or recurrent physical or psychological problem that is likely to have been caused or exacerbated by the substance 11. Craving or a strong desire or urge to use a specific substance.

Table 1. Tobacco-related Disorders according to DSM-IV-TR vs. DSM-V.

substance and thus needs ever increasing amounts to reach the desired state of intoxication (dose increase), however, also can tolerate higher doses than at the beginning of drug use (tolerance). In contrast, the *mental addiction* is characterized by behavioral patterns such as compulsive use, loss of control, addiction memory, craving and coping deficits. The term "addiction" refers more to the mental aspect of the dependency, i.e. to the continuing compulsive consumption of the drug despite negative effects and/or despite the wish to stop drug use. Whereas the somatic dependency syndrome is generally gone some weeks after the withdrawal, the addiction memory may remain active for years and decades and continue to trigger periodical craving or even relapses from time to time. Thus, a dependent smoker may have stopped to be dependent on tobacco after successful withdrawal therapy but he/she may remain addicted, possibly for his/her whole life.

Within the process for revising the Diagnostic and Statistical Manual of Mental Disorders (*DSM-V*) the work group which is responsible for addressing substance use disorders currently developed new recommendations to redefine these diagnostic categories. Among the work group's proposals are the following recommendations:

i.   To move the categories of 'abuse' and 'dependence' in one common diagnosis category named 'Substance-Related Disorders';

ii.   To include both substance use disorders and non-substance addictions (Gambling disorder, Internet addiction) in this new diagnostic category

iii. To tentatively re-title the category into the term 'Addiction and Related Disorders'.

In consequence, the diagnosis 'Nicotine Dependence' (305.1) should be replaced by *'Tobacco Use Disorder'* which includes 11 diagnostic criteria (s. table 1).

2.2 Epidemiology
2.2.1 Prevalence of cigarette smoking and nicotine dependence

The epidemiology of addictive smoking can be demonstrated by international *point prevalence* as well as *life-time prevalence* data of representative population-based health surveys. The rates of current smokers in adult population (> 14 years) are extremely varying by country and gender (figure 2).

Approximately one half of the smoking men and one-third of the women are classified as heavy smokers (>20 cig./day). However, not every chronic cigarette smoker will necessarily become addicted to nicotine or tobacco. A number of international epidemiological studies found that only a minority of persistent smokers become dependent according the diagnostic criteria for substance use disorders described above. In a currently conducted, well controlled population survey on nearly 8,000 representative participants in Germany, 6.3% participants among the total sample and 29.9% of all current smokers (smoking rate: 29,6%) met the DSM-IV criteria for a *nicotine dependence disorder* (Papst et al., 2010). Nevertheless, nicotine dependence has an outstanding significance from an epidemiological perspective since, with a lifetime prevalence of 17% and 21% (cf. Tab. 2), it is one of the most common mental disorders, compared to affective disorders (lifetime prevalence: 12-19%) or anxiety disorders (LT prevalence: 15%). By trend, nicotine dependence occurred more often in female smokers and in younger age groups compared with older cohorts. In Lifetime, 50% of all smokers succeed to quit, mostly after 5-10 ineffective attempts.

Approximately every second smoker who has tried to quit smoking reports somatic withdrawal symptoms that manifest themselves in psycho-vegetative conditions or cognitive-emotional adverse effects (cf. table 3). The *nicotine withdrawal syndrome* starts 2-4 hours after the last cigarette, reaches its intensity peak after 24-48 hours and gradually passes after 1-4 weeks. However, the primarily mental symptoms (craving, feeling of hunger, dysphoria) may persist for months.

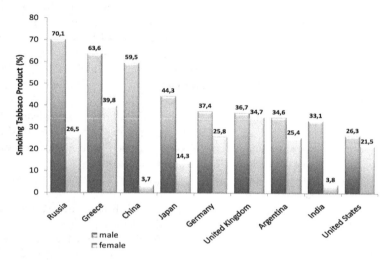

Fig. 1. WHO Report on the Global Tabacco Epidemic (2008)

	Total		Gender	
			Men	Women
Consumption prevalence (30 d)[1]	7,983		3,542	4,441
Non-Smokers	44.8%	(3,858)	38.8%	51.0%
Ex-smokers	26.0%	(1,771)	28.5%	23.6%
Smokers	29.2%	(2,354)	32.8%	25.5%
Consumption frequency (30 d)[2]	2,238		1,096	1,142
Not daily	29.6%	(714)	28.4%	31.0%
Daily up to 10	21.7%	(530)	17.4%	27.1%
Daily 11-19	23.5%	(517)	25.7%	20.9%
Daily more than 20	25.2%	(477)	28.5%	21.1%
DSM-IV (12M)[3]	7,984		3,521	4,427
Total sample	6.3%	(531)	6.8%	5.8%
Consumers[4]	19.9%	(531)	19.2%	20.9%

[1] Non-Smokers: have smoked a total of maximum 100 cigarettes; ex-smoker: have smoked more than 100 cigarettes, but not in the previous 30 days; smokers: smoked cigarettes in the previous 30 days.
[2] Referring to cigarette smokers during the previous 30 days.
[3] Nicotine dependence according to DSM-IV: unweighted number of cases regarding to total sample
[4] Referring to 12 months prevalence of smoking.

Table 2. Prevalence of smoking, of smoke frequency and nicotine dependence according to DSM-IV (Papst e al., 2010, p. 332)

- craving
- increased appetite, sensation of hunger, weight gain
- concentration problems
- nervousness, irritability, restlessness, insomnia
- feeling of frustration, unhappiness, depressive moods, depression, states of anxiety, anxieties
- circulation problems, sweating, digestive disorders

Table 3. Withdrawal symptoms during the smoke stop

The strength of the nicotine dependency can best be measured through specific withdrawal symptoms. The *Fagerstrom Test for Nicotine Dependence (FTND;* Heatherton et al., 1991; cf. table 4), which consists of six items, is recommended worldwide as a dimensional research tool for the measurement of nicotine dependency. This test has been validated in international studies and represents one of the best predictors for abstinence success.

Questions	Answers	Points
1 . How soon after you wake up do you smoke your first cigarette?	Within 5 minutes	3
	6 – 30 minutes	2
	31 – 60 minutes	1
	After 60 minutes	0
2. Do you find it difficult to refrain from smoking in places where it is forbidden, e.g., in church, at the library, in the cinema, etc.?	Yes	1
	No	0
3. Which cigarette would you hate most to give up?	The first one in the morning.	1
	Any other.	0
4. How many cigarettes/day do you smoke?	10 or less	0
	11 – 20	1
	21 – 30	2
	31 or more	3
5. Do you smoke more frequently during the first hours after awakening than during the rest of the day?	Yes	1
	No	0
6. Do you smoke if you are so ill that you are in bed most of the day?	Yes	1
	No	0
Score: Possible range is 0 – 10: Scores of 4 and greater indicating nicotine dependence Scores of 4 and greater indicating severe nicotine dependence		

Table 4. Fagerstrom Test for Nicotine Dependence (FTND; Heatherton et al., 1991)

2.2.2 Addiction and risk potential of the drug tobacco

The *'addiction potential'* of a drug describes the risk for developing a mental or physical dependence when using a drug and the subsequent failure to quit the use and to master a withdrawal. This addiction risk results from a) the pharmacological effects of the substance on the organism, b) the quality and intensity of the evoked subjective states of intoxication or well-being and c) the learned stimulus-response association between the drug use on the one hand and the 'kick' or flush response (positive reinforcement) and/or the avoidance of withdrawal symptoms on the other (negative reinforcement). The addiction potential of a psychotropic substance is not exclusively determined by its pharmacological characteristics and its potency for physical dependence but essentially, among other things, by the type of the substance intake (addiction potential decreasing with types of applications: injecting, sniffing, smoking and swallowing). This explains that smoked nicotine has a high addiction potential compared to nicotine patches at the same dose.

Alongside heroin, nicotine is seen as the substance with the highest *'pure addiction potential'*. This finding has been determined in animal studies wherein different substances are applied in standardised form (e.g. as an oral application). The measure for the addiction potential is typical addiction behaviour shown by the laboratory animals after a number of applications (e.g. number of lever actions or toleration of pain stimuli in order to get to the drug). However, the approaches for the determination of the addiction potential that are based on complex expert judgements on the addiction risk of persons under real using conditions seem to be more adequate. In a study conducted by the Swiss Institute for the Prevention of Alcohol and Drug Problems (SIPA), renowned addiction experts evaluated the addiction potential of seven different substances in direct comparison according to five evaluation criteria (cf., tab. 5). In the resulting ranking list heroin reached the highest addiction potential, followed by cocaine, alcohol and nicotine, whereby for nicotine especially a very high value for (mental) 'addiction' was declared (Fahrenkrug & Gmel, 1996).

Substance	Overall Evaluation	With-drawal Symptoms	Reinforce-ment	Increase of Tolerance	Addiction	Intoxication
Heroin	1	1	1	1	1	2
Cocaine	2	3	2	3	3	1
Alcohol	3	2	4	2	4	3
Nicotine	4	4	3	4	2	6
Caffeine	7	7	7	6	7	7
Ecstasy	5	5	5	5	5	4
Marihuana	6	6	6	7	6	5

1= highest addiction potential; 7= lowest addiction potential

Table 5. Addiction Potential of Different Psychotropic Substances (quoted in Fahrenkrug & Gmel, 1996).

The 'addiction potential' relates to the addiction risk, but does not state anything about the *overall biopsychosocial risk potential* of a drug. Nutt et al. (2007) determined three main factors of potential damage by a psychotropic substance: 1) physical damage, 2) addiction potential and 3) social effects. A three-dimensional risk categories matrix was derived from this, by means of which the different substances were evaluated by two independent expert groups regarding their overall risk potential. In this multi-dimensional evaluation of the biopsychosocial overall risks, tobacco smoking is positioned in the upper middle field (place 9).

2.2.3 Comorbidity: Tobacco smoking and mental disorders

Tobacco addiction is closely associated with the occurrence of *mental disorders* and their course of disease. Cigarette smoking is disproportionately prevalent amongst persons with mental disorders (population) and/or psychiatric patients (clinical populations; Breslau, 1995; Degenhardt & Hall, 2001; John et al., 2004; Meyer et al, 2004; Haug et al., Heinberg & Guarda, 2001; Kordon & Kahl, 2004). On the whole, prevalence of smoking in mentally comorbid persons is approximately twice as high (50%) when compared to the general population (25-30%) (Grant et al., 2004; Lasser et al., 2000). It even amounts to 71-90% in patients with addictions to other substances (Ker et al., 1996; Patten et al., 1996; Martin et al., 1997; Williams & Ziedonis, 2004); for other *severe types of disorders* such as schizophrenia and bipolar disorders prevalence is on average 80% (Hughes, 1993; Leon & Diaz, 2005). In the US, the market share of the overall cigarette consumption by persons with psychiatric diagnoses is currently between 44 and 46% (Lasser et al., 2000; Grant et al., 2004).

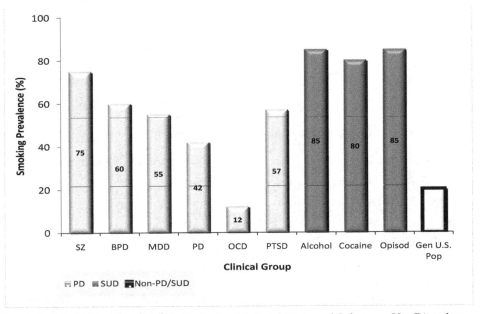

Fig. 2. Co-Morbidity of Smoking in Patients with Psychiatric and Substance Use Disorders (Kalman et al., 2005, p. 107)

Smokers with *mental comorbidity* mostly are heavy smokers, that means they are prone to smoke more cigarettes per day (days pack) and to smoke each cigagette more intensively (e.g. draws per cigarette, draw frequency, inhalation depth) (Lasser et al., 2000; Tidey et al., 2005). As a result, they do not only show increased physic long-term morbidity and mortality rates due to organic diseases associated with tobacco (Williams & Ziedonis, 2004), but they also have, amongst other things, a worse prognosis in relation to their mental disorder, a higher psychiatric lifetime-co-/multimorbidity, a more unfavourable course of disease (e.g. episodes in MDE that are more often, longer and more intensive), less successful therapy outcomes, a higher burden of disease, severe impairment of psychosocial functioning (Brown et al. 2000) as well as a lower *quality of life* (Schmitz et al., 2003). Smokers suffering from a mental disorder also show a lower self-efficacy and more negative attitudes towards a smoke stop (Carossella et al., 1999; Esterberg & Compton, 2005) as well as below average success rates for tobacco withdrawal that are often <15% (Glassman et al., 1993; Hall, Munoz, Reus, & Sees, 1993; Rohde et al., 2004; Ziedonis & George, 1997; Ziedonis et al., 1994). Moreover, smoking tobacco is a significant predictor for a *lifetime-suicidal tendency*, even when monitoring possible confounders (Breslau et al., 2005; Oquendo et al., 2004; Bronisch et al., 2009; Miller et al., 2000; figure 4).

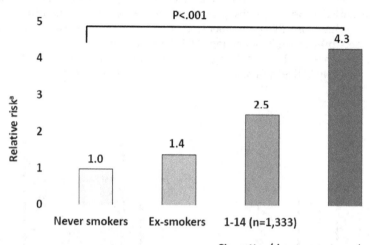

Adjusted for time period, age, alcohol, and marital status

Fig. 3. Smoking and suicide risk (Miller et al., 2000)

The *etiological causality* of this coincidence between smoking tobacco and mental disorders is largely unresolved. Three competing theoretical models are being discussed: 1) According to the *'primary disorder model'* smoking is a reaction to the mental disorder (Guidelines of the American Psychiatric Association, 1996; Kendler et al., 1993; Pomerleau et al., 1997). In the sense of the *'self treatment hypothesis'*, persons suffering from mental strain use nicotine for stress reduction (easing effect of nicotine) and for alleviating their subjective mental symptoms (effect of nicotine to soothe, enhance moods and improve the well-being of smokers) (Kendler et al., 1993; Hughes, 2004; Breslau, 2001). It is true that nicotine has specific anti-depressive effects (Tizabi et al., 1999; Balfour et al., 2000), since the serotonergic system is activated by nicotine similar to antidepressants (Vazquez-Palacios et al., 2005), and it is often used by psychiatric patients to specifically enhance their mood. According to this model, initial manifestation of the mental disorder would have to precede chronological tobacco smoking. 2) In contrast, the *'primary smoking model'* states that smoking can contribute to the development of a mental disorder. According to that, exposition to nicotine is a risk factor making individuals vulnerable to mental disorders due to the chronic impact on diverse transmitter systems that are involved in the development of mental disorders. This hypothesis is supported by the observation that the initial manifestation of mental symptoms often follows a longer break of regular smoking. Furthermore, for example, prenatal exposition to smoking is associated with the later occurrence of ADHD and depression in infancy and adolescence. 3) The *'bidirectional model'* assumes a long lasting interaction effect between smoking and mental disorders. Therefore, smoking triggers the development of mental symptoms in genetically disposed persons first and is later used for easing symptoms. In this way, regular nicotine consumption contributes to the chronification of the disorders in the long term (Mueser et al., 1998). It could be possible that smokers with mental disorders shy away from smoke stop because nicotine withdrawal symptoms contribute to an exacerbation of psychiatric symptoms and an increase of the relapse risk (Glassman, 2001; Balfour et al., 2000). Finally, it has been proven that e.g. schizophrenic patients often use nicotine to specifically counter regulate the effect of neuroleptics (Barnes et al., 2006; Glassman, 1994; Haring, Barnas, Saria, Humpel, & Fleischhaker, 1989; Hughes, 1993). 4) Finally, the *'common-factor model'* assumes a common etiology of nicotine dependence and other mental disorders (Breslau et al., 1998; Dierker, 2002; Covey, 1998). Since nicotine dependence itself is a mental disorder with manifold commonalities in terms of neurobiological, cognitive personal or social risk factors and mechanisms with a) other substance disorders (e.g. dopaminergic system) and also b) with other mental disorders (e.g. serotonergic system in MD), a common genetic disposition for e.g. depressions and susceptibility for the effects of nicotine positive seems likely (Kendler et al., 1993; Breslau et al., 1998).

2.3 Etiology: Neurobiological and psychological addiction mechanisms
2.3.1 Vulnerability and risk factors

Today, the average age of onset for smoking cigarettes ranges between eleven to thirteen years (Silagy et al., 1994; Nelson et al., 1998). The development of a tobacco addiction is dependent on a number of factors or causes. In addition to a *genetic disposition* (e.g. number of receptors, availability of specific enzymes, and function of transmitter systems), multiple acquired vulnerabilities and risk factors have been identified that comprise individual characteristics as well as specific environmental conditions (Brown et al., 1992; US Department of Health and Human Services, 1990). In the stage of initial or experimental use, despite of *availability of tobacco products* and *advertising influences, social factors like family models and the peer group* that are decisive for the start of one's smoking (Silagy et al., 1994). There are significant differences in *social classes* with the highest smoking rates in the lower social class, in unemployed people and social groups with lower educational achievement. Furthermore, an existing *psychiatric comorbidity* and unfavourable influences of the *family milieu* (parental psychopathology) primarily count towards the individual risk factors for the development of a tobacco addiction (WHO, 2001). Moreover, tobacco addiction and health risks towards smoking-related disorders correlate with the *early onset of smoking*. The physical addiction phenomena seem to develop especially rapidly in children and adolescents. In the stage of regular and dependent use, smokers try to manage their *psychosocial stress* or *daily hassles* by using nicotine ('self treatment'). In the long term run, the most important condition to maintain dependency is *negative reinforcement*, because every cigarette acts more and more to reduce withdrawal symptoms in the first line.

2.3.2 Neurobiological mechanisms

Like all psychotropic substances, nicotine stimulates the *mesolimbic dopamine system ('desire and reward system')* whose neurones are located in the area tegmentalis ventralis and project to the nucleus accumbens as well as the corpus striatum, among others. In contrast to other drugs, nicotine exposition initiates a particular long term potentiation of specific neurons in this area of the brain, which causes a persistent increase of the dopamine level even after short term nicotine exposition.

In order to compensate for the artificial biochemical flooding and to maintain the normal functions, the brain reacts on two levels: 1) with a neuroanatomical change of the number and responsiveness of specific receptors (*neuroplastic down or up regulation*) and 2) with an inhibiting feedback on the level of transmitters, restricting the effect of nicotine by releasing *counter-regulative molecules* (Kunze et al., 1998). Both reactions lead to a weakening of the effect of nicotine. If the smoker subsequently tries to compensate the diminishing effect by means of more intensive smoking, the brain respectively produce more inhibiting molecules in that ever-increasing doses of nicotine are necessary to achieve 'intoxication' (*tolerance*). If the organism is then suddenly deprived of the substance (*withdrawal*), the balance of the system is forcefully disturbed. On the one hand, too few bodily-owned transmitters are available since the body has limited its own production and, on the other hand, a surplus of compensatorily released inhibitory molecules, which further inhibit the normal remaining functions of the transmitter balance, exist for a number of weeks. A strong *state of deprivation* results thereof and causes torturing mental and physical acute withdrawal conditions (withdrawal syndrome). The body is now not able to exist without tobacco any more and, therefore, an *addiction* has formed.

2.3.3 Psychological and neuropsychological mechanisms

Addicted ex-smokers are still at *risk to relapse* in face of any smoking-associated cues which trigger an irresistible desire (craving) for nicotine, even many years and decades after the withdrawal, probably for their whole lifetime. This long time active *'addiction memory'* cannot be explained by mechanism of physical dependence, which normalise within a few weeks after quitting. In the first line, complex *learned conditioning processes* are responsible for the continuing sensitisation to nicotine and the ongoing high relapse rates.

Simultaneously to dopamine release in the *'desire and reward system'* nicotine stimulates specific *areas in the brain which are involved in association learning processes.* That is why smoking tobacco has a particularly strong link to *situational* (smoking break, coffee drinking, after work beer), *behavioural* (reaching for the box of cigarettes), *sensory* (smell, taste) or *affective* (mood) *cues* that are associated with smoking. Insofar, persistent addiction can be primarily traced back to *respondent* and *operant conditioning*. In the case of smoking *positive reinforcement* is generated by the fateful association between the inhalation (stimulus) and the subsequent state of well-being (response) that permanently becomes engraved in memory (*'addiction memory'*) within a short time. Despite the missing intensive intoxication, the high addiction potential of tobacco smoking results from the brain of a regular smoker being flooded with nicotine 200 to 400 times per day (per year: 73,000 to 146,000 times) — and the stimulus-response connection is thereby continuously enforced.

The high *risk of a relapse* and the actual *relapse process* after a smoke stop can be explained by means of *neuropsychological* and *cognitivepsychological models*. However, one of the main - questions, why the addiction behaviour and craving is not extinguished after a certain time was not resolved satisfactorily. The latest research in cognitive learning shows that the *extinction* of a respondent conditioning is, in a neurobiological sense, no unlearning in terms of a decoupling of synaptic links but a *new learning and/or re-learning* where new stimulus-reaction-links are generated while the old ones are principally still available (Conklin &

Tiffany, 2002). That is why old addiction conditionings can, if certain triggers emerge, be reactivated even after a long time (e.g. by reinstatement or spontaneous recovery).

Furthermore, the hypersensitivity to the addiction cues (*cue reactivity*), which is profoundly resistant against extinction and overwriting, can be explained with *neuroplastic changes* in the dopamine system. In the case of chronic substance intake a neurobiological hyper reactivity to the drug and their trigger cues develops in the mesolimbic dopamine system (*subcortical dysfunction*) and, at the same time, the areas that are responsible for executive control (*frontal cortical dysfunction*) are weakened. Finally, the relapse can be described by the different levels of information processing of addiction-related cues on the one hand, and by the intentional control of action on the other (Tiffany und Conklin, 2000). The addicts' reaction to drug-associated cues is an example of '*automatic processing*', i.e. it is made unconsciously quick, linked to certain trigger situations, with a low use of cognitive capacity and can only be influenced to a small degree. In contrast, abstinence demands an intentional regulation of action with conscious information processing and executive control functions ('*controlled processing*'), which is consciously, intention controlled and flexible, but relatively slow, cognitively demanding and limited by the processing capacity. In case of chronic substance abuse an increasing disequilibrium between the growing influence of automatic stimulus processing ('*implicit cognitions*'), as well as a weakening of executive control and regulation of emotions that makes the person trying to quit increasingly vulnerable to addiction triggers and, finally, relapse.

2.4 Treatment

Almost all smokes are aware of the smoke-related health risks and a majority of them repeatedly tries to stop smoking. The *willingness to quit* depends on the individual stage of motivation. According to the widely known *transtheoretical model* (Prochaska & DiClimente, 1993) smokers move through a discrete series of five motivational stages before they quit successfully: (i) *precontemplation* (no thoughts of quitting), (ii) *contemplation* (thinking about quitting), (iii) *preparation* (planning to quit in the next 30 days), (iv) *action* (quitting successfully for up to six months), and (v) *maintenance* (no smoking for more than six months). The transtheoretical theory has not been empirically supported, and some authors cast doubt its practical value (Etter & Sutton, 2002; Sutton, 2001).

However, most smokers will succeed to quit at one point in their life: There are more ex-smokers than current smokers to be found in the age cohort over 50 years old. However, tobacco withdrawal often requires a multitude of stop smoking trials to be successful when no professional help is sought. The success rate of unassisted smoke stop trials is at a mere 3-6% during the 12-months period. However, less than 5 % of all smokers willing to stop make use of professional help, despite the availability of effective smoking cessation therapies (WHO, 2001; Nelson & Wittchen, 1998).

Professional smoking cessation treatments include a wide range of interventions, from medical advice through to brief motivational interventions to complex withdrawal programs. In practice, less effective methods such as hypnosis and acupuncture are used alongside motivational interviewing, cognitive-behavioural therapy interventions (CBT) and medicinal approaches in withdrawal and substitution treatment. Professional smoking cessation treatment is first and foremost based on behavioural group interventions (cf. Box 1) and approaches of motivational interviewing, and often offered in combination with medicinal support (e.g. nicotine substitutes).

1. Psychoeducation: education, information and attitude change
2. Analysis of problem and behaviour: Analysis and documentation of smoking behaviour and the maintaining cognitive and situational or social conditions
3. Strengthening of motivation to change (motivational interview): Clear decision to quit smoking, determination of a deadline to stop smoking
4. Systematic preparation for abstinence, execution of smoke stop and modification of behaviour: Control of conditioning stimuli, development and training of alternative behaviour, contract management, self-reward, teaching of strategies of self-control
5. Activation of a supporting social network and teaching of health promotional behaviour
6. Relapse prevention: Dealing with risk situations, strategies against relapse risks (role play exercises)

Box 1. Components of complex behavioural therapy programmes for smoking cessation.

Primary goal in smoking cessation treatment is *total abstinence*. Controlled tobacco use leading to harm reduction is only aimed for in exceptional cases (in cases of severe disease or pregnancy with simultaneous inability to remain abstinent; Stead & Lancaster, 2007; Lumley et al., 2009). The medicinal treatment in smoking cessation primarily aims to soothe the somatic withdrawal symptoms and associated craving. The *pharmacological treatment* options are based on three different modes of action:

i.   In *nicotine replacement therapy* a patient is given nicotine doses, which substitute the nicotine the patient does not take in anymore by smoking, by means of drugs containing nicotine (nicotine patch, gum, inhaler, lozenge, nasal spray, sublingual tablet). By means of retaining an equal level of nicotine withdrawal symptoms are soothed and the withdrawal is made easier by stepwise downdosing the pharmacological nicotine.

ii. The nicotine-free drug *bupropion (Zyban®)*, originally developed as *anti-depressant*, inhibits the synaptic absorption of catecholamines (adrenalin, dopamine) in the mesolimbic dopamine system, thereby compensating the dopamine lack caused by the nicotine withdrawal and, in this way, soothes the withdrawal symptoms without supplying nicotine. Due to serious contra-indications, side-effects and pharmaceutical risks, bupropion may only be applied under medical supervision.

iii. The *partial agonist varenicline (Chantix®)* binds to specific nicotine receptors of the subtype that is responsible for one of the addictive effects of the nicotine. The active agent stimulates the receptors and thereby eases withdrawal symptoms. At the same time, it inhibits the effect of externally supplied nicotine by blocking the receptors. Also due to the serious side-effects and risks (nausea, headache, insomnia, abnormal dreams, suicidal ideation and occasional suicidal behavior, erratic behavior and drowsiness) there are similarly strict regulations for varenicline in terms of prescription and medical supervision.

Multi-modal smoking cessation programmes can be divided into three stages: (i) reinforcement of the abstinence motivation and the patient's commitment to quit smoking, (ii) preparation and realisation of smoke stop, (iii) maintenance of abstinence and using new coping strategies to avoid a return to use.

i.   Regular smokers generally are ambivalent towards quitting. Although almost every smoker is aware of the health risks and further disadvantages of smoking, most of them dread the burdens associated with smoke stop (fear of withdrawal symptoms and loss of positive reinforcement) and continually postpone their withdrawal, often for years. This is why it is necessary to make an explicit decision pro tobacco withdrawal at the beginning of the *withdrawal stage* (in case of smokers willing to stop) and/or to motivate in favor of a smoke stop (in case of smokers not yet willing to stop). For this purpose, *motivational interviewing* is a suitable approach (Miller & Rollnick, 2002 by which the motivation to quit smoking and the confidence to change can be analysed and systematically strengthened during the preparation stage. In smoking cessation practice, behavioural-therapeutic techniques (smoking diaries, behavioural analysis, CO-measurement, reinforcement plans, pros-cons lists, target hierarchies, aim in life analysis, short and long term benefits, strengthening of self-efficacy) as well as cognitive techniques (disputation of irrational ideas, worst case scenarios, development of rational alternatives) are applied for the preparation of the smoke stop. The explicit commitment of the smoker to his/her desire to quit smoking (importance) and his belief to being able to reach this goal (realisability) proves to be decisive in this stage.

ii. During the *quitting stage* the smoker is systematically prepared for the smoke stop and the time of abstinence. For this purpose, it is important, not only to create adequate commitment but also to enhance the optimism about one's ability to change and to strengthen self efficacy. Using the 'cold turkey method', a certain quit day is determined. In the sense of a stimulus control, all triggers (smoke utensils such as ashtray, cigarette boxes, lighter etc.) are removed from the immediate surrounding and/or typical smoke situations (e.g. local pub) are temporarily avoided for the time of the smoke stop preparation stage. The smoke stop can be supported by means of aversion therapy (excessive inhaling, retain smoke in lung, smelling of containers with cigarette butts and cold ash) or counter conditioning (presentation of unpleasant stimuli such as deterring photos of smoke-related diseases contingent to smoking).

iii. The treatment stage most important to keep long term abstinence is the *maintenance and relapse prevention*. The ex-smoker is supported in his/her self control management (response control) and self instruction in order for him/her to master craving and withdrawal symptoms and to successfully cope with high risky situation (refusal training). At the same time, positive alternatives to smoking (relaxation exercise, physical exercise, easy breathing, water drinking, pleasant activities and attentional distraction) are proposed and trained. Positive stimuli (e.g. appraisal, material rewards, amount of money saved, improvement of lung function, duration of abstinence) or contracting (written commitment, rewards vs punishment) are used to support abstinence and social resources are mobilised (workshop assistants, supporters). During abstinence a cognitive reframing shall be triggered in which the smokefree life comes to be seen as less unpleasant condition of withdrawal and loss but increasingly as an awarding situation in which a positive physical well-being and independence dominates. Finally, an individual emergency plan is drafted and structured relapse prevention management is trained (what to do when having a relapse).

2.5 Empirical evidence

Up to date, a large amount of professional and more or less *evidence-based smoking cessation treatments* have been developed, that range from minimal interventions (physician's advice to quit smoking) and medicinal withdrawal treatment (nicotine replacement therapy, psychotropic drugs such as bupropion or varenicline) to telephone counselling ('quit-line') and online quitting programmes as well as to multi-modal smoking cessation in behavioural group therapy described above. The efficacy of professional smoking cessation treatments is well determined. An impressive number of RCTs as well as several meta-analyses and *Systematic Cochrane Reviews* clearly proved the high efficacy of several cessation treatments towards the primary outcome of long-term abstinence.

In particular, *group behaviour therapy* programmes for smoking cessation yielded high effect sizes in many randomised controlled trials (RCT) and were found to be superior to self help, and other less intensive interventions (Stead & Lancaster, 2005). However, there is not enough evidence to evaluate whether groups are more effective, or cost-effective, than intensive individual counselling and only limited evidence that the addition of group therapy to other forms of treatment, such as advice from a health professional or nicotine replacement, produced extra benefit (Stead & Lancaster, 2005, p 2). *Individual behavioural counselling interventions* for smoking cessation have been well-proven, too (Lancaster & Stead, 2005). Individual counselling was more effective than control, but a greater effect of intensive counselling compared to brief counseling could not be found. *Aversion therapy*, which pairs the pleasurable stimulus of smoking a cigarette with some unpleasant stimulus in order to extinguish the urge to smoke, has been evaluated in a smaller number of RCT's that provide insufficient evidence to determine the efficacy of rapid smoking (Hajek & Stead, 2001).

Pharmaceutical treatment in smoking cessation is high efficient as well. All of the commercially available forms of *nicotine replacement therapy* (gum, transdermal patch, nasal spray, inhaler and sublingual tablets/lozenges) can help people who make a quit attempt to increase their chances of successfully stopping smoking by 50-70%, regardless of setting Stead et al., 2008). The empirical evidence show that the *antidepressants* bupropion and nortriptyline are equally effective and of similar efficacy to nicotine replacement therapy, but there is insufficient evidence that adding bupropion to nicotine replacement therapy provides an additional long-term benefit (Hughes et al., 2007, p 2). Also *varenicline* at standard dose increases the chances of successful long-term smoking cessation between two- and threefold compared with pharmacologically unassisted quit attempts (Cahill et al., 2011, p 2).

The trials to *internet-based interventions* for smoking cessation did not show consistent effects, but for some interventions there is evidence that online counselling can assist smoking cessation, especially if the information is appropriately tailored to the users and frequent automated contacts with the users are ensured (Civljak, Sheikh, Stead & Car, 2010, p 2). Similarly, proactive *telephone counselling* for smoking cessation can efficiently help smokers in quitting, but a minimum of three or more calls are required to increase the chances of quitting compared to a minimal intervention (providing standard self-help materials, brief advice), or compared to pharmacotherapy alone (Stead et al., 2006). *Motivational interviewing* for smoking cessation yielded a modest but significant increase in quitting compared to brief advice or usual care and was more effective, when delivered by primary care physicians and by counselors and when conducted in longer and multiple sessions (Lai et al., 2010).

In contrast, there is no consistent, bias-free evidence that *acupuncture, acupressure, laser therapy* or *electrostimulation* or *exercise interventions* for smoking cessation are effective for smoking cessation (White et al., 2011; Ussher et al., 2008). Also, the empirical evidence for *hypnotherapy* fails to show a greater effect on six-month quit rates than other interventions or no treatment (Barnes et al., 2010). *Standard self-help materials* may increase quit rates compared to no intervention, but the effect is likely to be small, and no additional benefit has been found alongside other interventions such as advice from a healthcare professional, or nicotine replacement therapy (Lancaster & Stead, 2005, p 2). Materials that are tailored for individual smokers are more effective than untailored materials, although the absolute size of effect is still small.

Smoking *reduction versus abrupt cessation* in smokers who want to quit makes no difference with regard to long-term abstinence (Lindson et al., 2010). According to the *transtheoretical model stage-based* self-help interventions (expert systems and/or tailored materials) and individual counselling were neither more nor less effective than their non-stage-based equivalents (Cahill et al., 2010, p 2).

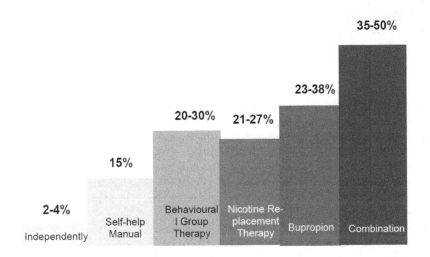

Fig. 4. Success rates (12-months abstinence) of measurements for tobacco withdrawal in clinical studies (efficacy) according to a meta-analysis of the US Department of Health and Human Services (Fiore et al., 2008)

In context of the *US Clinical Practice Guidelines*, sponsored by the U.S. Public Health Service, Guideline Panel conducted 2000 a large mega-metanalysis *'Treating Tobacco Use and Dependence'* which has been updated in 2008 (Fiore et al., 2008). The main results are shown in figure 7. In Detail, the effectiveness and abstinence rates of various interventions and medications in smoking cessation treatment are presented in table 6 and 7. In summary, the most effective smoking cessation treatment is a combination of group behavior therapy or individual counseling with pharmaceutical treatment, whereas a combination of more than one pharmaceutics has an extra benefit (e.g., NRT patch + NRT gum or NRT patch + oral medication).

Based on the empirical evidence of international trials in the field of smoking, tobacco dependence and smoking cessation in numerous countries specific clinical guidelines for treating tobacco addiction have been developed during the last decade, e.g. :

- The well-known US 'Clinical Practice Guideline for Treating Tobacco Use and Dependence' (Fiore et al., 2000, 2008) occurred as a result of an extraordinary partnership among Federal Government and nonprofit organizations;
- in UK the National Institute for Health and Clinical Excellence – NICE created a number of clinical guidelines:
  - Smoking cessation services in primary care, pharmacies, local authorities and workplaces, particularly for manual working groups, pregnant women and hard to reach communities (2008)
  - The Impact of Quitlines on Smoking Cessation (2007)
  - Economic Analysis of Interventions for Smoking Cessation Aimed at Pregnant Women (2007)
  - School-based interventions to prevent the uptake of smoking among children and young people: cost-effectiveness model (2010)
  - The effectiveness of smoking cessation interventions to reduce the rates of premature death in disadvantaged areas through proactive case finding, retention and access to services
  - Mass-media and point-of-sales measures to prevent the uptake of smoking by children and young people (2008)
  - Workplace health promotion: how to help employees to stop smoking (2007)
- Association of the Scientific Medical Societies in Germany co-ordinates the national programme of medical guidelines of its member organizations. In cooperation with numerous institutions and non-profit organizations (e.g. German Society of Addiction Research; German Association for Psychiatry and Psychotherapy) two smoking cessation guidelines have been developed:
  - Guidelines for Treating Substance Use Disorders (2004)
  - Smoking Cessation in COPD patients (2008)

These various national guidelines do explicitly consider the different conditions of the social, cultural or health care systems in each country and should be received by the health care professionals in the specific region they are developed for.

Various intensity levels of session length (n = 43 studies)[a]			
Level of contact	Number of arms	Estimated odds ratio (95% C.I.)	Estimated abstinence rate (95% C.I.)
No contact	30	1.0	10.9
Minimal counseling (< 3 minutes)	19	1.3 (1.01–1.6)	13.4 (10.9–16.1)
Low-intensity counseling (3–10 minutes)	16	1.6 (1.2–2.0)	16.0 (12.8–19.2)

Higher intensity counseling (> 10 minutes)	55	2.3 (2.0–2.7)	22.1 (19.4–24.7)

Total amount of contact time (n = 35 studies) [a]

Total amount of contact time	Number of arms	Estimated odds ratio (95% C.I.)	Estimated abstinence rate (95% C.I.)
No minutes	16	1.0	11.0
1–3 minutes	12	1.4 (1.1–1.8)	14.4 (10.3–17.5)
4–30 minutes	20	1.9 (1.5–2.3)	18.8 (15.6–22.0)
31–90 minutes	16	3.0 (2.3–3.8)	26.5 (21.5–31.4)
91–300 minutes	16	3.2 (2.3–4.6)	28.4 (21.3–35.5)
> 300 minutes	15	2.8 (2.0–3.9)	25.5 (19.2–31.7)

Various types of formats (n = 58 studies) [a]

Format Number	Number of arms	Estimated odds ratio (95% C.I.)	Estimated abstinence rate (95% C.I.)
No format	20	1.0	10.8
Self-help	93	1.2 (1.02–1.3)	12.3 (10.9–13.6)
Proactive tel. counseling	26	1.2 (1.1–1.4)	13.1 (11.4–14.8)
Group counseling	52	1.3 (1.1–1.6)	13.9 (11.6–16.1)
Individual counseling	67	1.7 (1.4–2.0)	16.8 (14.7–19.1)

Various types of counseling and behavioral therapies (n = 64 studies) [a]

Type of counseling and behavioral therapy	Number of arms	Estimated odds ratio (95% C.I.)	Estimated abstinence rate (95% C.I.)
No counseling/ behavioral therapy	35	1.0	11.2
Relaxation/breathing	31	1.0 (0.7–1.3)	10.8 (7.9–13.8)
Contingency contracting	22	1.0 (0.7–1.4)	11.2 (7.8–14.6)
Weight/diet	19	1.0 (0.8–1.3)	11.2 (8.5–14.0)
Cigarette fading	25	1.1 (0.8–1.5)	11.8 (8.4–15.3)
Negative affect	8	1.2 (0.8–1.9)	13.6 (8.7–18.5)
social support	50	1.3 (1.1–1.6)	14.4 (12.3–16.5)
Extratreatment social support	19	1.5 (1.1–2.1)	16.2 (11.8–20.6)
Practical counseling (problem solving/skills)	104	1.5 (1.3–1.8)	16.2 (14.0–18.5)
Other aversive smoking	19	1.7 (1.04–2.8)	17.7 (11.2–24.9)
Rapid smoking	19	2.0 (1.1–3.5)	19.9 (11.2–29.0)

[a] Go to www.surgeongeneral.gov/tobacco/gdinrefs.htm for the articles used in this meta-analysis.

Table 6. Meta-analysis (2000): Effectiveness and abstinence rates of various interventions in smoking cessation treatment

Various medications and medication compared to placebo at 6-months post quit (n = 83 studies) [a]			
Medication	Number of arms	Estimated odds ratio (95% C.I.)	Estimated abstinence rate (95% C.I.)
Placebo	80	1.0	13.8
Monotherapies			
Varenicline (2mg/day)	5	3.1 (2.5–3.8)	33.2 (28.9–37.8)
Nicotine Nasal Spray	4	2.3 (1.7–3.0)	26.7 (21.5–32.7)
Hig-Dose Nicotine Patch (> 25mg) (These include both standard or ling-term-duration)	4	2.3 (1.7–3.0)	26.5 (21.3–32.5)
Long-Term Nicotine Gum (>14 weeks)	6	2.2 (1.5–3.2)	26.1 (19.7–33.6)
Varenicline (1mg/day)	3	2.1 (1.5–3.0)	25.4 (19.6–32.2)
Nicotine Inhaler	6	2.1 (1.5–2.9)	24.8 (19.1–31.6)
Clonidine	3	2.1 (1.2–3.7)	25.0 (15.7–37.3)
Bupropion SR	226	2.0 (1.8–2.2)	24.2 (22.2–26.4)
Nicotine Patch (6–14 weeks)	632	1.9 (1.7–2.2)	23.4 (21.3–25.8)
Long-Term Nicotine Patch (> 14 weeks)	3102	1.9 (1.7–2.3)	23.7 (21.0–26.6)
Nortriptyline	5	1.8 (1.3–2.6)	22.5 (16.8–29.4)
Nicotine Gum (6–14 weeks)	15	1.5 (1.2–1.7)	19.0 (16.5–21.9)
Combination therapies			
Patch (long-term; > 14 weeks) + ad llb NRT (gum or spray)	3	3.6 (2.5–5.2)	36.5 (28.6–45.3)
Patch + Bupropion SR	3	2.5 (1.9–3.4)	28.9 (23.5–35.1)
Patch + Nortriptyline	2	2.3 (1.3–4.2)	27.3 (17.2–40.4)
Patch + Inhaler	2	2.2 (1.3–3.6)	25.8 (17.4–36.5)
Patch + Second generation antidepressants (paroxetine, venlafaxine)	3	2.0 (1.2–3.4)	24.3 (16.1–35.0)
Medications not shown to be effective			
Selective Serotonin Re-uptake Inhibitors (SSRIs)	3	1.0 (0.7–1.4)	13.7 (10.2–18.0)
Naltrexone	2	0.5 (0.2–1.2)	7.3 (3.1–16.2)

[a] Go to www.surgeongeneral.gov/tobacco/gdinrefs.htm for the articles used in this meta-analysis.

Table 7. Meta-analysis (2000): Effectiveness and abstinence rates of various medications in smoking cessation treatment

3. Conclusion

The *smoking rates* in the population vary from country to country with a range between approximately 25-60% of adult population. Although only every third smoker meets the diagnostic criteria for *nicotine dependence*, tobacco addiction is the *most prevalent mental disorder* worldwide. Besides the well-known impact of tobacco smoking on physical health, there is a growing body of evidence that smoking increases the *vulnerability for mental disorders*, too. Point prevalence of tobacco smoking amongst persons with mental disorders (MD) is 40-50% and thus, on average, twice as high as amongst the general population. Smokers with psychiatric comorbidity do not only show increased somatic morbidity and mortality rates, but also a significantly worse prognosis in relation to their MD, up to a significant increase of lifetime *suicide risks*.

The *addiction potential of tobacco smoking* as well as the difficulty to quit and to permanently remain abstinent is often highly underestimated by smokers themselves, but by many health care professionals as well. The high failure and relapse rates in smoking cessation, even in patients with life threatening smoking-associated disorders (e.g. myocardial infarction, pulmonary emphysema or lung transplantation) demonstrates that nicotine dependence is a serious mental disorder and an addiction comparable harmful like in case of illicit drugs. Overcoming smoking as a serious 'substance use disorder' in many cases calls for *professional cessation treatment*. Although every second smoker succeeds to quit at some point in his/her life without professional help, however, this is only achieved after many years and after a number of failed trials. During this long lasting period since smokers are successful in quitting, in many cases serious harm to their physical or mental health has already been caused. Therefore, in *routine care*, smokers should be *encouraged to quit smoking* at an *early stage* and they should be tested on a routine basis for a *tobacco addiction* and, if necessary, be referred to a *smoking cessation specialist* or an outpatient cessation clinic.

4. Acknowledgment

I acknowledge Ph.D. Stefanie Fuchs and Ph.D. Anja Sehl for their helpful support in the systematic evidence search and Ms. Christina Bernd for editing this manuscript.

5. References

Balfour, D. J. K. & Ridley, D. L. (2000). The effects of nicotine on neural pathways implicated in depression: A factor in nicotine addiction? *Pharmacology, Biochemistry and Behavior*, Vol. 66, No. 1, pp. 79-85, ISSN 0091-3057

Barnes, J., Dong, C. Y., McRobbie, H., Walker, N., Mehta. M. & Stead, L. F. (2010). Hypnotherapy for smoking cessation. *Cochrane Database of Systematic Reviews*, Vol. 10, (October 2010), ISSN 13616137

Breslau, N., Johnson, E. O., Hiripi, E. & Kessler, R. (2001). Nicotine dependence in the United States - Prevalence, trends, and smoking persistence. *Archives of General Psychiatry*, Vol. 58, No. 9, (September 2011), pp. 810-816, ISSN 0003-990X

Breslau, N., Novak, S. P. & Kessler, R. C. (2004). Psychiatric disorders and stages of smoking. *Biological Psychiatry*, Vol. 55, No. 1, pp. 69-76, ISSN 0006-3223

Breslau, N., Schultz, L. R., Johnson, E. O., Peterson, E. L. & Davis, G. C. (2005). Smoking and the risk of suicidal behavior: a prospective study of a community sample. *Archives of General Psychiatry*, Vol. 62, No. 3, (March 2005), pp. 328-34, ISSN 0003-990X

Brown, S. L. & Owen, N. (1992). Self-help smoking cessation materials. *Australian Journal of Public Health*, Vol. 16, No. 2, (June 1992), pp. 188-191, ISSN 1035-7319

Brown, S., Inskip, H. & Barraclough, B. (2000). Causes of the excess mortality of schizophrenia. *British Journal of Psychiatry*, Vol. 177, (September 2000), pp. 212-217, ISSN 0007-1250

Brown, R., Kahler, C., Niaura, R. S., Abrams, D. B., Sales, S., Ramsey, S., Goldstein, M. G., Burgess, E. S. & Miller, I. W. (2001). Cognitive-behavioral treatment for depression in smoking cessation. *Journal of Consulting and Clinical Psychology*, Vol. 69, No. 3, (June 2001), pp. 471–480, ISSN 0022-006X

Buchkremer, G., Bents, H., Horstmann, M., Opitz, K. & Tölle, R. (1989). Combination of behavioral smoking cessation with transdermal nicotine substitutution. *Addictive Behaviors*, Vol. 14, No. 2, pp. 229-238, ISSN 0306-4603

Buchkremer, G., Minneker, E. & Block, M. (1991). Smoking-cessation treatment combining transdermal nicotine substitution with behavioral therapy. *Pharmacopsychiatry*, Vol. 24, No. 3, (May 1991), pp. 96-102, ISSN 0176-3679

Cahill, K., Lancaster, T. & Green, N. (2010). Stage-based interventions for smoking cessation. *Cochrane Database of Systematic Reviews*, Vol. 11, (November 2010), ISSN 13616137

Cahill, K., Stead, L. F. & Lancaster, T. (2011). Nicotine receptor partial agonists for smoking cessation. *Cochrane Database of Systematic Reviews*, Vol. 2, (February 2011), ISSN 13616137

Civljak, M., Sheikh, A., Stead, L. F. & Car, J. (2010). Internet-based interventions for smoking cessation. *Cochrane Database of Systematic Reviews*, Vol. 9, (September 2010). ISSN 13616137

Conklin, C. A., & Tiffany, St. (2002). Applying extinction research and theory to cue-exposure addiction treatment. *Addiction*, Vol. 97, No. 2, pp. 155-167, ISSN 09652140

De Leon, J. & Diaz, F. J., (2005). A meta-analysis of worldwide studies demonstrates an association between schizophrenia and tobacco smoking behaviors. *Schizophrenia Research*, Vol. 76, No. 2/3, (July 2005), pp. 135-157, ISSN 09209964

El-Guebaly, N., Cathcart, J., Currie, S., Brown, D. & Gloster, S. (2002). Public health and therapeutic aspects of smoking bans in mental health and addiction settings. *Psychiatric Services*, Vol. 53, No. 12, (December 2002), pp. 1617–1622, ISSN 10752730

Etter, J. F. & Sutton, S. (2002). Assessing stage of change in current and former smokers. *Addiction*, Vol. 97, No. 9, pp. 1171-1182, ISSN 09652140

ENSH. (2007). Tobacco Force United, 30. 03. 2010, Available from: http://www. ensh. eu/ensh/racine/

Fagerström, K. O., Schneider, N. G. & Lunell, E. (1993). Effectiveness of nicotine patch and nicotine gum as individual versus combined treatment for tobacco withdrawal symptoms. *Psychopharmacology*, Vol. 111, No. 3, (June 1993), pp. 271-277, ISSN 00333158

Fahrenkrug, H. & Gmel, G. (1996) Addictiveness: How Swiss experts rate alcohol and other drugs. *Alcologia*, Vol. 8, No. 3, pp. 225-229

Fiore, M. C. (2000). US Public Health Practice Guideline: Treating tobacco use and dependence. *Respiratory Care*, Vol. 45, No. 10, (October 2000), pp. 1200–1262, ISSN 0020-1324

Fowler, J. S., Logan, J., Wang, G. J. & Volkow, N. D. (2003). Monoamine oxidase and cigarette smoking. *Neurotoxicology*, Vol. 24, No. 1, (January 2003), pp. 75–82, ISSN 0161813X

Gallinat, J., Meisenzahl, E., Jacobsen, L. K., Kalus, P., Bierbrauer, J., Kienast, T., Witthaus, H., Leopold, K., Seifert, F., Schubert, F. & Staedtgen, M. (2006). Smoking and structural brain deficits: a volumetric MR investigation. *The European Journal of Neuroscience*, Vol. 24, No. 6, (September 2006), pp. 1744-1750; ISSN 0953816X

Grant, B. F., Hasin, D. S., Chou, S. P., Stinson, F. S. & Dawson, D. A. (2004). Nicotine dependence and psychiatric disorders in the United States - Results from the National Epidemiologic Survey on Alcohol and Related Conditions. *Archives of General Psychiatry*, Vol. 61, No. 11, (November 2004), pp. 1107-1115, ISSN 15383636

Gubbay, J. (1992). *Smoking and the Workplace*. Centre for Health Policy Research, University of East Anglia.

Gulliver, S. B., Rohsenow, D. J. & Colby, S. M. (1995). Interrelationship of smoking and alcohol dependence, use and urges to use. *Journal of Studies on Alcohol*, Vol. 56, No. 2, (March 1995), pp. 202–206, ISSN 0096-882X

Gulliver, S. B., Kalman, D. & Rohsenow, D. J. (2000). Smoking and drinking among alcoholics in treatment: cross-sectional and longitudinal relationships. *Journal of Studies on Alcohol*, Vol. 61, No. 1, (January 2000), pp. 157–163, ISSN0096-882X

Gulliver, S. B., Kamholz, B. W., & Helstrom, A. W. (2006). Smoking Cessation and Alcohol Abstinence: What Do the Data Tell Us?. *Alcohol Research & Health*, Vol. 29, No. 3, pp. 208-212, ISSN 15357414

Hajek, P. & Stead, L. F. (2001). Aversive smoking for smoking cessation. *Cochrane Database of Systematic Reviews*, Vol. 3, ISSN 13616137

Haug, N. A., Heinberg, L. J. & Guarda, A. S. (2001). Cigarette smoking and its relationship to other substance use among eating disordered inpatients. *Eating and weight disorders*, Vol. 6, No. 3, (September 2001), pp. 130-139, ISSN 1124-4909

Haustein, K. O. (2000). Pharmacotherapy of nicotine dependence. *Int J Clin Pharmacol Ther*, Vol. 38, No. 6, (June 2000), pp. 273-290, ISSN 0946-1965

Heatherton, T. F., Kozlowski, L. T., Frecker, R. C. & Fagerström, K. O. (1991). The Fragerström Test for Nicotine Dependence: a revision of the Fagerstrom Tolerance Questionaire. *British Journal of Addiction*, Vol. 86, No. 9, (September 1991), pp. 1119-1127, ISSN 0952-0481

Hughes, J. R., Oliveto, A. H., Riggs, R., Kenny, M., Liguori, A., Pillitteri, J. L. & MacLaughlin, M. A. (2004). Concordance of different measures of nicotine dependence: Two pilot studies. *Addictive Behaviors*, Vol. 29, No. 8, (November 2004), pp. 1527-1539, ISSN 03064603

Hughes, J. R., Stead, L. F. & Lancaster, T. (2007). Antidepressants for smoking cessation. *Cochrane Database of Systematic Reviews*, Vol. 1, (January 2007), ISSN 13616137

Hurt, R. D., Sachs, D. P., Glover, E. D., Offord, K. P., Johnston, J. A., Dale, L. C., Khayrallah, M. A.,Schroeder, D. R., Glover, P. N., Sullivan, C. R., Croghan, I. T. & Sullivan, P. M. (1997). A comparison of substained-release bupropion and placebo for smoking cessation. *New England Journal of Medicine,* Vol. 337, No. 17, (October 1999), pp. 1195-1202, ISSN 0028-4793

Jochelson, K. & Majrowski, W. (2006). *Clearing the Air: Debating Smoke-Free Policies in Psychiatric Units* (Vol. 1), King's Fund, ISBN 978 1 85717 550 9, London

John, U., Meyer, C., Rumpf, H-J. & Hapke, U. (2004). Smoking, nicotine dependence and psychiatric comorbidity – a population-based study including smoking cessation after three years. *Drug and Alcohol Dependence,* Vol. 76, No. 3, (December 2004), pp. 287-295, ISSN 03768716

Jorenby, D. E., Leischow, J. J., Nides, M. A., Rennard, S. I., Johnston, J. A., Hughes, A. R., Smith, S. S., Muramoto, M. L., Daughton, D. M., Doan, K., Fiore, M. C. & Baker, T. B. (1999). A controlled trial of substained-release Bupropion, a nicotine patch, or both for smoking cessation. *New England Journal of Medicine,* Vol. 340, No. 9, (March 1999), pp. 685-691, ISSN 0028-4793

Kalman, D., Baker Morissette, S. & George, T. P. (2005). Co-Morbidity of Smoking in Patients with Psychiatric and Substance Use Disorders. *The American Journal on Addictions,* Vol. 14, No. 2, (March-April 2005), pp. 106–123, ISSN 1055-0496

Keltner, N. L. & Grant, J. S. (2006). Smoke, smoke, smoke that cigarette. *Perspectives Psychiatric Care,* Vol. 42, No. 4, (November 2006), pp. 256-261, ISSN 00315990

Koenen, K. C., Hitsman, B., Lyons, M. J., Niaura, R., McCaffery, J., Goldberg, J., Eisen, S. A., True, W. & Tsuang, M. (2005). A twin registry study of the relationship between posttraumatic stress disorder and nicotine dependence in men. *Archives of General Psychiatry,* Vol. 62, No. 11, (November 2005), pp. 1258-1265, ISSN 15383636

Kunze, U., Schmeiser-Rieder, A. & Schoberberger, R. (1998). European Medical Association Smoking for Health (EMASH) – Consensus on smoking cessation: guidelines for physicians. *Sozial und Präventivmedizin,* Vol. 4, No. 3, pp. 167-172, ISSN 0303-8408

Lai, D. T. C., Cahill, K., Qin, Y. & Tang, J. L. (2010). Motivational interviewing for smoking cessation. *Cochrane Database of Systematic Reviews,* Vol. 1, (January 2010), ISSN 13616137

Lancaster, T. & Stead, L. F. (2005). Self-help interventions for smoking cessation. *Cochrane Database of Systematic Reviews,* Vol. 3, (July 2005), ISSN 13616137

Lasser, K., Boyd, J. W., Woolhandler, S., Himmelstein, D. U., McCormick, D. & Bor, D. H. (2000). Smoking and Mental Illness – A Population-Based Prevalence Study. *JAMA: Journal of the American Medical Association,* Vol. 284, No. 20, (November 2000), pp. 2606-2610, ISSN 15383598

Lawn, S., Pols, G. & Barber, J. (2002). Smoking and quitting: a qualitative study with community-living psychiatric clients. *Social Science and Medicine,* Vol. 54, No. 1, (January 2002), pp. 93- 104, ISSN 0277-9536

Lawn, S. & Condon, J. (2006). Psychiatric nurses' ethical stance on cigarette smoking by patients: Determinants and dilemmas in their role in supporting cessation. *International Journal of Mental Health Nursing,* Vol. 15, No. 2, (June 2006), pp. 111-118, ISSN 14458330

Levin, E. D., Wilson, W., Rose, J. E. & McEvoy, J. (1996). Nicotine-haloperidol interactions and cognitive performance in schizophrenics. *Neuropsychopharmacology,* Vol. 15, No. 5, (November 1996), pp. 429-436, ISSN 0893133X

Lindson, N., Aveyard, P. & Hughes, J. R. (2010). Reduction versus abrupt cessation in smokers who want to quit. *Cochrane Database of Systematic Reviews*, Vol. 3, (March 2010), ISSN13616137

Lumley, J., Chamberlain, C., Dowswell, T., Oliver, S., Oakley, L. & Watson, L. (2009). Interventions for promoting smoking cessation during pregnancy. *Cochrane Database of Systematic Reviews*, Vol. 3, (July 2009), ISSN 13616137

McChargue, D. E., Gulliver, S. B., & Hitsman, B. (2002a). A reply to the commentaries on schizophrenia and smoking treatment: more research is needed. *Addiction*, Vol. 97, No. 7, (July 2002), pp. 799-800, ISSN 09652140

McChargue, D. E., Gulliver, S. B., & Hitsman, B. (2002b). Would smokers with schizophrenia benefit from a more flexible approach to smoking treatment? *Addiction*, Vol. 97, No. 7, (July 2002), pp. 785-793, ISSN 09652140

McChargue, D. E., Collins, F. L., & Cohen, L. M. (2002). Effect of non-nicotinic moist snuff replacement and lobeline on withdrawal symptoms during 48-hour smokeless tobacco deprivation. *Nicotine and Tobacco Research*, Vol. 4, No. 2, (May 2002), pp. 195-200, ISSN 014622203

McCloughen, A. (2003). The association between schizophrenia and cigarette smoking: a review of the literature and implications for mental health nursing practice. *International Journal of Mental Health Nursing*, Vol. 12, No. 2, (June 2003), pp. 119-129, ISSN 14458330

Mester, R., Toren, P., Ben-Moshe, Y. & Weizman, A. (1993). Survey of smoking habits and attitudes of patients and staff in psychiatric hospitals. *Psychopathology*, Vol. 26, No. 2, (March-April 1993), pp. 69-75, ISSN 02544962

Meyer, C., Rumpf, H. -J., Hapke, U., & John, U. (2004). Impact of psychiatric disorders in the general population: satisfaction with life and the influence of comorbidity and disorder duration. *Social Psychiatry and Psychiatric Epidemiology*, Vol. 39, No. 6, pp. 435 – 441, ISSN 09337954

Miller, M., Hemenway, D., & Rimm, E. (2000). Cigarettes and suicide: a prospective study of 50,000 men. *American Journal of Public Health*, Vol. 90, No. 5, (May 2000), pp. 768-773, ISSN 00900036

Miller, W. R., & Rollnick, S. (2002). *Motivational interviewing: Preparing people for change (2nd ed.)*. New York, NY US: Guilford Press

Morrell, H. E. R., & Cohen, L. M. (2006). Cigarette smoking, anxiety, and depression. *Journal of Psychopathology and Behavioral Assessment*, Vol. 28, No. 4, (December 2006), pp. 281–295, ISSN 08822689

Moxham, J. (2001). Mental health and smoking – an opening address. *Symposium report – smoking and mental health*, Royal Pharmaceutical Society, London, 9 November 2001

Mühlig, S. (2008). Smoking cessation in patients with COPD: the status of routine care in Germany. *Pneumologie, Vol. 62*, No. 10, (October 2008), pp. 616-622, ISSN 09348387

Nelson, C. B. & Wittchen, H. U. (1998). Smoking and nicotine dependence: Results from a sample of 14-24-years olds in Germany. *European Addiction Research*, Vol. 4, No. 1-2, (March 1998), pp. 42-49, ISSN 1022-6877

Nutt, D., King, L. A., Saulsbury, W. & Blakemore, C. (2007) Development of a rational scale to assess the harm of drugs of potential misuse. *The Lancet*, Vol. 369, No. 9566, (March 2007), pp. 1047-1053, ISSN 01406736

Oquendo, M. A., Lizardi, D., Greenwald, S., Weissman, M. M. & Mann, J. J. (2004). Rates of lifetime suicide attempt and rates of lifetime major depression in different ethnic groups in the United States. *Acta Psychiatrica Scandinavica*, Vol. 110, No. 6, (December 2004), pp. 446-451, ISSN 0001690X

Pabst, A., Piontek D., Kraus L. & Müller, S. (2010). Substance Use and Substance Use Disorders. Results of the 2009 Epidemiological Survey of Substance Abuse. *Sucht*, Vol. 56, No. 5, (October 2010), pp. 327–336, ISSN 0939-5911

Patkar, A. A., Gopalakrishnan, R., Lundy, A., Leone, F. T., Certa, K. M. & Weinstein, S. P. (2002). Relationship between tobacco smoking and positive and negative symptoms in schizophrenia. *Journal of Nervous and Mental Disease*, Vol. 190, No. 9, (September 2002), pp. 604-610, ISSN 00223018

Patten, C. A., Martin, J. E. & Owen, N. (1996). Can psychiatric and chemical dependency treatment units be smoke free? *Journal of Substance Abuse Treatment*, Vol. 13, No. 2, (March-April 1996), pp. 107-118, ISSN 07405472

Pelkonen, M. & Kankkunen, P. (2001). Nurses' competence in advising and supporting clients to cease smoking: a survey among Finnish nurses. *Journal of Clinical Nursing*, Vol. 23, No. 4, (July 2001), pp. 189-200, ISSN 09621067

Prochaska, J. O., DiClemente, C. C., Velicer, W. F. & Rossi, J. S. (1993). Standardized, individualized, interactive, and personalized self-help programs for smoking cessation. *Health Psychol*, Vol. 12, No. 5, (September 1993), pp. 399-405, ISSN 02786133

Prochaska, J., Butterworth, S., Redding, C. A., Burden, V., Perrin, N., Leo, M., Flaherty-Robb, M. & Prochaska, J. M. (2008). Initial efficacy of MI, TTM tailoring and HRI's with multiple behaviors for employee health promotion. *Preventive Medicine*, Vol. 46, No. 3, (March 2008), pp. 226-31, ISSN 00917435

Prochaska, J., Fromont, S. C. & Hall, S. M. (2005). How prepared are psychiatry residents for treating nicotine dependence? *Academic Psychiatry*, Vol. 29, No. 3, (August 2005), pp. 256-261, ISSN 10429670

Prochaska, J., Fletcher, L., Hall, S. E. & Hall, S. M. (2006). Return to smoking following a smoke-free psychiatric hospitalisation. *American Journal on Addictions*, Vol. 15, No. 1, (January 2006), pp. 15–22; ISSN 10550496

Prochaska, J., Fromont, S. C., Louie, A. K., Jacobs, M. H. & Hall, S. M. (2006). Training in Tobacco Treatments in Psychiatry: A National Survey of Psychiatry Residency Training Directors. *Academic Psychiatry*, Vol. 30, No. 5, (September 2006), pp. 372-379, ISSN 10429670

Prochaska, J., Gill, P. & Hall, S. M. (2004). Treatment of Tobacco Use in an Inpatient Psychiatric Setting. *Psychiatric Services*, Vol. 55, No. 11, (November 2004), pp. 1265-1270, ISSN 10752730

Rosen-Chase, C. & Dyson, V. (1999). Treatment of nicotine dependence in the chronically mentally ill. *Journal of Substance Abuse Treatment*, Vol. 16, No. 4, pp. 315-320, ISSN 07405472

Rowe, K. & Clark, J. M. (2000). The incidence of smoking amongst nurses: a review of the literature. *Journal of Advanced Nursing*, Vol. 31, No. 5, (May 2000), pp. 1046–1053, ISSN 03092402

Schmitz, N., Kruse, J. & Kugler, J. (2003). Disabilities, quality of life, and mental disorders associated with smoking and nicotine dependence. *The American Journal of Psychiatry*, Vol. 160, No. 9, (September 2003), pp. 1670-1676, ISSN 15357228

Schneider, B., Schnabel, A., Wetterling, T., Bartusch, B., Weber, B. & Georgi, K. (2008). How do personality disorders modify suicide risk?. *Journal of Personality Disorders*, Vol. 22, No. 3, (June 2008), pp. 233-245, ISSN 0885579X

Silagy, C., Mant, D., Fowler, G. & Lodge, M. (1994). Meta-analysis on efficacy of nicotine replacement therapies in smoking cessation. *The Lancet*, Vol. 343, (January 1994), pp. 139–142, ISSN 0140-6736

Stead, L. F. & Lancaster, T. (2005). Group behaviour therapy programmes for smoking cessation. *Cochrane Database of Systematic Reviews*, Vol. 2, (April 2005), ISSN 13616137

Stead, L. F., Perera, R. & Lancaster, T. (2006). Telephone counselling for smoking cessation. *Cochrane Database of Systematic Reviews*, Vol. 3, (July 2006), ISSN 13616137

Stead, L. F. & Lancaster, T. (2007). Interventions to reduce harm from continued tobacco use. *Cochrane Database of Systematic Reviews*, Vol. 3, (July 2008), ISSN 13616137

Stead, L. F., Perera, R., Bullen, C., Mant, D. & Lancaster, T. (2008). Nicotine replacement therapy for smoking cessation. *Cochrane Database of Systematic Reviews*, Vol. 1, (January 2008), ISSN 13616137

Sutton, S. (2001). Back to the drawing board? A review of applications of the transtheoretical model to substance use. *Addiction*. Vol. 96, No. 1, pp. 175-186, ISSN 09652140

Tiffany, S. T, & Conklin, S. A. (2000). A cognitive processing model of alcohol craving and compulsive alcohol use. *Addiction*, Vol. 95, No. 2, (August 200), pp. 145-154, ISSN 09652140

Tizabi, Y., Getachew, B., Rezvani, A., Hauser, S. R. & Overstreet, D. H. (2009). Antidepressant-like effects of nicotine and reduced nicotinic receptor binding in the Fawn-Hooded rat, an animal model of co-morbid depression and alcoholism. *Progress in Neuro-Psychopharmacology and Biological Psychiatry*, Vol. 33, No. 3, (April 2009), pp. 398-402, ISSN 02785846

Ussher, M. H., Taylor, A. & Faulkner, G. (2008). Exercise interventions for smoking cessation. *Cochrane Database of Systematic Reviews*, Vol. 4, (October 2008), ISSN 13616137

Vazquez-Palacios, G., Bonilla-Jaime, H. & Velazquez-Moctezuma, J. (2005). Antidepressant effects of nicotine and fluoxetine in an animal model of depression induced by neonatal treatment with clomipramine. *Progress in Neuro-Psychopharmacology and Biological Psychiatry*, Vol. 29, No. 1, (January 2005), pp. 39-46, ISSN 02785846

White, A. R., Rampes, H., Liu, J. P., Stead, L. F. & Campbell, J. (2011). Acupuncture and related interventions for smoking cessation. *Cochrane Database of Systematic Reviews*, Vol. 1, (January 2011), ISSN 13616137

WHO. (2001). Evidence based Recommendations on the treatment of tobacco dependence, In: *WHO-recommendations*, Available from:
http://www. bvsde. paho. org/bvsacd/cd16/whoevidence. pdf

WHO. (2008). WHO Report on the Global Tobacco Epidemic, *The MPOWER package*. World Health Organization, ISBN 978 92 4 159628 2, Geneva

Wiesbeck, G. A., Kuhl, H. -C., Yaldizli, Ö. & Wurst, F. M. (2008). Tobacco smoking and depression - Results from the WHO/ISBRA study. *Neuropsychobiology*, Vol. 57, No. 2, (June 2008), pp. 26-31, ISSN 14230224

Wilhelm, K., Wedgwood, L., Niven, H. & Kay-Lambkin, F. (2006). Smoking cessation and depression: current knowledge and future directions. *Drug Alcohol Review*, Vol. 25, No. 1, (October 2005), pp. 97-107, ISSN 09595236

Williams, J. M. & Ziedonis, D. (2004). Addressing tobacco among individuals with a mental illness or an addiction. *Addictive Behaviors*, Vol. 29, No. 6, pp. 1067-1083, ISSN 03064603

Wye, P. M., Bowman, J. A., Wiggers, J. H., Baker, A., Knight, J., Carr, V. J., Terry, M. & Clancy, R. (2009). Smoking Restrictions and Treatment for Smoking: Policies and Procedures in Psychiatric Inpatient Units in Australia. *Psychiatric Services*, Vol. 60, No. 1, (January 2009), pp. 100-107, ISSN 10752730

Ziedonis, D. M. & George, T. P. (1997). Schizophrenia and nicotine use: report of a pilot smoking cessation programme and review of neurobiological and clinical issues. *Schizophrenia Bulletin*, Vol. 23, No. 2, pp. 247-254, ISSN 0586-7614

Ziedonis, D. M. & Williams, J. (2003). Management of smoking in people with psychiatric disorders. *Current Opinion in Psychiatry*, Vol. 16, No. 3, (May 2003), pp. 305-15, ISSN 0951-7367

4

Substance Use and Abuse Among Older Adults: A State of the Art

Marja Aartsen
VU-University Amsterdam
The Netherlands

1. Introduction

Substance abuse, defined here as the abuse of alcohol, cannabis, cocaine and heroin, in older adults is often neglected, both in science and in practice. Substance abuse is a serious public health issue as it not only affects physical and mental health of the abusers, it also leads to increased costs for society (Adams et al., 1993). Older adults with addiction problems deserve special attention. Compared to younger people, smaller amounts of substance may lead to intoxication and organ damage because of greater use of contraindicated medications, less efficient liver metabolism and decreases in lean body mass and total body water (Dufour & Fuller, 1995).

Substance use and abuse among people aged 50 and over is rapidly increasing in Europe and the United States (Beynon, 2009). For Europe, the number of older people with substance use problems is estimated to more than double between 2001 and 2020 (Gossop, 2008). This is partly due to the size of the baby-boom cohort (born between 1946 and 1964) and the higher rate of substance use among this group (Gfroerer et al., 2003). Estimates from the United States suggest that the number of adults aged 50 and over will double from 2.8 million (annual average) in 2002–06 to 5.7 million in 2020 (Han et al., 2009).

To reduce the negative trend in substance abuse, effective prevention is required. Cuijpers and Willemse (2005) distinguish four types of prevention in this context; universal prevention, selective prevention, indicated prevention and care based prevention. For each level of prevention, specific knowledge is needed. For universal prevention, targeted at the entire population regardless of the risk of addiction, knowledge about the prevalence, causes and adverse consequences of risk-full use are important. In selective prevention, aimed at groups at risk of becoming addicted, knowledge of risk factors is essential to identify the groups. For indicated prevention, aimed at people with limited symptoms, it is important to recognize signs of addiction and have knowledge of appropriate treatments. Finally, care based prevention, referring to people with an addiction according to DSM criteria, it is important to have insight into factors that influence the course of the disease. Insufficient knowledge of one or more levels of prevention can lead to under-recognition of addiction problems by social workers (Adams et al., 1992), lack of agreement between doctors on the causes and treatment of addiction (Brown, 1982), and people are still insufficiently aware of the importance and effects of proper treatment (McInnes & Powell, 1994).

In this chapter, an overview is given of what is known about the prevalence and the bio-psycho-social characteristics of older people who abuse substances. In addition, we will describe the known risk factors for the development and course of substance abuse.

2. Methods

2.1 Review

In addressing the aim of this chapter, three databases (PubMed, PsychINFO, and Socindex) were investigated for potentially relevant studies using the following keywords: "Alcohol", "drug abuse", "heroin", "cocaine", "cannabis", "substance abuse" each combined with AND (elderly OR older adults). Based on the title and abstract of each retrieved article the potential relevance for the current study was investigated. We selected only articles that were written in English, have appeared in peer-reviewed journals, were based on original quantitative empirical research, aiming at the older population (aged 50 years or older). Relevant information for answering the research questions was extracted from each selected article. For information on the prevalence and the bio-psycho-social characteristics of older people who abuse substances, studies containing information on one or more of the following characteristics were selected: prevalence, trends in use with age, bio-psycho-social characteristics of users, and risk-full use or addiction. For information on risk factors for the development and course of substance abuse, only longitudinal studies or case-control studies were selected.

2.2 Definitions

Substance abuse is defined in accord with the Diagnostic and Statistical Manual of Mental Disorders (DSM) if three or more of the following criteria were met: 1) tolerance, as defined by either a need for markedly increased amounts of the substance to achieve intoxication or the desired effect or markedly diminished effect with continued use of the same amount of the substance; 2) withdrawal, as manifested by the characteristic withdrawal syndrome for the substance or the same (or closely related) substance is taken to relieve or avoid withdrawal symptoms; 3) the substance is often taken in larger amounts or over a longer period than intended; 4) there is a persistent desire or unsuccessful efforts to cut down or control substance use; 5) a great deal of time is spent in activities necessary to obtain the substance, use the substance, or recover from its effects; 6) important social, occupational, or recreational activities are given up or reduced because of substance use; and 7) the substance use is continued despite knowledge of having a persistent physical or psychological problem that is likely to have been caused or exacerbated by the substance.

A limitation of the DSM classification is that it does not take account of the specific circumstances and life stage in which older people reside. The consequences of substance abuse are more visible in people who are still employed than in people who live alone, which is more prevalent among older people. Also milder forms of abuse or risky use can significantly affect the physical, cognitive and mental health of older adults. Therefore, also risk-full substance use will be addressed in this study.

3. Results

The literature search resulted in 432 studies potentially relevant to this investigation. Based on the title and abstract 81 studies were subsequently selected for further study and data extraction. Of the 81 selected studies, 75 studies were on alcohol consumption, 7 studies on alcohol use in combination with medicines and one study on cocaine and heroin use. Only a small fraction of all studies (n = 10) focused on addiction according to DSM-IV criteria. The results will be summarized around 6 themes: recognition of alcohol abuse, prevalence, changes in substance use with aging, bio-psycho-social characteristics of older substance users, risk factors, and consequences of abuse. In addition, also study results for risk-full of alcohol that does not fit the DSM criteria for an addiction will be summarized. The results will be described separately for alcohol, cannabis, heroin and cocaine.

3.1 Recognition of alcohol abuse

Assessing correct diagnosis regarding alcohol abuse is complicated (Aartsen et al., 2009). This is partly due to the reluctance of abusers and health care practitioners to discuss the drinking behavior. However, even without explicitly asking, there are signs that may indicate an underlying alcohol problem. For example, in some cases the breath of people can smell like alcohol, there may be complaints from the social environment of people about alcohol consumption, there may be convictions for driving with to much previous alcohol intake, and people may become annoyed once the subject is brought up to alcohol. Also, certain physical problems may indicate alcohol problems, such as hypertension, gastrointestinal problems, unexplained falls and psychological symptoms as anxiety and depression. There are screening instruments especially developed for older people that can help professionals to make a more deliberated diagnose. A simple, but not always adequate way is to ask how much alcohol is consumed on average per day. Besides the danger of under-reporting (people tend to underestimate their own drinking behavior), the average number of drinks per day is not always informative. Whether you drink two glasses a day, or once a week, 14 units, the average remains the same, but the social and physical consequences can vary widely. Moreover, one factor that affects the harmful effects of alcohol intake is the fat-moisture balance, and whether there are any concurrent medications or other chronic diseases that does not tolerate alcohol intake. A good alternative is the Alcohol Related Problem Survey (ARPS: Fink et al., 2002). The ARPS is a comprehensive questionnaire which not only questions drinking behavior, but also assesses health, life style, drug use and risky behaviors such as driving after alcohol use. Other screenings instruments are the Alcohol Use Disorders Identification Test (AUDIT), the Short Michigan Alcohol Screening Test-Geriatric (SMAST-G) and the Cut down, Annoyed, Guilty, Eye-opener test (CAGE).

3.2 Prevalence of substance use and abuse

Prevalence of risk-full alcohol consumption in the community ranged from 3 to 22% in men and 1 to 4% in women (Table 1). Men are two to five times more often risk-full alcohol consumers. The number of cannabis, heroin and cocaine users in the U.S. population is low (Blazer & Wu, 2009), of which the use of cannabis was the most prevalent. The annual prevalence of cannabis for people aged 50-64 year was 3,9%, and for people aged 65 0.7%. The annual prevalence of cocaine use by 50-64 year olds and 65 + was, respectively 0.68% and 0.04%. Heroin was used by 0.08% of 50-64 year old people. Heroin use is not observed among people aged 65 and over.

Prevalence rates of substance abuse, however, should be taken with caution. Taking into account that substance abuse among older adults is often under-diagnosed (Stewart & Oslin, 2001), and given the fact that only a small fraction of those with disorders related to substance abuse seek treatment, the actual number of older people with an alcohol use disorder in the general population must be much higher.

Alcohol First author and year of publication		**Country**
Breslow 2003	Prevalence of heavy drinking ranged from 9 to 10% in men and from 2% to 3% in women	US
Merrick 2008	16% of the men and 4% of the women are risk-full users	US
Du 2009	15% risk-full drinking, and 8% benzodiazepine and alcohol use	DE
Ganry 2001	3% of the 75+ women drank more than 30 grams per day	FR
Halme 2009	20% of the men and 1% of the women are heavy drinkers (more than 8 standard glasses per week)	FI
La Greca 1988	6% heavy users	US
Lang 2007	22% of the men and 4% of the women are heavy drinkers	GB
Rodgers 2005	7% of the men and 6% of the women drink hazardous amounts of alcohol	AU
Mirand 1996	13% of the men and 2% women were heavy drinkers	US
Cannabis, Cocaine, Heroin		
Blazer 2009	Prevalence of cannabis use: 3,9% for people aged 50-64 Prevalence of cannabis use: 0,7% 65 year old people Prevalence of cocaine use: 0,7% for people aged 50-64 Prevalence of cocaine use: 0,04% for 65 year old Prevalence of heroin use: 0,08% for people aged 50-64 Prevalence of heroin use: 0,0% 65 year old people	US

Table 1. Prevalence of alcohol, cannabis, cocaine and heroin use in society

In patient populations, prevalence rates of alcohol use were higher (Table 2). Estimates of the incidence of risk-full drinking range from 2% in women to 17% in men. Alcohol addiction in France varies in different patient populations from 3% in women and 18% in men (Lejoyeaux et al., 2003). Also Speckens et al., (1991) found high prevalence of alcohol in a university hospital in the Netherlands.

3.3 Developments in alcohol use with aging
Trends in alcohol use with aging were estimated in a number of longitudinal studies. Research in the United States (Adams et al., 1990) shows that older people generally reduce the number of drinks as they become older (each year a decrease of 2% drinkers). There is an indication for a gender effect. Men who drink heavily, but continue to drink, reduce drinking as opposed to heavily drinking women whose alcohol consumption remained stable (Breslow et al., 2003).

First author and year of publication		Country
Adams 1992	Prevalence of lifetime alcohol abuse: 24% Prevalence of current alcohol abuse: 14%.	US
Blow 2000	Prevalence of risk-full drinkers: 7%	US
Kahn 2001	Prevalence of risk-full alcohol use: 5%. Prevalence of lifetime alcohol abuse: men 37%, women 12%. Prevalence for last year alcohol abuse: 0.5%	NZ
Ganry 2000	Prevalence of risk-full alcohol use: men 17%, women 3%	FR
Kirchner 2007	Prevalence of risk-full drinkers: 5%	US
Lawley 1996	Prevalence of risk-full use: 12% Prevalence of abuse: 3%	GB
Lejoyeux 2003	Prevalence of alcohol abuse: 18% men and 3% women	FR
Onen 2005	Prevalence in Emergency Departments of alcohol abuse: 5,3%	BE
Speckens 1991	Prevalence of alcohol abuse: men 13%, women 7% women	NL

Table 2. Prevalence of alcohol abuse in patient population

3.4 Bio-psycho-social characteristics of older substance users
3.4.1 Alcohol
Older adults who are addicted to alcohol constitute a heterogeneous group consisting of people who have been addicted to alcohol before the age of 25 (early onset), people whose addiction started between the 25th and 45th year of life (late onset), and people who could remain at moderate levels of drinking till the age of 45, and became addicted at higher ages (very late onset). It is currently believed that the etiology and the course of alcohol disorders or risk-full drinking is complex and includes both genetic and environmental factors and the interaction of the two (Edenberg & Foroud, 2006). Genetic factors leading to differential risk for alcoholism were demonstrated using twin and family studies. In addition, functional polymorphisms of alcohol dehydrogenase (ADH2) and aldehyde dehydrogenase (ALDH2) genes have been shown to have a significant impact on alcohol metabolism in the liver, and thus, may contribute to vulnerability to alcohol abuse and dependence (Yokoyama & Omori, 2003). Antisocial personality is found to be a frequent cause of early onset (Watson et al., 1997), whereas very late onset seems to be more often induced by stressful life events (Hurt, 1988). Furthermore, early onset is more often seen among people who are homeless, who have family members with alcohol problems, and who have low socio-economic status, and people with very late onset often show better social functioning, have normal family lives and professional careers, rarely have a criminal history; furthermore, the course of very late onset is more favorable compared to early onset or late onset (Liberto & Oslin, 1995; Rigler, 2000).
Studies consistently show that there is a U-shaped relationship between alcohol use and mental and physical health. Abstainers, high-risk users and addicts have a poorer physical and mental health than moderate users (Blow et al., 2000; Brideveaux et al., 2004, Mukamal et al., 2001; Rodgers et al., 2005). Alcohol use appears to be related to prevailing beliefs about alcohol (Akers et al., 1989, Preston & Goodfellow, 2006; Graham & Braun, 1999).

Catholics, white people and non religious people drink significantly more than other ethnic groups or religions (Breslow et al., 2003; Forster et al., 1993, Merrick et al., 2008; Ruchlin, 1997). Higher education is associated with more, but also risk-full alcohol use (Breslow et al., 2003, Forster et al., 1993; Goodwin et al., 1987; Merrick et al., 2008; Ruchlin, 1997). Alcohol consumers smoke more than non-users (Mirand & Welte, 1996; Ganry et al., 2001), and alcoholics often live alone (Brennan, 2005; Onen et al., 2002).

First author	Main findings
Adlaf 1995	Men report more alcohol related problems then women
Aira 2005	Most alcohol drinkers used medications on a regular basis (86.9%) or as needed (87.8%).
Akers 1989	Drinking is related to the norms and behavior of one's primary groups, one's own attitudes toward (definitions of) alcohol, and the balance of reinforcement for drinking
Blow 2000	Low-risk drinkers were significantly better off than abstainers on the following domains: general health, physical functioning, bodily pain, vitality, mental health, emotional role, and social functioning. At-risk drinkers had significantly poorer mental health functioning than low-risk drinkers.
Brennan 2005	Nursing home residents with alcohol use disorders were more likely to have lived alone before admission and to have obtained mental health and social services. Residents with alcohol use disorders had somewhat better performance of basic activities than did residents in the demographically-matched sample group. Men with alcohol use disorders had shorter lengths of stay than did men without alcohol use disorders; women with alcohol use disorders had longer lengths of stay than did women without such disorders.
Breslow 2003	White people had the highest prevalence of moderate and heavier drinking compared with other racial/ethnic groups. Higher education was related to higher drinking levels. Moderate drinking was related to living with a partner.
Brideveaux 2004	Drinkers have a better health status than nondrinkers. Problem drinkers had lower health status than drinkers without drinking problems
Christie 2008	Controlling for age, gender, and vascular health, global Cerebral Blood Flow was greater in the lightest alcohol consumption group (<1 per week) and lower in the heaviest (>15 per week).
Forster 1993	Drinking is related to male gender, higher education, Catholic or no organized religious affiliation.
Ganry 2001	Smoking, good health status, higher socioeconomic status or single marital status are related to higher levels of alcohol use.
Gao 2009	Moderate current and lifetime alcohol consumption were found to be associated with reduced chronic atrophic arthritis compared to alcohol.
Geroldi 1994	Male gender, poorer cognitive function, and income dissatisfaction were significantly associated with alcohol problems.

First author	Main findings
Goodwin 1987	Alcohol intake was positively associated with male gender, income, cognitive functioning and amount of education and negatively associated with age.
Graham & Schmidt 1999	Depression was correlated with heavier drinking.
Graham & Braun 1999	Having a drinking spouse (versus an abstinent spouse) was associated with higher levels of drinking.
Kirchner 2007	Heavy drinking showed significant positive association with depressive/anxiety symptoms and less social support. Heavy drinking combined with binging was similarly positively associated with depressive/anxiety symptoms and perceived poor health.
Lang 2007	For both men and women, better cognition and subjective well-being, and fewer depressive symptoms, were associated with moderate levels of alcohol consumption than with never having drunk any.
Mattace-Raso 2005	Moderate alcohol consumption is associated with lower arterial stiffness in women but not in men independently of cardiovascular risk factors and atherosclerosis
Merrick 2008	Unhealthy drinking Is associated with higher education and income; better health status; male sex; younger age; smoking; being white; and being divorced, separated, or single. were associated with higher likelihood of unhealthy drinking. Among drinkers, in addition to socio-demographic variables, self reported depressive symptoms were positively associated with unhealthy drinking. Among unhealthy drinkers, race and ethnicity variables were associated with likelihood of heavy episodic drinking.
Midanik 1992	Sense of Coherence was a significant negative predictor of alcohol problems while controlling for alcohol consumption level, frequency of drunkenness and demographic characteristics.
Mirand 1996	Positive associations between heavy drinking and being male, having suburban residency, and currently using cigarettes. Negative relationships between heavy drinking and socioeconomic status, rural residency, and degree of health orientation.
Mukamal 2001	Moderate alcohol consumption is associated with a lower prevalence of white matter abnormalities and infarcts, thought to be of vascular origin, but with a dose-dependent higher prevalence of brain atrophy on MRI among older adults.
Mukamal 2004	Alcohol intake is associated with lower levels of inflammatory markers in older adults free of cardiovascular disease
Musick 2000	Alcohol use had no effect on depressive symptoms. One exception to this latter finding was that among rural Baptists who rarely attended religious services, using alcohol was associated with more depressive symptoms.

First author	Main findings
Onen 2002	Being homeless, living alone, being divorced and never married and being a man was associated with alcohol use disorders. Drinkers more commonly presented with gastrointestinal disorders.
Oslin 2005	Among people with alcohol use disorders, 22,3% has current depressive disorder, 44,9 physical disabilities, 13,6 anxiety disorder, 70,8% have college or higher education, 57% married. Compared to younger patients, they have less mental health problems, less severe alcohol use, and less outpatient treatment experience.
Preston 2006	Frequency of drinking and abuse is positively associated with personal approval of daily alcohol use and number of peers who use alcohol.
Rapuri 2000	Moderate alcohol intake was associated with higher bone mineral density in postmenopausal elderly women.
Rice 1995	Alcohol consumption was negatively associated with General Practitioners visits, controlling for gender and health
Riserus 2007	In men: self-estimated alcohol intake was not related to insulin sensitivity, early insulin response, or BMI, but was positively related to Waist Circumference.
Rodgers 2005	Abstainers have poorer cognitive function than light drinkers.
Ruchlin 1997	Everyday drinkers are more likely to being male, white, higher educated, living in the city centre and less likely to be in less than in excellent health, having diabetes, and believing that drinking has negative health consequences.
Schuckit 1978	Compared to younger alcoholics, older alcoholics had relatively more stable lives in early years and had developed alcohol-related problems in later years
Sheahan 1995	Alcohol use is not related to falls
Steunenberg 2008	Depression and alcohol use are not related in this very old, mostly female population. Alcohol use was related to extraversion and openness to experience. Chronic diseases was related to non-alcohol use and parental problem drinking was found to be a risk factor for late life problem drinking.
Sulander 2004	Higher alcohol use was more common among retired office workers than other former employees.
Westerterp 2004	Alcohol intake does not lead to increased body weight, probably due to the higher physical activity level

Table 3. Bio-Psycho-Social chraracteristics of older people who (ab)use alcohol

The relationship between cognitive functioning, cognitive pathology and drinking is more complicated. Risk-full use seems to be associated with worse cognitive function (Geroldi et al., 1994) and moderate use with better cognitive function (Goodwin et al., 1987; Lang et al., 2007; Rodgers et al., 2005). There are indications that the relationship is actually spurious, as the relation disappears when controlling for other potential influences (Cooper et al., 2009; Goodwin et al., 1987).

Several studies found a relationship with physical characteristics. Women who drink moderate levels of alcohol have a higher density of mineral in bone (Ilich et al., 2002; Rapuri et al., 2000). A positive correlation between alcohol use, reduced inflammation, lower prevalence of strokes and white matter pathology, and the quality of blood vessels is found by Christie et al. (2008), Gao et al.(2009), Mattace-Raso et al. (2005) and Mukamal et al. (2001, 2004).

Risk-full drinkers appear to be more often depressed (Blow et al., 2000, Graham & Schmidt, 1999; Oslin et al., 2005), while moderate drinkers have fewer levels of depressive symptoms (Blow et al., 2000, Graham & Schmidt, 1999; Kirchner et al., 2007; Lang et al., 2007, Merrick et al, 2008). A relationship between alcohol and depression was however not found in very old nursing home residents (Steunenberg et al., 2008) and older Baptists (Musick, 2000).

3.4.2 Cannabis, cocaine and heroin

One study reported information on older cannabis, cocaine and heroin users. These users are more often male, single, and have depressive symptoms, but no differences in educational background are observed (Blazer & Wu, 2009).

3.5 Risk factors for substance abuse

Only one longitudinal study examined risk factors for risk-full drinking (Moos et al., 2010). The study revealed that a lower quality of marriage, lower participation in social activities, approval of drinking by friends and larger financial resources lead to an increased risk of risky alcohol use.

3.6 Consequences of substance use

In general, moderate consumption of alcohol has beneficial effects on physical and mental health, while risk-full use entails negative effects. Moderate alcohol use leads to higher bone density (Felson et al., 1995), longer life (Brideveaux et al., 2004; Colditz et al., 1985; Simons et al., 2000;), and reduced risk of Type 2 Diabetes (Djousse et al., 2007). Moderate alcohol consumption may also have some negative consequences as it may increase blood pressure, glycemia and body weight (Buja et al., 2010). Risk-full alcohol use leads to an increased risk of mental health problems (Friedman et al., 1999) and mortality (Gronbaek et al., 1998) and possibly an increased risk of acute pneumonia (Van der Horst Graat et al., 2007).

4. Conclusions

This study provides an overview of scientific knowledge in the field of substance abuse (alcohol, cannabis, heroin, and cocaine) in people aged 55 and older. Three databases were searched for relevant literature. There is useful information on alcohol use and risk-full use, but large gaps in knowledge about substance abuse exists. Research on alcohol addiction is limited and use of cannabis, cocaine and heroin in older adults is virtually absent. Moreover, many of the studies had a cross-sectional design, which limits conclusions about causes and effects. An additional problem is that most of the studies were conducted in the United States, while that information not necessarily applies to other countries because of cultural differences is (Vaz De Almeida et al., 2005).

Nevertheless, an outline of people who use risk-full amounts of alcohol became visible. First, there is a U-shaped relationship between amount of alcohol use and health. Moderate users are healthier than high-risk users and abstainers. The fact that abstainers were worse of than moderate users is possibly explained on the basis of the great heterogeneity in the non-using group. Not drinking is associated with certain medications and thus indicates the presence of disease, previous alcohol dependence, but also a healthy lifestyle.

High-risk alcohol users were more often male (2-5 times more), live in social environments where alcohol is not condemned, are higher educated, smoke more often, are more often single or depressed and may have poorer cognitive function. With age, the average consumption of alcohol decreases, except for risk-full drinking women. The consequences of risk-full alcohol use are decreased mental health and increased mortality. Very little is known about causes of alcohol addiction.

For information about use of cannabis, heroin and cocaine in older adults, we can only rely on one study conducted in the US. Of the three, cannabis is most often used, particularly 50-64 year olds (year prevalence 3.89% and 0.69% at 65). Less than 1 percent of older people use cocaine, while heroin use is not seen in people over 65 (Blazer & Wu, 2009).

In sum, it appears that knowledge of substance abuse in older adults is still mainly limited to the description of bio-psycho-social characteristics of older adults with alcohol abuse. Knowledge of prevalence, causes, consequences and characteristics of the elderly who according to DSM criteria are addicted to any of the tested agents is still virtually absent. The design of effective prevention of substance abuse in older adults, as well as effective therapies is therefore strongly hampered. With respect to universal and selective prevention at the population level, more research is required into causes and consequences of substance abuse. For effective care-oriented prevention research into the effects of treatments in patients populations such as in addiction clinics is needed in order to improve the effect of treatment programs.

5. Acknowledgements

The literature review was supported by The Netherlands Organization for Scientific Research NWO/ZonMW (project number 31160205).

6. References

Aartsen, M., Van Etten, D. & Spitsbaard, A. (2009). Older people and substance abuse [Ouderen en verslavingsproblematiek]. In: *Addiction, handbook for care, support and prevention*, Rutten, R., Loth, C. & Hulshof, A., pp.255-267, Elseviers gezondheidszorg, ISBN 978 90 352 3071 2, Maarssen, The Netherlands.

Adams, W. L., Garry, P. J., Rhyne, R., Hunt, W. C., & Goodwin, J. S. (1990). Alcohol intake in the healthy elderly. Changes with age in a cross-sectional and longitudinal study. *J.Am.Geriatr.Soc.*, 38, 211-216.

Adams, W. L., Magruder-Habib, K., Trued, S., & Broome, H. L. (1992). Alcohol abuse in elderly emergency department patients. *J.Am.Geriatr.Soc.*, 40, 1236-1240.

Adams, W. L., Yuan, Z., Barboriak, J. J., & Rimm, A. A. (1993). Alcohol-related hospitalizations of elderly people. Prevalence and geographic variation in the United States. *JAMA*, 270, 1222-1225.

Adlaf, E. M. & Smart, R. G. (1995). Alcohol use, drug use, and well-being in older adults in Toronto. *Int.J.Addict.*, 30, 1985-2016.

Aira, M., Hartikainen, S., & Sulkava, R. (2005). Community prevalence of alcohol use and concomitant use of medication. A source of possible risk in the elderly aged 75 and older? *Int.J.Geriatr.Psychiatry*, 20, 680-685.

Akers, R. L., La Greca, A. J., Cochran, J., & Sellers, C. (1989). Social learning theory and alcohol behavior among the elderly. *The Sociological Quarterly*, 30, 625-638.

Blazer, D. G. & Wu, L. T. (2009). The epidemiology of substance use and disorders among middle aged and elderly community adults: national survey on drug use and health. *Am.J.Geriatr.Psychiatry*, 17, 237-245.

Blow, F. C., Walton, M. A., Barry, K. L., Coyne, J. C., Mudd, S. A., & Copeland, L. A. (2000). The relationship between alcohol problems and health functioning of older adults in primary care settings. *J.Am.Geriatr.Soc.*, 48, 769-774.

Brennan, P. L. (2005). Functioning and health service use among elderly nursing home residents with alcohol use disorders: findings from the National Nursing Home Survey. *Am.J.Geriatr.Psychiatry*, 13, 475-483.

Breslow, R. A., Faden, V. B., & Smothers, B. (2003). Alcohol consumption by elderly Americans. *J.Stud.Alcohol*, 64, 884-892.

Bridevaux, I. P., Bradley, K. A., Bryson, C. L., McDonell, M. B., & Fihn, S. D. (2004). Alcohol screening results in elderly male veterans: association with health status and mortality. *J.Am.Geriatr.Soc.*, 52, 1510-1517.

Brown, B. B. (1982). Professionals' perceptions of drug and alcohol abuse among the elderly. *Gerontologist*, 22, 519-525.

Buja, A., Scafato, E., Sergi, G., Maggi, S., Suhad, M. A., Rausa, G. et al. (2010). Alcohol consumption and metabolic syndrome in the elderly: results from the Italian longitudinal study on aging. *Eur.J.Clin.Nutr.*, 64, 297-307.

Christie, I. C., Price, J., Edwards, L., Muldoon, M., Meltzer, C. C., & Jennings, J. R. (2008). Alcohol consumption and cerebral blood flow among older adults. *Alcohol*, 42, 269-275.

Colditz, G. A., Branch, L. G., Lipnick, R. J., Willett, W. C., Rosner, B., Posner, B. et al. (1985). Moderate alcohol and decreased cardiovascular mortality in an elderly cohort. *Am.Heart J.*, 109, 886-889.

Cooper, C., Bebbington, P., Meltzer, H., Jenkins, R., Brugha, T., Lindesay, J. E. et al. (2009). Alcohol in moderation, premorbid intelligence and cognition in older adults: results from the Psychiatric Morbidity Survey. *J.Neurol.Neurosurg.Psychiatry*, 80, 1236-1239.

Cuijpers, P., & Willemse, G. (2005) Preventie van depressie bij ouderen: Een overzicht van interventies. Trimbos Instituut, Utrecht 2005.

Djousse, L., Biggs, M. L., Mukamal, K. J., & Siscovick, D. S. (2007). Alcohol consumption and type 2 diabetes among older adults: the Cardiovascular Health Study. *Obesity.(Silver.Spring)*, 15, 1758-1765.

Du, Y., Scheidt-Nave, C., & Knopf, H. (2008). Use of psychotropic drugs and alcohol among non-institutionalised elderly adults in Germany. *Pharmacopsychiatry*, 41, 242-251.

Dufour, M & Fuller, R.K. (1995) Alcohol in the elderly. Annual Review of Medicine, 46, 123-132

Edenberg, H.J. & Foroud, T. (2006). The genetics of alcohol disorder: Identifying specific genes through family studies. *Addiction Biology*, 11, 386-396.

Felson, D. T., Zhang, Y., Hannan, M. T., Kannel, W. B., & Kiel, D. P. (1995). Alcohol intake and bone mineral density in elderly men and women. The Framingham Study. *Am.J.Epidemiol.*, 142, 485-492.

Fink, A., Morton, S.C., Beck, J.C., e.a. (2002). The alcohol-related problems survey: Identifying hazardous and harmful drinking in older primary care patients. *Journal of American Geriatrics Society*, 50, 1717-1722.

Forster, L. E., Pollow, R., & Stoller, E. P. (1993). Alcohol use and potential risk for alcohol-related adverse drug reactions among community-based elderly. *Journal of Community Health,* 18, 225-239.

Friedmann, P. D., Jin, L., Karrison, T., Nerney, M., Hayley, D. C., Mulliken, R. et al. (1999). The effect of alcohol abuse on the health status of older adults seen in the emergency department. *Am.J.Drug Alcohol Abuse,* 25, 529-542.

Ganry, O., Joly, J. P., Queval, M. P., & Dubreuil, A. (2000). Prevalence of alcohol problems among elderly patients in a university hospital. *Addiction,* 95, 107-113.

Ganry, O., Baudoin, C., Fardellone, P., & Dubreuil, A. (2001). Alcohol consumption by non-institutionalised elderly women: the EPIDOS Study. *Public Health,* 115, 186-191.

Gao, L., Weck, M. N., Stegmaier, C., Rothenbacher, D., & Brenner, H. (2009). Alcohol consumption and chronic atrophic gastritis: population-based study among 9,444 older adults from Germany. *Int.J.Cancer,* 125, 2918-2922.

Geroldi, C., Rozzini, R., Frisoni, G. B., & Trabucchi, M. (1994). Assessment of alcohol consumption and alcoholism in the elderly. *Alcohol,* 11, 513-516.

Gfroerer, J., Penne, M., Pemberton, M., & Folson, R. (2003). Substance abuse treatment need among older adults in 2020. The impact of the aging baby-boom cohort. *Drug and Alcohol Dependence,* 69, 127-135.

Goodwin, J. S., Sanchez, C. J., Thomas, P., Hunt, C., Garry, P. J., & Goodwin, J. M. (1987). Alcohol intake in a healthy elderly population. *Am.J.Public Health,* 77, 173-177.

Gossop, M (2008) *Substance Use among Older Adults: A Neglected Problem.* Lisbon: European Monitoring Centre for Drugs and Drug Addiction; 2008. Available from http://www.emcdda.europa.eu/attachements.cfm/att_50566_EN_TDAD08001EN C_web.pdf

Graham, K. & Schmidt, G. (1999). Alcohol use and psychosocial well-being among older adults. *J.Stud.Alcohol,* 60, 345-351.

Graham, K. & Braun, K. (1999). Concordance of use of alcohol and other substances among older adult couples. *Addictive Behaviors,* 24, 839-856.

Gronbaek, M., Deis, A., Becker, U., Hein, H. O., Schnohr, P., Jensen, G. et al. (1998). Alcohol and mortality: is there a U-shaped relation in elderly people? *Age Ageing,* 27, 739-744.

Halme, J. T., Seppa, K., Alho, H., Poikolainen, K., Pirkola, S., & Aalto, M. (2010). Alcohol consumption and all-cause mortality among elderly in Finland. *Drug Alcohol Depend.,* 106, 212-218.

Han, B, Gfroerer, J.C., Colliver, J.D. & Penne, M.A. (2009) Substance use disorder among older adults in the United States in 2020. *Addiction,* 104, 88-96

Hurt, R.D., Finlayson, R.E. Morse, R.M., & Davis, L.J. (1988), *Alcoholism in elderly persons: Medical aspects and prognosis of 216 inpatients,* in: Mayo Clinic Procedures, 63, 8, 761-768.

Ilich, J. Z., Brownbill, R. A., Tamborini, L., & Crncevic-Orlic, Z. (2002). To drink or not to drink: how are alcohol, caffeine and past smoking related to bone mineral density in elderly women? *J.Am.Coll.Nutr.,* 21, 536-544.

Khan, N., Wilkinson, T. J., Sellman, J. D., & Graham, P. (2001). Patterns of alcohol use and misuse among elderly rest home residents in Christchurch. *N.Z.Med.J.,* 114, 58-61.

Kirchner, J. E., Zubritsky, C., Cody, M., Coakley, E., Chen, H., Ware, J. H. et al. (2007). Alcohol consumption among older adults in primary care. *J.Gen.Intern.Med.,* 22, 92-97.

La Greca, A., Akers, R. L., & Dwyer, J. W. (1988). Life events and alcohol behavior among older adults. *Gerontologist*, 28, 552-558.

Lang, I., Wallace, R. B., Huppert, F. A., & Melzer, D. (2007). Moderate alcohol consumption in older adults is associated with better cognition and well-being than abstinence. *Age Ageing*, 36, 256-261.

Lawley, D. I., Reham, H., & Kendrick, D. (1996). The misuse of alcohol in elderly psychiatric patients. *Psychiatric Bulletin*, 20, 310.

Liberto, J.G. & Oslin, D.W. (1995). Early versus late onset alcohol disorder in the elderly. International Journal of Addiction, 30, 1799-1818.

Lejoyeux, M., Delaroque, F., McLoughlin, M., & Ades, J. (2003). Alcohol dependence among elderly French inpatients. *Am.J.Geriatr.Psychiatry*, 11, 360-364.

Mattace-Raso, F. U., van der Cammen, T. J., van den Elzen, A. P., Schalekamp, M. A., Asmar, R., Reneman, R. S. et al. (2005). Moderate alcohol consumption is associated with reduced arterial stiffness in older adults: the Rotterdam study. *J.Gerontol.A Biol.Sci.Med.Sci.*, 60, 1479-1483.

McInnes, E. & Powell, J. (1994). Drug and alcohol referrals: are elderly substance abuse diagnoses and referrals being missed? *BMJ*, 308, 444-446.

Merrick, E., Horgan, C. M., Hodgkin, D., Garnick, D. W., Houghton, S. F., Panas, L. et al. (2008). Unhealthy Drinking Patterns in Older Adults: Prevalence and Associated Characteristics. *Journal of American Geriatrics Society*, 56, 214-223.

Midanik, L. T., Soghikian, K., Ransom, L. J., & Polen, M. R. (1992). Alcohol problems and sense of coherence among older adults. *Soc.Sci.Med.*, 34, 43-48.

Mirand, A. L. & Welte, J. W. (1996). Alcohol consumption among the elderly in a general population, Erie County, New York. *Am.J.Public Health*, 86, 978-984.

Moos, R. H., Brennan, P. L., Schutte, K. K., & Moos, B. S. (2010). Social and financial resources and high-risk alcohol consumption among older adults. *Alcohol Clin.Exp.Res.*, 34, 646-654.

Mukamal, K. J., Longstreth, W. T., Jr., Mittleman, M. A., Crum, R. M., & Siscovick, D. S. (2001). Alcohol consumption and subclinical findings on magnetic resonance imaging of the brain in older adults: the cardiovascular health study. *Stroke*, 32, 1939-1946.

Mukamal, K. J., Cushman, M., Mittleman, M. A., Tracy, R. P., & Siscovick, D. S. (2004). Alcohol consumption and inflammatory markers in older adults: the Cardiovascular Health Study. *Atherosclerosis*, 173, 79-87.

Mukamal, K. J., Chung, H., Jenny, N. S., Kuller, L. H., Longstreth, W. T., Jr., Mittleman, M. A. et al. (2005). Alcohol use and risk of ischemic stroke among older adults: the cardiovascular health study. *Stroke*, 36, 1830-1834.

Musick, M. A. (2000). Religious Activity, Alcohol Use, and Depression in a Sample of Elderly Baptists. *Research on Aging*, 22, 91.

Onen, S.H., Onen, F., Mangeon, J. P., Abidi, H., Courpron, P., & Schmidt, J. (2005). Alcohol abuse and dependence in elderly emergency department patients. *Archives of Gerontology and Geriatrics*, 41, 191-200.

Oslin, D. W., Slaymaker, V. J., Blow, F. C., Owen, P. L., & Colleran, C. (2005). Treatment outcomes for alcohol dependence among middle-aged and older adults. *Addict.Behav.*, 30, 1431-1436.

Preston, P. & Goodfellow, M. (2006). Cohort comparisons: social learning explanations for alcohol use among adolescents and older adults. *Addict.Behav.*, 31, 2268-2283.

Rapuri, P. B., Gallagher, J. C., Balhorn, K. E., & Ryschon, K. L. (2000). Alcohol intake and bone metabolism in elderly women. *Am.J.Clin.Nutr.*, 72, 1206-1213.

Rice, C. & Duncan, D. F. (1995). Alcohol use and reported physician visits in older adults. *Preventive Medicine*, 24, 229-234.

Rigler, S.K. (2000), Alcoholism in the elderly. *American Family Physician* 61, 1710-1725.

Riserus, U. & Ingelson, E. (2007). Alcohol intake, insulin resistance, and abdominal obesity in elderly men. *Obesity*, 15, 1766-1773.

Rodgers, B., Windsor, T. D., Anstey, K. J., Dear, K. B., Jorm, F., & Christensen, H. (2005). Non-linear relationships between cognitive function and alcohol consumption in young, middle-aged and older adults: the PATH Through Life Project. *Addiction*, 100, 1280-1290.

Ruchlin, H. S. (1997). Prevalence and correlates of alcohol use among older adults. *Prev.Med.*, 26, 651-657.

Schuckit, M. A., Morrissey, E. R., & O'Leary, M. R. (1978). Alcohol problems in elderly men and women. *Addictive Diseases*, 3, 405-416.

Sheahan, S. L., Coons, S. J., Robbins, C. A., & Martin, S. S. (1995). Psychoactive medication, alcohol use, and falls among older adults. *Journal of Behavioral Medicine*, 18, 127-140.

Simons, L. A., McCallum, J., Friedlander, Y., Ortiz, M., & Simons, J. (2000). Moderate alcohol intake is associated with survival in the elderly: the Dubbo Study. *Med.J.Aust.*, 173, 121-124.

Speckens, A. E., Heeren, T. J., & Rooijmans, H. G. (1991). Alcohol abuse among elderly patients in a general hospital as identified by the Munich Alcoholism Test. *Acta Psychiatr.Scand.*, 83, 460-462.

Steunenberg, B., Yagmur, S., & Cuijpers, P. (2008). Depression and alcohol use among the Dutch residential home elderly: Is there a shared vulnerability? *Addiction Research & Theory*, 16, 514-525.

Stewart, D., & Oslin, D.W. (2001). Recognition and treatment of late-life addictions in medical settings. *Journal of Clinical Geropsychology*, 7, 145-158.

Sulander, T., Helakorpi, S., Rahkonen, O., Nissinen, A., & Uutela, A. (2004). Smoking and alcohol consumption among the elderly: trends and associations, 1985-2001. *Prev.Med.*, 39, 413-418.

Van der Horst Graat JM, Terpstra, J. S., Kok, F. J., & Schouten, E. G. (2007). Alcohol, smoking, and physical activity related to respiratory infections in elderly people. *J.Nutr.Health Aging*, 11, 80-85.

Vaz De Almeida, M. D., Davidson, K., De Morais, C., Marshall, H., Bofill, S., Grunert, K. G. et al. (2005). Alcohol consumption in elderly people across European countries: Results from the food in later life project. *Ageing International*, 30, 377-395.

Watson, C.G., Hancock,M.B.A., Gearhart, L.P.M., Malovrh, P., Mendez, C.B.S. & Raden, M.B.A (1997). A comparison of the symptoms associated with early and late onset alcohol dependence. *The Journal of Nervous and Mental Disease*, 185, 507-509.

Westerterp, K.R., Meijer, E.P., Goris, A.H.C., & Kester, A.D.M. (2004). Alcohol energy intake and habital physical activity in older adults. *British Journal of Nutrition*, 91, 149-152.

5

Contributions of Non-Human Primates to the Understanding of Cocaine Addiction

Rafael S. Maior, Marilia Barros and Carlos Tomaz
University of Brasilia
Brazil

1. Introduction

In this review, we aim to highlight the importance of neuropharmacological data, originated in non-human primate studies, towards our understanding of the mechanisms of cocaine addiction. Most studies in this field are undertaken with rodents as animal models, having provided over the years important knowledge on the behavioral, neurological and pharmacological mechanisms of drug addiction. There are, nonetheless, significant hormonal, neurochemical and neuroanatomical discrepancies between rodents and primates, particularly in reference to humans. Although the phylogenetic distance between humans-rodents, as opposed to humans-non-human primates may seem obvious, the impact this has on research findings is not always very evident. The gap in brain chemistry, neuronal organization and development, as well as behavioral diversity has serious implications in rodent models and limits somewhat their significance and generalization potential when trying to understand cocaine addiction – a phenomenon typical in humans. Due to ethical and important methodological restrictions on human testing, non-human primate (NHP) models are not only insightful, but also crucial to further the current scientific knowledge on this topic.

2. Addiction and cocaine

Cocaine is one of the most prevalent drugs of abuse. Data from the World Health Organization (WHO) estimated that, until 2008, approximately 19 million people worldwide had made use of cocaine (WHO, 2010). While the illicit retail market of cocaine is deemed to be worth around US$ 88 billions per year (WHO, 2009), its economic burden is difficult to measure. In terms of health treatment costs, there were 31,800 drug-related deaths in the United States alone in 2007 – a rate twice as high as that for murder in that year – with cocaine being related to about 40% of this toll. From 2002 to 2007, the WHO estimates that these premature deaths cost around 33 billion dollars. The American Drug Control program's budget for all drug-related control efforts in 2011 corresponds to US$15 billion, including treatment, prevention and illicit trade combat (National Drug Control Budget, 2011). Most of this will be spent on cocaine control, as the USA is the major destination of cocaine exports (WHO). On the other hand, the global cost of cocaine is less clear, considering that data from several countries are less reliable or regular.

Cocaine addiction is a psychological substance dependence where addicts have great difficulty in abstaining from drug-seeking, even at the cost of evident negative consequences (Vanderschuren & Everitt, 2004). It is a relapsing disorder with pervading effects on the human brain (O'Brien, 1997). Repeated use of cocaine leads to sensitization, i.e. enhanced response to the stimulus. In this case, repeated cocaine intake induces increased motor response and motivation (Robinson & Berridge, 2008). Sensitization is a long-lasting behavioral phenomenon with several implications to addiction (Paulson et al., 1991). The enduring sensitization induced by cocaine is linked to the relapsing properties of this disorder. Relapse or reinstatement is the return of drug-seeking or drug-taking behavior after a drug-free interval. In animal models, reinstatement has been shown to take place with priming injections of the drug (de Wit & Stewart, 1981), other compounds (Crombag et al., 2002), re-exposure to environmental cues associated with drug-taking (Meil & See, 1996) or even by stressful events (Anker & Carroll, 2010). In fact, cocaine relapse is one of the most difficult obstacles for the rehabilitation of addicts (O'Brien, 1997), possibly being related to cocaine sensitization of motivation or stimulus salience and not sensitization of locomotor activity (Robinson & Berridge, 2008).

Although progress in understanding the function of the brain and addiction has been made, there is still no pharmacological treatment that effectively blocks cocaine dependence, even after 30 years or so of research. Therefore, it is evident that cocaine addiction is a lingering and crippling health issue that warrants continued attention from the scientific community.

3. The case for non-human primates as models

As in the case of most biomedical fields, rodent models stand as the primary source of data in the study of addiction. Their small size and short reproductive cycle makes them easy to maintain, handle and reproduce, as well as relatively inexpensive in up keeping in laboratories around the world. Nevertheless, rats and mice did not reach this ubiquity in biomedical research on these merits alone. Rodent models have proved reliable in a wide range of topics, from drug screening to cognitive tests (eg. Fouquet et al., 2010; Heinrichs, 2010; Schmidt et al., 2011). Naturally, the versatility of these subjects has reflected on the enormous amount of scientific literature and experimental apparatus that have been generated over the course of the last five decades. The extensive amount of rodent research also spurs a faster refinement of the techniques, which in turn, makes rodents an even more practical and useful model. In terms of cocaine addiction, rats have been employed in several paradigms (self-administration, conditioned place-preference, open field; Mello & Negus, 1996; Ator & Griffiths, 2003) and also make up the majority of cocaine-related studies. Unfortunately, there is a significant genetic gap between humans and rodents: the actual figure being 66-82% homology (Nilsson et al., 2001). This difference has several implications in the understanding of cocaine abuse in humans.

NHP have been employed in addiction paradigms for approximately 40 years (Thompson and Schuster, 1964; Griffiths et al., 1980; Mello and Negus, 1996). Although the primate database on addiction is less abundant than that of rodents', there is considerable information available for comparison and interpretation. The genetic homology between NHP and human falls within 95%, depending on the species considered (Hacia et al., 1998). A greater phylogenetic proximity reflects on a more similar anatomy, physiology and behavior. In the sections below, we will examine the most important discrepancies between rodents and NHP and the contributions of primate research to the understanding of cocaine addiction. The importance of NHP however does not lie solely on their genetic distance to rodents. There is rather a powerful tool in primate research that allows for a greater and more refined analysis of the intricacies of cocaine effects: primate behavior.

In this sense, one of the most widespread and reliable tests for cocaine addiction is the self-administration paradigm (Griffiths et al., 1980; Ator & Griffiths, 2003). In this model, the animal subject is trained to press a lever or push a button to receive a rewarding stimulus (e.g. electrical stimulation to "rewarding centers" in the brain or a direct infusion of an addictive substance). There are several schemes under which this paradigm may work for both rodents and NHP. Nevertheless, there is a limit to how many response parameters one may expect to gather from rats and mice. The great advantage of primate research is the plethora of behaviors that may be drawn upon, ranging from simple self-directed behaviors, to very complex social behaviors. All apes and monkey species present high cognitive indices and good manipulatory skills (Pouydebat et al., 2009, 2011). They may form large social structures, including even non-kin members. As a result, there are quite complex social situations that entail a variety of social cues and behaviors. For instance, they display (and react appropriately to) facial expressions signaling emotional states or intentions beyond only aggressiveness, as in the case of most non-primates species (Schimidt & Cohn, 2001). They may even engage in very cognitively demanding behaviors such as deception (Reader et al., 2011). Thus, the use of a species-appropriated ethogram may add a wealth of new data even to simple reaction time experiments. Models may be improved to resemble very closely human social conditions or complex cognitive tasks that models human drug-seeking behavior. As pointed out by Nader and coworkers (2008), "…all animal models are, as a minimum, predictive of some clinical outcome… When social behaviors of NHP and cocaine self-administration (for example) are included, these models are homologous models of human drug abuse." Indeed, some paradigms have included social variables in the study of cocaine abuse (Czoty et al., 2005; Morgan et al. 2002).

Furthermore, physical reactions to compounds or the abstinence thereof mirrors very closely those of humans. For example, NHP demonstrate all key signs of opioid withdrawal seen in humans, including retching, hiccups, pallor and abdominal cramps (see Weerts et al., 2007). Rodents, on the other hand, lack those and several other symptoms. Likewise, more subtle and yet relevant drug effects, such as hallucinatory behavior, are only clearly discernible in NHP (Castner & Goldman-Rakic, 2003; Ellison et al., 1981).

In the case of addiction, NHP longevity is also another advantage. Most ape and monkey species tend to live quite long; a few may even live beyond the age of 40 (Judge & Carey, 2000). This has important implications for the study of long-term effects of drug abuse. It means, among other aspects, that long-term effects of cocaine consumption may be more easily modeled for a specific developmental stage, such as adolescence. It also allows studies of a drug's cumulative effects or cross-drug comparisons in the same subject (Ator & Griffiths, 2003). Together with their greater physiological similarities and behavioral diversity, longevity makes NHP models key for addiction research.

At this point, it is important to add a caveat to our argument. Although NHP might prove crucial to research in most biomedical fields, for several reasons it may not always be the ideal model for many laboratories worldwide. First, primates require appropriate facilities that cater to their size, locomotion, habits and social needs. This makes primate research considerably more expensive than working with rats or mice. Longer reproductive cycles and development stages also reduce the pace of any experimental output. Even small species offers difficulty in handling and training. Another restriction refers to the lack of background research on the behavior and/or physiology for several primate species. Behavioral ethograms, for instance, are not always readily available in the literature. Lastly, ethical considerations regarding the availability of specimens and the threat of extinction for some species may also limit the use of primates. Therefore, we are not advocating the use of primates as the primary source of scientific data. Biomedical research will still rely heavily on rodent studies, and rightly so. One of the aims of the present review is to advise that caution should be taken before generalizing rodent findings to human and to show how NHP research may help bridge the gap between them.

3.1 Dopamine

The primary focus of cocaine research, as well as most drug of abuse, is the brain's dopaminergic system. Dopamine (DA) is a neurotransmitter produced in the substantia nigra, ventral tegmental area (VTA) and hypothalamus. The projection of VTA dopaminergic neurons reaches two main targets in the brain: the prefrontal cortex (mesocortical pathway) and the ventral striatum (mesolimbic pathway). Both comprise what is called the reward system, with the mesolimbic pathway playing a major role (see Berridge, 2007 and Wise, 1996 for review). Not surprisingly, the rewarding and psychostimulant effects of cocaine are mediated by its ability to enhance dopaminergic activity within the meso-cortico-limbic circuit (Roberts et al., 1977). Briefly, cocaine binds to and blocks the pre-synaptic transporter responsible for DA re-uptake (Heikkila et al., 1975; Ritz et al., 1987,). This dopamine transporter is referred to as DAT. As DA reuptake is inhibited, the synaptic cleft is overflown with DA that will bind to post-synaptic receptors, inducing a prolonged or enhance signaling effect.

The DA receptors are classically divided into 5 subtypes, classified as: D_1, D_2, D_3, D_4 and D_5. These subtypes have been further divided and organized into two main groups, the 'D_1-like' receptors: D_1/D_{1a}, D_5/D_{1b}, D_{1c} and D_{1d}; and the 'D_2-like' receptors: $D_{2long\ and\ short}$, D_3, D_4 or $D_{2al\ and\ s}$, D_{2b} and D_{2c} (Sibley and Monsma, 1992). D_1-like and D_2-like are traditionally involved in the rewarding properties of stimuli such as cocaine (Hummel & Unterwald, 2002; Di Chiara et al., 2004). In this regard, several studies have reported critical differences between rodents and primates. NHP post-synaptic D_1-like receptors show higher levels and their laminar distribution is more complex than in rodents, but similar to humans (Smiley et al., 1994). Regarding the densities of D_2-like receptors, Lidow and coworkers (1989) showed a distinct pattern of distribution in the primate cortex: a rostro-caudal gradient, with the prefrontal cortex showing the highest concentration and the occipital cortex the lowest. Rats, on the other hand, were found to have a more diffuse distribution of these receptors. More specifically, the ratio between D_1-like and D_2-like receptors in the NHP striatum is almost 1:1 (Madras et al, 1988; Weed et al, 1998), whereas D_1-like receptors are three times more prevalent than D_2-like (Hyttel and Arnt, 1987; Weed et al, 1998). The density ratio in humans seems to follow the same pattern as that observed in NHP (Hall et al, 1994; Piggott et al, 1999). There is also greater similarity between humans and NHP in the distribution of D_1-like (Hersi et al., 1996) and D_2-like receptors in the hippocampal formation (Kohler et al., 1991). These are also reflected in low ligand efficacy of D_1-like receptor agonists in the primate brain (Izenwasser & Katz, 1993; Pifl et al., 1991; Vermeulen et al., 1994).

The distribution and the organization of DA receptors are not the only discrepancies concerning the DA system. An early review from Berger and coworkers (1991) noted important differences in the organization of primate and rodent DA cells. They indicated larger and differentially organized terminal fields in the DA mesocortical pathway in primates. DA cells arriving in the rat striatum are clearly organized into two tiers, ventral and dorsal, whereas no such distinction is found in monkeys (Joel & Weiner, 2000). Cytoarchitecture of midbrain DA cells in monkeys and humans is noticeably different with large and dense dendritic plexuses (Gonzalez-Hernandez et al., 2004). The primate cortex shows a higher density of DA innervation, as compared to rodents (Goldman-Rakic et al., 1992; Goldman-Rakic et al., 1989). Goldman-Rakic and coworkers (1992) emphasized that the cortical DA system in rhesus monkeys is near identical to that of humans. Both species show a bi-laminar innervation of the prefrontal cortex with projections reaching upper and deep cortical areas. These discrepancies bear important consequences for cocaine addiction studies. For instance, the development of compounds that may block cocaine addictive effects will probably depend on receptor specificity.

It is noteworthy that greater focus is generally given to rodent pathways that show high homology with humans. Nevertheless, a few promising options may remain unexplored if NHP are not employed. For instance, the rat thalamus is very poorly innervated by DA neurons (Groenewegen, 1988). Only recently has some attention been given to the multiple DA projections to the thalamus in the monkey and human brain (Sanchez-Gonzalez et al., 2005). Likewise, drug screening may be severely restricted by results in rodents. As pointed out by Weerts and coworkers (2007), "unacceptable performance in the rat can result in termination of further examination of a compound or an entire chemical series".

All the physiological and anatomical dissimilarities between primates and rodents seem to bear on the dynamics of DA circuits and its associated metabolism. Cocaine infusion in NHP was shown to reduce glucose metabolism in several brain regions, including the prefrontal cortex and the ventral striatum, in a manner similar to that reported in human studies (London et al., 1990; Pearlson et al., 1993; Lyons et al. 1996). The effect seems to reduce metabolism also in cortical areas projecting to the ventral striatum (Lyons et al. 1996; Porrino et al., 2002). This is in clear opposition to rodent findings, where metabolic activity is increased, not decreased, being also restricted to dopaminergic circuits (Hammer & Cooke, 1994; Porrino et al., 1988).

The pharmacokinetics of the DA system also shows important differences in behavioural profiles. In NHP, rate-increasing effects of cocaine seem not to be important for the reinstatement of behavior after extinction (Banks et al. 2007). Odum and Shahan (2004) had found earlier that also the psychostimulant amphetamine significantly increased extinguished responding. Lile and co-workers also reported that cocaine and DA agonists induce different behavioural effects in monkeys and challenged the accepted influence of neurotransmitters transporters in reinforcement, as previously established in rats (Lile et al. 2003; Roberts et al. 1999). This became clearer when Letchworth and coworkers (2001) found long-term cocaine-induced increases in DAT densities in monkey striatum, which is not seen in rodents but is quite similar to human studies.

Regarding drug abuse in general, the DA system has been the most extensively investigated pathway. Despite this, its causal role in the reward system is still under debate. In short, three competing hypotheses have been put forward: (1) DA mediates the hedonic aspects of reward (i.e. 'liking'; Wise, 1980); (2) DA mediates the prediction of rewards concordant with associative learning (Schultz, 2004); and (3) DA mediate the motivational aspect of drug-seeking behavior by attributing incentive salience to reward-related stimuli (i.e. 'wanting'; Berridge & Robinson, 1998). In a detailed review of mostly rodent literature, Berridge (2007) examined the findings from the last 30 years and concluded that there is more support for the incentive salience hypothesis. However, there is also support from a few electrophysiological studies in monkeys showing that DA neurons cease to fire after reward-related cues have been learned (Schultz, 2006).

Nonetheless, primate studies have yielded a few other contributions. The study of cocaine-induced response sensitization also showed striking differences between primate and rodents. Rats generally display a dose-dependent sensitization of DA reinforcing responses (Liu et al., 2005). Chronic exposure to cocaine or amphetamine, on the other hand, has failed to produce sensitization in NHP (Castner et al., 2000; Bradberry & Rubino, 2006; Castner & Williams, 2007), which is in agreement with human imaging studies (Volkow et al. 1997; Martinez et al. 2003). Similarly, cocaine-associated cues have been shown to induce DA release in the rat striatum (Ito et al., 2002; Weiss et al. 2000). Similar studies with monkeys were unable to produce significant increases in extracellular DA in either the striatum or cortex (Bradberry, 2000; Kimmel et al. 2005). Human findings, via imaging studies, seem to agree with NHP results, although DA release was not measured directly (see Bradberry, 2007 for review). It is beyond the scope of the present review to try to settle the issue of DA causal role in drug abuse. Instead, the data shown here underscores critical NHP findings that put rodent studies in perspective.

Overall, the data reviewed above indicates that rodent DA system differs significantly from humans'. This is important to keep in mind when analyzing results from rats and mice studies. Although rodent studies provide the initial step of investigation, data obtained from such models are not easily generalized to humans. In some cases they may even bias investigation towards rodent-related issues. As we shall see further, there are also important differences concerning serotonin (5-HT), neuropetides and hormones. However, these systems have been studied less extensively in the framework of cocaine abuse, but their importance is gradually becoming clearer.

3.2 Serotonin

Serotonin or (5-hydroxytryptamine [5-HT]) is an important neurotransmitter in the brain. It is mostly synthesized in the raphe nuclei in the midbrain and from there 5-HT neurons project to several regions in the brain (Kazakov et al., 1993). There are at least 14 types of 5-HT receptors grouped into seven families (see Roth, 2006), with $5-HT_1$ and $5-HT_2$ being the most relevant and widespread in the human brain (Glennon et al., 2000). The release of 5-HT is modulated by the inhibition of two types of 5-HT auto-receptors: cell body and fiber terminal (Price et al., 1996).

As in the case of DA receptors, discrepancies between rodent and primate 5-HT auto-receptor distribution have been reported. $5-HT_{1A}$ distribution in rats and humans seem to be highly congruent (Hartig et al., 1992). Autoradiographic assays, however, have shown an abundance of $5-HT_{1A}$ mRNA expression in the superficial layers of monkeys' prefrontal cortex (de Almeida & Mengod, 2008; Marazziti et al. 1994; Mengod et al. 1996). This suggests that raphe nuclei efference may modulate high-level cortico-cortical communication in primates. In rodents, $5-HT_{1A}$ mRNA seems to be restricted to the deeper layers of the prefrontal cortex (Pompeiano et al., 1992; Santana et al., 2004) and therefore would not exert the same influence on cortical activity.

Although data on $5-HT_{1A}$ distribution throughout the brain is still lacking for NHP, there is little reason to suppose it differs much from humans and rodents. The same does not hold true, for example, in the case of $5-HT_{2A}$ receptors. High densities of this receptor were found in the rat caudate, putamen and accumbens nuclei, as well as 5-HT_{2A} mRNA in the caudate, putamen and substantia nigra (Lopez-Gimenez et al., 2001). This may reflect the fact that 5-HT neurons in the rat striatum are not as evenly distributed as in NHP (Ikemoto et al., 1996; Van Bockstaele et al. 1993). A similar pattern emerges from immunohistochemical assays on 5-HT transporting proteins (SERT), where rats show a more heterogeneous distribution than primates (Owashi et al., 2004). In spite of some efforts, there is as serious lack of data regarding the distribution specific 5-HT receptors in NHP brains. At this point, the involvement of 5-HT in cocaine behavioral effects still seems quite complicated (eg. Dic Dhonnchadha & Cunningham, 2008) and unfolding the intricacies of serotonergic system in the primate brain may prove crucial.

Nevertheless, the basic interaction between cocaine and 5-HT seems to be the same as DA. Besides its effects on DAT, cocaine is also a potent inhibitor of 5-HT reuptake: it binds strongly to SERT, thereby preventing their reuptake by pre-synaptic cells (Heikkila et al., 1975; Ritz et al., 1987; Ritz et al., 1990). There are, once again, discrepancies in how cocaine affects rodent and primate serotonergic transmission. Work from Miller and coworkers (2001) showed that although both rodents and NHP share a high similarity in DAT sequence homology with humans ($\cong 98.9\%$). In the case of SERT, NHP to human homology is slightly lower (98.3%), and even lower in for rodents (95%). Not surprisingly, SERT inhibition has an inverted effect on rats and primates, where it strengthens the discriminative stimulus of cocaine and has no impact on self-administration on the former (Tella, 1995), while it reduces the discriminative stimulus and self-administration in the latter (Howell & Byrd, 1995; Spealman, 1995).

Although the effects of cocaine on 5-HT inhibition were already well established by the early 1990s (Cunningham & Lakoski, 1990; Cunningham et al., 1992), it was only more recently that 5-HT neurotransmission was implicated in the cocaine-increased locomotor activity in rats (Hergers & Taylor, 1998). These findings were further explored by Carey and coworkers (2000, 2001 and 2005) showing that cocaine-induced locomotor activity in rats was mediated more specifically by 5-HT_{1A} receptors. Although self-administration of cocaine seems unaffected by 5-HT_{1A} manipulations in rats (Parsons, Weiss, & Koob, 1998), low doses of highly selective 5-HT_{1A} antagonist WAY100635 were shown to block cocaine-induced hyperlocomotion, whereas pre-treatment with 8-OHDPAT (5-HT_{1A} partial agonist) enhanced it. These findings were corroborated in NHP, where WAY100635 also blocked increases in locomotion induced by diethylpropion, an amphetamine-like drug (Mello Jr. et al., 2005). Pharmacological antagonism of this particular subtype of receptor showed conflicting results in rodent stress and anxiety tests (Fletcher et al., 1996; Griebel et al., 2000; Bell et al., 1999; Groenink et al., 1996). In monkeys, WAY100635 reduced anxiety behaviors in a confrontation model (Barros et al., 2003). These results are important if one considers the fact that stress and anxiety may trigger relapse in cocaine addicts (Steketee & Kalivas, 2011). Also 5-HT_{1A} agonism has been shown to enhance cocaine's reinforcing effects in NHP (Czoty et al., 2002).

The role of 5-HT on cocaine relapse seems to be related not only to its involvement in anxiety and stress processes. 5-HT may influence cocaine relapse due to its role in memory retrieval (Molodtsova, 2008). In rodents, the non-selective $5\text{-HT}_{1B/1A}$ agonist RU24969 was shown to reduce the retrieval of cocaine induced cues (Acosta et al., 2005). This effect was reversed by 5-HT_{1B} antagonism which indicates prevalence of 5-HT_{1B} receptor in this case. Antagonism of 5-HT_{1B} receptors receptors seems to have no effect of their own on cocaine-related memories or behavior reinstatement. There are no reports on the effects of 5-HT_{1A}

agonists on retrieval of cocaine operant behavior *per se*, but one study found a reinstatement of cocaine-induced locomotor behavior (Carey et al., 2009). Retrieval of cocaine-associated memories in rats was also shown to be impaired by $5\text{-}HT_{2A}$ antagonism (Burmeister et al., 2004; Fillip, 2005) and $5\text{-}HT_{2C}$ agonism (Burbassi & Cervo, 2008; Fletcher et al., 2008; Neisewander & Acosta, 2007).

Although the understanding of 5-HT receptor's modulation of cocaine-related memory is still inceptive, Nic Dhonnchadha & Cunningham (2008) argued that future research should focus on $5\text{-}HT_{1B}$, $5\text{-}HT_{2A}$ and $5\text{-}HT_{2C}$. To our knowledge, the effects of $5\text{-}HT_{1A/1B}$ and $5\text{-}HT_{2A/2C}$ pharmacological manipulation on cocaine-associated memories have yet to be tested. Nevertheless, disparities of primate and rodent serotonergic system warrant a broader stance for future research. Although $5\text{-}HT_{1B}$ and $5\text{-}HT_{2A/2C}$ modulation enhance self-administration in both species (Bubar & Cunningham, 2006; Czoty et al., 2005; Fletcher et al., 2002; Howell & Byrd, 1995; Parsons, Weiss, & Koob, 1998), $5\text{-}HT_{1A}$ agonism has shown to enhance the reinforcing properties of cocaine only in primates (Gold & Balster, 1992; Nader and Barrett, 1990). Therefore, differences in 5-HT reinforcing effects between rodents and NHP may very well transpose to cocaine-associated memories or even provide a entirely distinct pattern.

3.3 Peptides

Compared to DA and 5-HT, the role of neuropeptides in the effects of cocaine remains largely unknown. Nonetheless the past 20 years have witnessed important advances, especially in two fronts: tachykinin receptors and cocaine-and-amphetamine regulated transcript (CART). As shown below, the differences in primate and rodent brain regarding these two neuropeptides should exact caution from researchers.

Tachykinins comprise a group of neuropeptides that share a common C-terminal sequence (Phe-X-Gly-Leu-Met-NH2), with five known mammalian tachykinins: substance P - SP, neurokinin A (NKA), neurokinin B (NKB), neuropeptide K and neuropeptide g. They have been shown to bind to three specific tachykinin receptors: NK1, NK2 and NK3. NK1-Rs and NK3-Rs are widely distributed in the brain, while the NK2-Rs are found only in restricted areas. Although SP, NKA and NKB have a high binding affinity to the NK1-R, NK2-R and NK3-R, respectively, all tachykinins bind to all three receptor types (Severini et al., 2002).

In rats, cocaine administration induced the expression of tachykinin-related mRNA in the striatum (Adams et al., 2001; Arroyo et al., 2000; Johansson et al., 1994; Hurd et al., 1992; Mathieu-Kia & Besson, 1998). It also increased SP immunoreactivity in the striatum, substantia nigra and frontal cortex (Alburges et al., 2000). Nevertheless, results from NK1 manipulations on cocaine effects in rodents have been controversial so far. NK1 antagonism was shown to block cocaine-induced hyperlocomotion (Kraft et al., 2001), reverse sensitization (Davidson et al., 2004) and reduce cocaine-induced DA increases in the striatum (Loonam et al., 2003). NK1 agonism reinstated cocaine operant behaviors, yet SP – which binds preferentially to NK1 – failed to replace cocaine (Ukai et al., 1995). NK1 knockout mice showed no difference in cocaine self-administration and sensitization, as compared to controls (Ripley et al., 2002).

In the case NK3 receptors, there are a few reports implicating its activity in alcohol addiction in rats (Ciccocioppo et al., 1998; Massi et al., 2000). Also, NK3 activation in the VTA has been shown to reinstate cocaine-seeking behavior (Placenza et al., 2004) and its antagonism seems to block cocaine sensitization (Nwaneshiudu & Unterwald, 2010). In a joint effort from Huston and Tomaz's groups, a series of comparative studies regarding the involvement of

NK3 receptors in the effects of cocaine in rats and marmoset monkeys has been carried out. In rats, NK3 antagonist SR142801 reduced behavioral effects of cocaine, but increased DA action in the ventral nucleus accumbens and showed no significant effect on conditioned place preference (Jocham et al., 2006). It also had no individual effect on DA content in the striatum. In monkeys, the same antagonist blocked cocaine-induced effects in a range of behaviors, including locomotion and vigilance (De Souza Silva et al., 2006b). It also had no effect *per se*. In contrast, NK3 agonist senktide showed discrepancies between the two species. In rats, senktide increased both cocaine-induced hyperlocomotion and the DA response in the nucleus accumbens (Jocham et al., 2007). Senktide alone induced a brief increase in activity but no neurochemical changes. On the other hand, this same compound blocked cocaine-induced hyperlocomotion in monkeys, although it enhanced cocaine's effects on exploratory activity and some vigilance behaviors dose-dependently (Fig. 1; De Souza Silva et al., 2006a). Furthermore, unlike rats, senktide did not induce significant

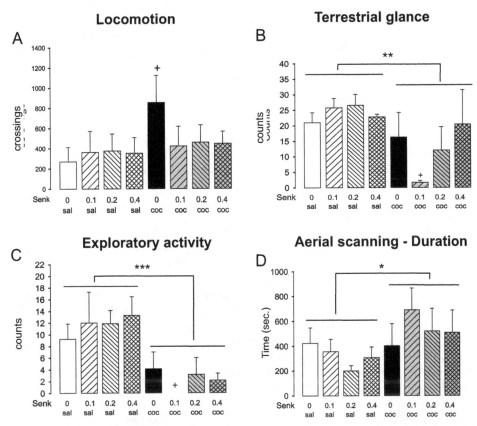

Fig. 1. The effects of cocaine (10 mg/kg, i.p.) on marmoset locomotor activity (A), terrestrial glance (B), exploratory activity (C) and aerial scanning duration (D; mean ± S.E.M.) and its modulation by the NK3-receptor agonist, senktide (0.1–0.4 mg/kg, s.c.), during a 20 min test trial ($n = 8$). +$p < 0.05$ vs. saline–saline, *$p < 0.05$, **$p < 0.01$, ***$p < 0.001$, two-way ANOVA (Modified from de Souza Silva et al., 2006a).

behavioral changes on its own (Fig 1A). These conflicting findings may be due to relevant differences in NK3 receptor distribution between rodents and NHP (Langlois et al., 2001). Despite that, NK3 receptor seems to be an interesting target for investigation and future therapeutic intervention of cocaine addiction.

CART is an mRNA identified in 1995, whose transcription seems to be modulated by psychostimulants (Douglas et al., 1995). It encodes two proteins in the rat (short and long CART), but only one in humans (short). In CART knockout mice, cocaine and amphetamine locomotor and reinforcing effects were reduced (Couceyro et al., 2005). The literature on CART research in primates, however, is scarce. There is one recent comparative report on the cocaine-induced expression of CART in the rat and monkey brain (Fagergren & Hurd, 2007). They report a higher expression of CART mRNA in the primate frontal and temporal cortices, positive labeling confined to the shell-like region of the striatum, different distribution in the hippocampal formation and more markedly differences in the thalamus. These aspects are different from those in rats, yet seem to be in agreement with human studies. Limbic distribution of CART mRNA was overall very similar to that of rodents'. However, the authors point that they were unable to investigate the nucleus accumbens where cocaine had been shown to induce increases in CART mRNA in humans (Albertson et al., 2004).

In summary, neuropeptidic involvement in cocaine-induced effects is beginning to provide important insights. The scarcity of primate studies on the subject is unsettling, considering that the discrepancies with rodents' anatomy and physiology are not trivial. There is, for instance, an absence of co-localization of several neuropeptides with DA in primates (Gaspar et al., 1990; Oeth & Lewis, 1992). Although the discovery of CART is fairly recent, compounds acting on NK1- and NK3-receptors have been under investigation for quite some time. Regardless, the understanding of tachykinins' influence on cocaine addiction seems to be progressing in a very slow pace.

3.4 Hypothalamic-pituitary-adrenal (HPA) axis

Another key aspect of psychostimulant effects concerns the neuroendocrine system. Stressful stimuli or situations trigger a series of neuroendocrine steps in the HPA axis; i.e., the release of corticotropin-releasing factor (CRF) from the hypothalamus, adrenocorticotropic hormone (ACTH) from the pituitary gland and finally glucocorticoids from the adrenal cortex. There is increasing evidence that this physiological response to stress is related to several aspects of drug addiction (Piazza & Le Moal, 1997; Sinha, 2001; Spealman et al., 2004). The work from Piazza and coworkers revealed that glucocorticoids were implicated in the DA response to cocaine and opioids (Marinelli et al., 1998; Marinelli et al., 1997; Piazza &Le Moal, 1997) and, therefore, the HPA axis was a possible target for addiction treatment. Glucocorticoid stress response seems to be essential for the acquisition, maintenance and reinstatement of stimulant self-administration (Goeders, 2002; Piazza et al., 1991; Piazza and Le Moal, 1998).

There are major and pervasive differences in the rodent and primate HPA system. First, the activation of the HPA in rodents relies predominantly on corticosterone, as opposed to cortisol in humans and NHP. There also seems to be discrepant age-related influences on hormones and cocaine. Rats display an increase in basal glucocorticoids as they age (Haugert et al., 1994; Meany et al., 1992), whereas no such difference was observed in NHP or humans (Goncharova & Lapin, 2002). More importantly, the distribution of corticotropin-releasing-factor (CRF) reactivity and that of corticoid receptors in the brain show great discrepancies in the amygdala (Bassett & Foote, 1992; Sanchez et al., 1999), hippocampus and pre-frontal cortex (PFC; Sanchez et al., 2000). The discrepancies in the amygdala and hippocampus are similar to the differences in the distribution of norepinephrine in those regions (Smith et al., 2006). These structures are important for learning and memory (McGaugh 2002; Tomaz et al., 1992) which, in turn, are also implicated in addictive behaviors (Garavan et al., 2000; Kilts et al., 2001; O'Brien et al., 1998). The amygdala also sends critical inputs to the striatum and PFC.

The discrepancies in receptor distribution in the PFC are of particular interest. The PFC is another area relevant for cocaine effects. It is a critical structure in decision-making and is involved in stress responses (Weinberg et al., 2010). It has undergone a massive expansion in primates, with NHP sharing a high similarity with humans in terms of structure, neurochemistry and connections (Carmichael and Price, 1994, 1996; Hardman et al., 2002; Ongur et al., 2003; Porrino & Lyons, 2000). The predominance of glucocorticoid receptors in the primate PFC, compared to the hippocampus, suggests that in humans and NHP this structure plays an important role in the HPA negative feedback through GR-mediated mechanisms (Sanchez et al., 2000). Furthermore, increasing evidence has implicated PFC asymmetry with stimulant use and hormonal changes. Activity in the right PFC was positively correlated with elevated levels of cortisol and cocaine craving (Kalin et al., 1998; Volkow et al., 1999). Chronic use of cocaine was also correlated with greater volume loss of the right PFC (Liu et al., 1998).

Despite these differences, cocaine-induced effects have shown a considerably similar response in rodents and primates. Plasma levels of ACTH, endorphin and corticosterone in rats increase in response to cocaine administration (Forman & Estilow, 1988; Levy et al., 1991; Moldow & Fischman, 1987; Saphier et al., 1993) as also seen in NHP (Lima et al., 2008; Sarnyai et al., 1996). This same pattern is seen in humans, where ACTH and adrenaline levels were increased with cocaine infusions, along with its subjective effects such as euphoria (Mendelson et al., 2002). On the other hand, glucocorticoids show reinforcing properties of their own in rodents, whereas no such effect has been observed in primates (Broadbear et al., 1999). Broadbear and coworkers (2004) also reported that increases in ACTH and cortisol in NHP in response to cocaine infusion were in line with rodents studies, but the same did not hold true for opioid drugs, which induced an inhibition of HPA activity in monkeys.

Although rodent and primate research presents direct mechanisms for the cocaine-induced activation of HPA axis, the impact that stress may have on the maintenance and relapse into drug seeking behavior is not so clear (Sinha, 2001). Initial studies with footshock paradigms in rodents have suggested that corticosterone may play a role in relapse (Deroche et al. 1997; Shaham et al. 1998; Mantsch and Goeders 1999). Rodent studies on reinstatement, however, yielded conflicting results (Erb et al., 1998; Goeders, 2003; Lu et al., 2001). Studies with squirrel monkeys by Spealman and coworkers suggest that the HPA axis is not involved in cocaine relapse (Lee et al., 2003). Rather, their following work indicated that the noradrenergic system is more likely to mediate stress response in cocaine reinstatement (Lee et al., 2004; but see Platt et al., 2007). Nevertheless, a recent study with rats suggests that cocaine reinstatement may be dependent on the interplay of both the HPA and noradrenergic systems (Graf et al., 2011).

4. Current and future strategies against cocaine addiction

As mentioned above, an effective pharmacological treatment for cocaine addiction is still lacking. A recent study has attempted to implement a novel cocaine vaccine trial, with limited results (Martell et al., 2009), yet other trials are currently under way (Kinsey et al., 2010). There are, nonetheless, several ongoing efforts to develop pharmacological strategies in primates to block or reduce the reinforcing properties of cocaine. From the findings discussed above, DA and 5-HT receptors and their respective transporters seem to currently be the most likely candidates for such an endeavor. In fact, the co-administration of DAT and SERT inhibitors has yielded encouraging results in primates (Howell, 2008), with such joint infusion leading to a better outcome, when compared to DAT alone. Strategies that influence CART transcription may also exert an important modulatory effect on stimulant-seeking behavior and thus should not be overlooked in primate studies. On the other hand, NK1 and NK3 receptors seem to be more involved in the hyperlocomotor property of cocaine, even if the present lack of studies limits such a prediction, while the interaction of the stress response, via HPA axis, with the noradrenergic system seems promising in terms of preventing a relapse.

The development of drugs with such mechanisms will require confirmation and further testing in NHP models. Well-established testing paradigms are just now being combined with neuroimaging techniques in monkeys, such as PET scans (Howell, 2008; Howell & Murnane, 2011) and fMRI (Jenkins et al., 2004; Brevard et al., 2006). Besides the several aspects already pointed out in this chapter, other advantages for using NHP (specifically related to imaging studies) are worth mentioning, including a similar cerebral metabolism and pharmacokinetics profile between humans and NHP, as opposed to rodents (Banks et al., 2007; Lyons et al., 1996; Porrino et al., 2002). Therefore, the translational value of NHP neuroimaging is unparallel to any other animal model.

In summary, there is compelling evidence for the importance of NHP in cocaine research. In all neural pathways analyzed, the discrepancies detected between rodents and humans warrant some caution when generalizing the results observed in the former. Nevertheless, there are several lines of research related to cocaine that have few or no corresponding studies being held with primates. Besides the difficulty in handling and research costs, this may also be due to restrictions in the use of these animals for research, especially for large primates. The findings discussed in this chapter indicate that NHP will remain crucial for biomedical research for several years to come, as substitutes have not yet been made available. Therefore, the development of a clinically effective anti-cocaine or anti-relapse drug/vaccine will very likely depend on our ability to cope with the lack of studies and ever-mounting pressure against the use of animals in research.

5. Acknowledgements

The writing of this chapter was supported by CAPES/DAAD/PROBAL (324/09). CNPq/Brazil provided RSM with a doctoral fellowship and MB with a researcher fellowship (311621/2009-0).

6. References

Acosta, J.I., Boynton, F.A., Kirschner, K.F. & Neisewander, J.L. (2005). Stimulation of 5- HT$_{1B}$ receptors decreases cocaine- and sucrose-seeking behavior. *Pharmacology Biochemistry and Behaviour*, Vol.80, pp. 297–307.

Adams, D.H., Hanson, G.R. & Keefe KA. (2001). Differential effects of cocaine and methamphetamine on neurotensin/neuromedin N and preprotachykinin messenger RNA expression in unique regions of the striatum. *Neuroscience*, Vol.102, pp. 843–851.

Albertson, D.N., Pruetz, B., Schmidt, C.J., Kuhn, D.M., Kapatos, G. & Bannon, M.J. (2004). Gene expression profile of the nucleus accumbens of human cocaine abusers: evidence for dysregulation of myelin. *Journal of Neurochemistry*, Vol.88, pp. 1211–1219.

Alburges, M.E., Ramos, B.P., Bush, L. & Hanson, G.R. (2000). Responses of the extrapyramidal and limbic substance P systems to ibogaine and cocaine treatments. *European Journal Pharmacology*, Vol.390, pp. 119–126.

Anker, J.J. & Carroll, M.E. (2010). Reinstatement of cocaine seeking induced by drugs, cues, and stress in adolescent and adult rats. *Psychopharmacology*, Vol.208, pp. 211-222.

Arroyo, M., Baker, W.A. & Everitt BJ. (2000). Cocaine self-administration in rats differentially alters mRNA levels of the monoamine transporters and striatal neuropeptides. *Molecular Brain Research*, Vol.83, pp. 107–120.

Ator, N.A. & Griffiths, R.R. (2003). Principles of drug abuse liability assessment in laboratory animals. *Drug and Alcohol Dependence*, Vol.70, No.3, pp. S55–S72.

Banks, M.L., Czoty, P.W. & Nader, M.A. (2007). The influence of reinforcing effects of cocaine on cocaine-induced increases in extinguished responding in cynomolgus monkeys. *Psychopharmacology*, Vol.192, pp. 449-456.

Barros, M., Mello, E.L., Maior, R.S., Muller, C.P., De Souza-Silva, M.A., Carey, R.J., Huston, J.P. & Tomaz, C. (2003). Anxiolytic-like effects of the selective 5-HT$_{1A}$ receptor antagonist WAY 100635 in non-human primates. *European Journal of Pharmacology*, Vol.482, pp. 197–203.

Bassett, J.L. & Foote, S.L. (1992). Distribution of corticotropin-releasing factor-like immunoreactivity in squirrel-monkey (saimiri-sciureus) amygdala. *Journal of Comparative Neurology*, Vol.323, pp. 91-102.

Bell, R., Lynch, K. & Mitchell, P. (1999). Lack of effect of the 5-HT1A receptor antagonist WAY-100635 on murine agonistic behaviour. *Pharmacology Biochemistry and Behavior*, Vol.64, pp. 549–554.

Berger, B., Gaspar, P & Verney, C. (1991). Dopaminergic innervation of the cerebral cortex: unexpected differences between rodents and primates. *Trends in Neuroscience*, Vol.14, pp. 21–27.

Berridge, K.C. (2007). The debate over dopamine's role in reward: the case for incentive salience. *Psychopharmacology*, Vol.191, 391-431.

Berridge, K.C. & Robinson, T.E. (1998). What is the role of dopamine in reward: hedonic impact, reward learning, or incentive salience? *Brain Research Reviews*, Vol.28, pp. 309–369.

Bradberry, C.W. (2000). Acute and chronic dopamine dynamics in a nonhuman primate model of recreational cocaine use. *Journal of Neuroscience*, Vol.20, pp. 7109–7115.

Bradberry, C.W. (2007). Cocaine sensitization and dopamine mediation of cue effects in rodents, monkeys, and humans: areas of agreement, disagreement, and implications for addiction. *Psychopharmacology*, Vol191, pp. 705-717.

Bradberry, C.W. & Rubino, S.R. (2006). Dopaminergic responses to self-administered cocaine in rhesus monkeys do not sensitize following high cumulative intake. *European Journal of Neuroscience*, Vol.23, pp. 2773-2778.

Brevard, M.E., Meyer, J.S., Harder, J.A. & Ferris, C.F. (2006). Imaging brain activity in conscious monkeys following oral MDMA ("ecstasy"). *Magnetic Resonance Imaging*, Vol.24, pp. 707-714.

Broadbear, J.H., Winger, G. & Woods, J.H. (1999). Glucocorticoid-reinforced responding in the rhesus monkey. Psychopharmacology, Vol.147, pp. 46-55.

Broadbear, J.H., Winger, G. & Woods, J.H. (2004). Self-administration of fentanyl, cocaine and ketamine: effects on the pituitary-adrenal axis in rhesus monkeys. *Psychopharmacology*, Vol.176, pp. 398-406.

Bubar, M.J. & Cunningham, K.A. (2006). Serotonin 5-HT$_{2A}$ and 5-HT$_{2C}$ receptors as potential targets for modulation of psychostimulant use and dependence. *Current Topics on Medical Chemistry*, Vol.6, pp. 1971-1985.

Burbassi, S. & Cervo L. (2008). Stimulation of serotonin(2C) receptors influences cocaine-seeking behavior in response to drug-associated stimuli in rats. *Psychopharmacology* (Berl), Vol.196, pp. 15-27.

Burmeister, J.J., Lungren, E.M., Kirschner, K.F. & Neisewander JL. (2004). Differential roles of 5-HT receptor subtypes in cue and cocaine reinstatement of cocaine-seeking behavior in rats. *Neuropsychopharmacology*, Vol.29, pp. 660-668.

Carey, R.J., Damianopoulos, E.N. & DePalma G. (2000). The 5-HT1A antagonist WAY 100635 can block the low dose locomotor stimulant effects of cocaine. *Brain Research*, Vol.862, pp. 242-246.

Carey, R.J., Damianopoulos, E.N. & Shanahan, A.B. (2009). Cocaine conditioning: Reversal by autoreceptor dose levels of 8-OHDPAT. *Pharmacology Biochemistry and Behavior*, Vol.91, pp. 447-452.

Carey, R.J., DePalma, G. & Damianopoulos, E. (2001). Cocaine and serotonin: a role for the 5-HT$_{1A}$ receptor site in the mediation of cocaine stimulant effects. *Behavioural Brain Research*, Vol.126, pp. 127-133.

Carey, R.J., DePalma, G., Damianopoulos, E., Shanahan, A., Muller, C.P. & Huston, J.P. (2005). Evidence that the 5-HT$_{1A}$ autoreceptor is an important pharmacological target for the modulation of cocaine behavioral stimulant effects. *Brain Research*, Vol.1034, pp. 162-171.

Carmichael, S.T. & Price, J.L. (1994). Architectonic subdivision of the orbital and medial prefrontal cortex in the macaque monkey. *Journal of Comparative Neurology*, Vol.346, pp. 366-402.

Castner, S.A. & Goldman-Rakic, P.S. (2003). Amphetamine sensitization of hallucinatory-like behaviors is dependent on prefrontal cortex in nonhuman primates. *Biological Psychiatry*, Vol.54, pp. 105-110.

Castner, S.A. & Williams, G.V. (2007). From vice to virtue: Insights from sensitization in the nonhuman primate. *Progress in Neuro-Psychopharmacology & Biological Psychiatry*, Vol.31, pp. 1572-1592.

Castner, S.A., al-Tikriti, M.S., Baldwin, R.M., Seibyl, J.P., Innis, R.B. & Goldman-Rakic, P.S. (2000). Behavioral changes and [123I]IBZM equilibrium SPECT measurement of amphetamine-induced dopamine release in rhesus monkeys exposed to subchronic amphetamine. *Neuropsychopharmacology*, Vol.22, pp. 4–13.

Ciccocioppo, R., Panocka, I., Polidori, C., Froldi, R., Angeletti, S. & Massi, M. (1998). Mechanism of action for reduction of ethanol intake in rats by the tachykinin NK-3 receptor agonist aminosenktide. *Pharmacology Biochemistry and Behaviour*, Vol.61, pp. 459–464.

Couceyro, P.R., Evans, C., McKinzie, A., Mitchell, D., Dube, M., Hagshenas. L., White, F.J., Douglass, J., Richards, W.G. & Bannon, A.W. (2005). Cocaine- and amphetamine-regulated transcript (CART) peptides modulate the locomotor and motivational properties of psychostimulants. *Journal of Pharmacology and Experimental Therapeutics*, Vol.315, pp. 1091–1100.

Crombag, H.S., Grimm, J.W. & Shaham, Y. (2002). Effect of dopamine receptor antagonists on renewal of cocaine seeking by reexposure to drug-associated contextual cues. *Neuropsychopharmacology*, Vol.27, pp. 1006–1015.

Cunningham, K.A. & Lakoski, J.M. (1990). The interaction of cocaine with serotonin dorsal raphe neurons. *Neuropsychopharmacology*, Vol.3, pp. 41–50.

Cunningham, K.A., Paris, J.M. & Goeders, N.E. (1992). Chronic cocaine enhances serotonin autoregulation and serotonin uptake binding. *Synapse*, Vol.11, pp. 112–123.

Czoty, P.W., Ginsburg, B.C. & Howell, L.L. (2002). Serotonergic attenuation of the reinforcing and neurochemical effects of cocaine in squirrel monkeys. *Journal of Pharmacology and Experimental Therapeutics*, Vol.300, pp. 831–837.

Czoty, P.W., McCabe, C. & Nader, M.A. (2005). Assessment of the relative reinforcing strength of cocaine in socially housed cynomolgus monkeys using a choice procedure. *Journal of Pharmacology and Experimental Therapeutics*, Vol.312, pp. 96–102.

Davidson, C., Lee, T.H. & Ellinwood, E.H. (2004). NK1 receptor antagonist WIN51708 reduces sensitization after chronic cocaine. *European Journal of Pharmacology*, Vol.499, pp. 355–356.

de Almeida, J. & Mengod, G. (2008). Serotonin 1A receptors in human and monkey prefrontal cortex are mainly expressed in pyramidal neurons and in a GABAergic interneuron subpopulation: implications for schizophrenia and its treatment. *Journal of Neurochemistry*, Vol.107, pp. 488-496.

de Souza Silva, M.A.D., Mello, E.L., Muller, C.P., Jocham, G., Maior, R.S., Huston, J.P., Tomaz, C. & Barros, M. (2006a). Interaction of the tachykinin NK3 receptor agonist senktide with behavioral effects of cocaine in marmosets (Callithrix penicillata). *Peptides*, Vol.27, pp. 2214-2223.

de Souza Silva, M.A.D., Mello, E.L., Muller, C.P., Jocham, G., Maior, R.S., Huston, J.P., Tomaz, C. & Barros, M. (2006b). The tachykinin NK3 receptor antagonist SR142801 blocks the behavioral effects of cocaine in marmoset monkeys. *European Journal of Pharmacology*, Vol.536, pp. 269-278.

de Wit, H. & Stewart, J. (1981). Reinstatement of cocaine-reinforced responding in the rat. *Psychopharmacology*, Vol.75, pp. 134–143.

Deroche, V., Caine, S., Heyser, C., Polis, I., Koob, G., & Gold, L. (1997). Differences in the liability to self-administer intravenous co- caine between C57BL/6 and BALB/cByJ mice. *Pharmacology Biochemistry and Behavior*, Vol.57, pp. 429–440.

Di Chiara, G., Bassareo, V., Fenu, S., De Luca, M., Spina, L., Cadoni, C., Acquas, E., Carboni, E., Valentini, V. & Lecca, D. (2004). Dopamine and drug addiction: the nucleus accumbens shell connection. *Neuropharmacology*, Vol.47, Suppl 1, pp. 227–41.

Douglass, J., McKinzie, A.A. & Couceyro, P. (1995). PCR differential display identifies a rat brain mRNA that is transcriptionally regulated by cocaine and amphetamine. *Journal of Neuroscience*, Vol.15, 2471–2481.

Ellison, G., Nielsen, E.B. & Lyon, M. (1981). Animal-model of psychosis-hallucinatory behaviors in monkeys during the late stage of continuous amphetamine intoxication. *Journal of Psychiatric Research*, Vol.16, pp. 13-22.

Erb, S., Shaham, Y. & Stewart, J. (1998). The role of corticotropin-releasing factor and corticosterone in stress- and cocaine-induced relapse to cocaine seeking in rats. *Journal of Neuroscience*, Vol.18, pp. 5529– 5536.

Fagergren, P. & Hurd, Y. (2007). CART mRNA expression in rat monkey and human brain: Relevance to cocaine abuse. *Physiology & Behavior*, Vol.92, pp. 218-225.

Filip, M. (2005). Role of serotonin (5-HT)2 receptors in cocaine self-administration and seeking behavior in rats. *Pharmacological Report*, Vol.57, pp. 35–46.

Filip, M., Bubar, M.J. & Cunningham, K.A. (2006). Contribution of serotonin (5-HT) 5-HT$_2$ receptor subtypes to the discriminative stimulus effects of cocaine in rats. *Psychopharmacology*, Vol.183, pp. 482-489.

Fletcher, A., Forster, E.A., Bill, D.J., Brown, G., Cliffe, I.A., Hartley, J.E., Jones, D.E., McLenachan, A., Stanhope, K.J., Critchley, D.J., Childs, K.J., Middlefell, V.C., Lanfumey, L., Corradetti, R., Laporte, A.M., Gozlan, H., Hamon, M. & Dourish, C.T. (1996). Electrophysiological, biochemical, neurohormonal and behavioural studies with WAY- 100635, a potent, selective and silent 5-HT$_{1A}$ receptor antagonist. *Behavioural Brain Research*, Vol.73, pp. 337–353.

Fletcher, P.J., Grottick, A.J. & Higgins, G.A. (2002). Differential effects of the 5-HT(2A) receptor antagonist M100907 and the 5-HT(2C) receptor antagonist SB242084 on cocaine-induced locomotor activity, cocaine self-administration and cocaine-induced reinstatement of responding. *Neuropsychopharmacology*, Vol.27, pp. 576–586.

Fletcher, P.J., Rizos, Z., Sinyard, J., Tampakeras, M. & Higgins, G.A. (2008). The 5-HT(2C) receptor agonist Ro60-0175 reduces cocaine self-administration and reinstatement induced by the stressor yohimbine, and contextual cues. *Neuropsychopharmacology*, Vol.33, pp. 1402–1412.

Forman, L.J. & Estilow, S. (1988). Cocaine influences beta-endorphin levels and release. *Life Sciences*, Vol.43, pp. 309–315.

Fouquet, C., Tobin, C. & Rondi-Reig, L. (2010). A new approach for modeling episodic memory from rodents to humans: The temporal order memory. *Behavioural Brain Research*, Vol.215, pp. 172-179.

Garavan, H., Pankiewicz, J., Bloom, A., Cho, J.K., Sperry, L., Ross, T.J., Salmeron, B.J., Risinger, R., Kelley, D. & Stein, E.A. (2000). Cue-induced cocaine craving:

neuroanatomical specificity for drug users and drug stimuli. *American Journal of Psychiatry*, Vol.157, pp. 1789-1798.

Gaspar, P., Berger, B. & Febvret, A. (1990). Neurotensin innervation of the human cerebral-cortex - lack of colocalization with catecholamines. *Brain Research* 530, pp. 181-195.

Gaspar, P., Berger, B., Febvret, A., Vigny, A. & Henry, J.P. (1989). Catecholamine innervation of the human cerebral-cortex as revealed by comparative immunohistochemistry of tyrosine-hydroxylase and dopamine-beta-hydroxylase. *Journal of Comparative Neurology*, Vol.279, pp. 249-271.

Glennon, R.A., Dukat, M., & Westkaemper, R.B. (2000). Serotonin receptor subtypes and ligands. In F. E. Bloom & D. J. Kupfer (Eds.), *Psychopharmacology: The fourth generation of progress* (4th rev. ed.). Philadelphia: Lippincott Williams & Wilkins.

Goeders, N.E. (2002). The HPA axis and cocaine reinforcement. *Psychoneuroendocrinology*, Vol.27, pp. 13-33.

Goeders, N.E. (2003). The impact of stress on addiction. *European Neuropsychopharmacology*, Vol.13, pp. 435-441.

Gold, L.H. & Balster, R.L. (1992). Effects of buspirone and gepirone on IV cocaine self-administration in rhesus monkeys. *Psychopharmacology*, Vol.108, pp. 289-294.

Goldman-Rakic, P.S., Leranth, C., Williams, S.M., Mons, N. & Geffard, M. (1989). Dopamine synaptic complex with pyramidal neurons in primate cerebral cortex. *Proceedings of the National Academy of Sciences of the United States of America*, Vol.86, No.22, pp. 9015-9019.

Goldman-Rakic, P.S., Lidow, M.S., Smiley, J.F. & Williams, M.S. (1992). The anatomy of dopamine in monkey and human prefrontal cortex. *Journal of Neural Transmission-General Section*, pp. 163-177.

Goncharova, N.D. & Lapin, B.A. (2002). Effects of aging on hypothalamic-pituitary-adrenal system function in non-human primates. *Mechanisms of Ageing and Development*, Vol,123, pp. 1191-1201.

Gonzalez-Hernandez, T., Barroso-Chinea, P., De La Cruz Muros, I., Del Mar Perez-Delgado, M. & Rodriguez, M. (2004). Expression of dopamine and vesicular mono- amine transporters and differential vulnerability of mesostriatal dopaminergic neurons. *Journal of Comparative Neurology*, Vol.479, pp. 198–215.

Graf, E.N., Hoks, M.A., Baumgardner, J., Sierra, J., Vranjkovic, O., Bohr, C., Baker, D.A. & Mantsch, J.R. (2011). Adrenal Activity during Repeated Long-Access Cocaine Self-Administration is Required for Later CRF-Induced and CRF-Dependent Stressor-Induced Reinstatement in Rats. *Neuropsychopharmacology*, Vol.36, pp. 1444-1454.

Griebel, G., Rodgers, R.J., Perrault, G. & Sanger, D.J. (2000). The effects of compounds varying in selectivity as 5-HT(1A) receptor antagonists in three rat models of anxiety. *Neuropharmacology*, Vol.39, pp. 1848–1857.

Griffiths, R.R., Bigelow, G.E. & Henningfield, J.E. (1980). Similarities in animal and human drug-taking behavior. In N. K. Mello (Ed.), *Advances in substance abuse* (pp. 1–90). Greenwich, CT: JAI Press.

Groenewegen, H.J. (1988). Organization of the afferent connections of the mediodorsal thalamic nucleus in the rat, related to the mediodorsal-prefrontal topography. *Neuroscience*, Vol.24, pp. 379–431.

Groenink, L., Mos, J., van der Gugten, J., Schipper, J. & Olivier, B. (1996). The 5-HT1A receptor is not involved in emotional stress-induced rises in stress hormones. *Pharmacology Biochemistry and Behavior*, Vol.55, pp. 303-308.

Hacia, J.G., Makalowski, W., Edgemon, K., Erdos, M.R., Robbins, C.M., Fodor, S.P., Brody, L.C. & Collins, F.S. (1998). Evolutionary sequence comparisons using high-density oligonucleotide arrays. *Nature Genetics*, Vol.18, pp. 155–158.

Hall, H., Sedvall, G., Magnusson, O., Kopp, J., Halldin, C. & Farde, L. (1994). Distribution of D_1- and D_2-dopamine receptors, and dopamine and its metabolites in the human brain. *Neuropsychopharmacology*, Vol.11, pp. 245–256.

Hammer, R.P. & Cooke, E.S. (1994). Gradual tolerance of metabolic-activity is produced in mesolimbic regions by chornic cocaine treatment, while subsequent cocaine challenge activates extrapyramidal regions of rat-brain. *Journal of Neuroscience*, Vol.14, pp.4289-4298.

Hardman, C.D., Henderson, J.M., Finkelstein, D.I., Horne, M.K., Paxinos, G. & Halliday, G.M. (2002). Comparison of the basal ganglia in rats, marmosets, macaques, baboons, and humans: volume and neuronal number for the output, internal relay, and striatal modulating nuclei. *Journal of Comparative Neurology*, Vol.445, pp. 238–255.

Hartig, P.R., Adham, N., Zgombick, J., Weinshank, R. & Branchek, T. (1992).Molecular biology of the 5-HT$_1$ Receptor family. *Drug Development Research*, Vol.26, pp. 215-224.

Haugert, B.L., Thrivikraman, K.V. & Plotsky, P.M. (1994). Age-related alterations of hypothalamic-pituitary–adrenal axis function in male Fischer 344 rats. *Endocrinology*, Vol.134, pp. 1528–1536.

Heikkila, R.E., Orlansky, H. & Cohen, G. (1975). Studies on distinction between uptake inhibition and release of h-3 dopamine in rat-brain tissue-slices. *Biochemical Pharmacology*, Vol.24, pp. 847-852.

Heinrichs, S.C. (2010). Neurobehavioral consequences of stressor exposure in rodent models of epilepsy. *Progress in Neuro-Psychopharmacology & Biological Psychiatry*, Vol.34, pp. 808-815.

Herges, S. & Taylor, D.A. (1998). Involvement of serotonin in the modulation of cocaine-induced locomotor activity in the rat. *Pharmacology Biochemistry and Behaviour*, Vol.59, pp. 595 – 611.

Hersi, A.I., Jacques, D., Gaudreau, P. & Quirion, R. (1996). Comparative distribution of D1-like receptors in the hippocampal formation of rat, monkey and human brains. Retrieved July 7, 2007, from http://www.neuroscience.com/manuscripts-1996/1996-005-quirion/1996-005-quirion.html

Howell, L.L. (2008). Nonhuman primate neuroimaging and cocaine medication development. *Experimental and Clinical Psychopharmacology*, Vol.16, pp. 446-457.

Howell, L.L. & Byrd, L.D. (1995). Serotonergic modulation of the behavioral effects of cocaine in the squirrel monkey. *Journal of Pharmacology and Experimental Therapeutics*, Vol.275, pp. 1551–1559.

Howell, L.L. & Murnane, K.S. (2011). Nonhuman Primate Positron Emission Tomography Neuroimaging in Drug Abuse Research. *Journal of Pharmacology and Experimental Therapeutics*, Vol.337, pp. 324-334.

Hummel, M. & Unterwald, E. (2002). D_1 dopamine receptor: a putative neurochemical and behavioral link to cocaine action. *Journal of Cell Physiology*, Vol.191, No.1, pp. 17–27.

Hurd, Y.L., Brown, E.E., Finlay, J.M., Fibiger, H.C. & Gerfen, C.R. (1992). Cocaine self-administration differentially alters messenger-RNA expression of striatal peptides. *Molecular Brain Research*, Vol.13, pp. 165–170.

Hyttel, J. & Arnt, J. (1987). Characterization of binding of 3*H*-SCH 23390 to dopamine D-1 receptors. Correlation to other D-1 and D-2 mea- sures and effect of selective lesions. *Journal of Neural Transmission*, Vol.68, pp. 171–189.

Ikemoto, K., Kitahama, K., Maeda, T. & Satoh, K. (1996). The distribution of noradrenaline, serotonin and gamma-aminobutyric acid in the monkey nucleus accumbens. *Progress in Neuro-Psychopharmacology & Biological Psychiatry*, Vol.20, pp. 1403-1412.

Ito, R., Dalley, J.W., Robbins, T.W. & Everitt, B.J. (2002). Dopamine release in the dorsal striatum during cocaine-seeking behavior under the control of a drug-associated cue. *Journal of Neuroscience*, Vol.22, pp. 6247–6253.

Izenwasser, S. & Katz, J.L. (1993). Differential efficacies of dopamine D1 receptor agonists for stimulating adenylyl cyclase in squirrel monkey and rat. *European Journal of Pharmacology*, Vol.246, pp. 39–44.

Jenkins, B.G., Sanchez-Pernaute, R., Brownell, A.L., Chen, Y.C. & Isacson, O. (2004). Mapping dopamine function in primates using pharmacologic magnetic resonance imaging. *Journal of Neuroscience*, Vol24, pp. 9553–9560.

Jocham, G., Lauber, A.C., Muller, C.P., Huston, J.P. & de Souza Silva, M.A. (2007). Neurokinin(3) receptor activation potentiates the psychomotor and nucleus accumbens dopamine response to cocaine, but not its place conditioning effects. *European Journal of Neuroscience*, Vol.25, pp. 2457-2472.

Jocham, G., Lezoch, K., Mueller, C.P., Kart-Teke, E., Huston, J.P. & de Souza Silva, M.A. (2006). Neurokinin(3) receptor antagonism attenuates cocaine's behavioural activating effects yet potentiates its dopamine-enhancing action in the nucleus accumbens core. *European Journal of Neuroscience*, Vol.24, pp. 1721-1732.

Joel, D. & Weiner, I. (2000). The connections of the dopaminergic system with the striatum in rats and primates: an analysis with respect to the functional and compartmental organization of the striatum. *Neuroscience*, Vol.96, pp. 451–74.

Johansson, B., Lindstrom, K. & Fredholm, B.B. (1994). Differences in the regional and cellular-localization of c-Fos messenger-RNA induced by amphetamine, cocaine and caffeine in the rat. *Neuroscience*, Vol.59, pp. 837–849.

Judge, D.S. & Carey, J.R. (2000). Postreproductive Life Predicted by Primate Patterns. *Journal of Gerontology: Biological Sciences*, Vol.55A, No.4, pp. B201–B209.

Kalin, N.H., Larson, C., Shelton, S.E. & Davidson, R.J. (1998). Asymmetric frontal brain activity, cortisol, and behavior associated with fearful temperament in rhesus monkeys. *Behavioural Neuroscience*, Vol.112, pp. 286–292.

Kazakov, V.N., Kravtsov, P.Y., Krakhotkina, E.D. & Maisky, V.A. (1993). Sources of cortical, hypothalamic and spinal serotonergic procjections – Topical organization within the nucleus-raphe-dorsalis. *Neuroscience*, Vol.56, pp. 157-164.

Kilts, C.D., Schweitzer, J.B., Quinn, C.K., Gross, R.E., Faber, T.L., Muhammad, F., Ely, T.D., Hoffman, J.N. & Dexter, K.P.G. (2001). Neural activity related to drug craving in cocaine addiction. *Archives of General Psychiatry*, Vol.58, pp. 334-341.

Kimmel, H.L., Ginsburg, B.C. & Howell, L.L. (2005). Changes in extracellular dopamine during cocaine self-administration in squirrel monkeys. *Synapse*, Vol.56, pp. 129-134.

Kinsey, B.M., Kosten, T.R. & Orson, F.M. (2010). Anti-cocaine vaccine development. *Expert Review of Vaccines*, Vol.9, pp. 1109-1114.

Kohler, C., Ericson, H., Hogberg, T., Halldin, C. & Chan-Palay, V. (1991). Dopamine D2 receptors in the rat, monkey and the post-mortem human hippocampus. An autoradiographic study using the novel D2-selective ligand 125I-NCQ 298. *Neuroscience Letters*, Vol.125, pp. 12-14.

Kraft, M., Ahluwahlia, S. & Angulo, J.A. (2001) Neurokinin-1 receptor antagonists block acute cocaine-induced horizontal locomotion. *Annual Reviews of the New York Academy of Sciences*, Vol.937, pp. 132-139.

Langlois, X., Wintmolders, C., te Riele, P., Leysen, J.E. & Jurzak, M. (2001). Detailed distribution of neurokinin 3 receptors in the rat, guinea pig and gerbil brain: a comparative autoradiographic study. *Neuropharmacology*, Vol.40, pp. 242-253.

Lee, B., Tiefenbacher, S., Platt, D.M. & Spealman, R.D. (2003). Role of the hypothalamic-pituitary-adrenal axis in reinstatement of cocaine-seeking behavior in squirrel monkeys. *Psychopharmacology*, Vol.168, pp. 177-183.

Lee, B., Tiefenbacher, S., Platt, D.M. & Spealman, R.D. (2004). Pharmacological blockade of alpha(2)-adrenoceptors induces reinstatement of cocaine-seeking behavior in squirrel monkeys. *Neuropsychopharmacology*, Vol.29, pp. 686-693.

Letchworth, S.R., Nader, M.A., Smith, H.R., Friedman, D.P. & Porrino, L.J. (2001). Progression of changes in dopamine transporter binding site density as a result of cocaine self-administration in rhesus monkeys. *Journal of Neuroscience*, Vol.21, pp. 2799-2807.

Levy, A.D., Li, Q., Kerr, J.E., Rittenhouse, P.A., Milonas, G., Cabrera, T.M., Battaglia, G., Alvarez Sanz, M.C. & Van De Kar, L.D. (1991). Cocaine-induced elevation of plasma adrenocorticotropic hormone and corticosterone is mediated by serotonergic neurons. *Journal of Pharmacology and Experimental Therapeutics*, Vol.259, pp. 495-500.

Lidow, M.S., Goldman-rakic, P.S., Rakic, P. & Innis, R.B. (1989). Dopamine-D_2 receptors in the cerebral-cortex – Distribution and pharmacological characterization with H-3 raclopride. *Proceedings of the National Academy of Sciences of the United States of America*, Vol.86, pp. 6412-6416.

Lile, J.A., Wang, Z.X., Woolverton, W.L., France, J.E., Gregg, T.C., Davies, H.M.L. & Nader, M.A. (2003). The reinforcing efficacy of psychostimulants in rhesus monkeys: The role of pharmacokinetics and pharmacodynamics. *Journal of Pharmacology and Experimental Therapeutics*, Vol.307, pp. 356-366.

Lima, D., Spindola, D.B., Dias, L.O., Tomaz, C. & Barros, M. (2008). Effects of acute systemic cocaine administration on the cortisol, ACTH and prolactin levels of black tufted-ear marmosets. *Psychoneuroendocrinology*, Vol.33, pp. 321-327.

Liu, X., Matochik, J.A., Cadet, J.L. & London, E.D. (1998). Smaller volume of prefrontal lobe in poly substance abusers: a magnetic resonance imaging study. *Neuropsychopharmacology*, Vol.18, pp. 243-252.

Liu, Y., Roberts, D.C. & Morgan, D. (2005). Sensitization of the reinforcing effects of self-administered cocaine in rats: effects of dose and intravenous injection speed. *European Journal of Neuroscience*, Vol.22, pp. 195-200.

London, E.D., Cascella, N.G., Wong, D.F., Phillips, R.L., Dannals, R.F., Links, J.M., Herning, R., Grayson, R., Jaffe, J.H. & Wagner, H.N. (1990). Cocaine-induced reduction of glucose utilization in human brain. *Archives in General Psychiatry*, Vol.47, pp. 567-574.

Loonam, T.M., Noailles, P.A.H., Yu. J., Zhu, J.P.Q. & Angulo, J.A. (2003). Substance P and cholecystokinin regulate neurochemical responses to cocaine and methamphetamine in the striatum. *Life Sciences*, Vol.73, pp. 727-739.

Lopez-Gimenez, J. F., Vilaro, M. T., Palacios, J. M. & Mengod, G. (2001). Mapping of 5-HT$_{2A}$ receptors and their mRNA in monkey brain: [3H]MDL100,907 autoradiography and in situ hybridization studies. *Journal of Comparative Neurology*, Vol.429, pp. 571-589.

Lu, L., Liu, D. & Ceng, X. (2001). Corticotropin-releasing factor receptor type 1 mediates stress-induced relapse to cocaine-conditioned place preference in rats. *European Journal of Pharmacology*, Vol.415, pp. 203-208.

Lyons, D., Friedman, D.P., Nader, M.A. & Porrino, L.J. (1996). Cocaine alters cerebral metabolism within the ventral striatum and limbic cortex of monkeys. *Journal of Neuroscience*, Vol.16:, pp. 1230-1238.

Madras, B.K., Fahey, M.A., Canfield, D.R. & Spealman, R.D. (1988). D$_1$ and D$_2$ dopamine receptors in caudate-putamen of nonhuman primates *Macaca fascicularis*. *Journal of Neurochemistry*, Vol.51, pp. 934-943.

Mantsch, J.R. & Goeders, N.E. (1999). Ketoconazole blocks the stressor-induced reinstatement of cocaine-seeking behavior in rats: relationship to the discriminative stimulus effects of cocaine. *Psychopharmacology*, Vol.142, pp. 399-407.

Marazziti, D., Marracci, S., Palego, L., Rotondo, A., Mazzanti, C., Nardi, I., Ladinsky, H., Giraldo E., Borsini, F. & Cassano, G.B. (1994). Localization and gene expression of serotonin 1A (5HT$_{1A}$) receptors in human brain postmortem. *Brain Research*, Vol.658, pp. 55-59.

Marinelli, M., Aouizerate, B., Barrot, M., Le Moal, M. & Piazza, P.V. (1998). Dopamine-dependent responses to morphine depend on glucocorticoid receptors. *Proceedings of the National Academy of Sciences of the United States of America*, Vol.95, pp. 7742-7747.

Marinelli, M., RougePont, F., DeJesusOliveira, C., LeMoal, M. & Piazza, P.V. (1997). Acute blockade of corticosterone secretion decreases the psychomotor stimulant effects of cocaine. *Neuropsychopharmacology*, Vol.16, pp. 156-161.

Martell, B.A., Orson, F.M., Poling, J., Mitchell, E., Rossen, R.D., Gardner, T. & Kosten, T.R. (2009). Cocaine Vaccine for the Treatment of Cocaine Dependence in Methadone-Maintained Patients A Randomized, Double-blind, Placebo-Controlled Efficacy Trial. *Archives of General Psychiatry*, Vol.66, pp. 1116-1123.

Martinez, D., Foltin, R., Kegeles, L., Hwang, D., Huang, Y., Hackett, E., Frankle, G & Laruelle, M. (2003). PET imaging of dopamine transmission in the striatal substructures of humans and predictors of relapse. *Society for Neuroscience Abstracts*, Vol.29, pp. 354.8

Massi, M., Panocka, I. & de Caro, G. (2000). The psychopharmacology of tachykinin NK-3 receptors in laboratory animals. *Peptides*, Vol.21, pp. 1597–1609.

Mathieu-Kia, A.M. & Besson, M.J. (1998). Repeated administration of cocaine, nicotine and ethanol: effects on preprodynorphin, preprotachykinin A and preproenkephalin mRNA expression in the dorsal and the ventral striatum of the rat. *Molecular Brain Research*, Vol.54, pp. 141–151.

McGaugh, J.L. (2002). Memory consolidation and the amygdala: a systems perspective. *Trends Neuroscience*, Vol.25, pp. 456-461.

Meany, M.J., Aitken, D.H., Sharma, S. & Viau, V. (1992). Basal ACTH, corticosterone, and corticosterone-binding globulin levels over the diurnal cycle, and age-related changes in hippocampal type I and type II corticosteroid receptor binding capacity in young and aged, handled and nonhan- dled rats. *Neuroendocrinology*, Vol.55, pp. 204–213.

Meil, W.M. & See, R.E. (1996). Conditioned cued recovery of responding following prolonged withdrawal from self-administered cocaine in rats: an animal model of relapse. *Behavioural Pharmacology*, Vol.7, pp. 754–763.

Mello Jr., E.L., Maior, R.S., Carey, R.C., Huston, J.P., Tomaz, C. & Muller, C.P. (2005). Serotonin$_{1A}$-receptor antagonism blocks psychostimulant properties of diethylpropion in marmosets (*Callithrix penicillata*). *European Journal of Pharmacology*, Vol.511, pp. 43-52.

Mello, N.K., & Negus, S.S. (1996). Preclinical evaluation of pharmacotherapies for treatment of cocaine and opioid abuse using drug self-administration procedures. *Neuropsychopharmacology*, Vol.14, pp. 375–424.

Mendelson, J.H., Mello, N.K., Sholar, M.B., Siegel, A.J., Mutschler, N. & Halpern, J. (2002). Temporal concordance of cocaine effects on mood states and neuroendocrine hormones. *Psychoneuroendocrinology*, Vol.27, pp. 71-82.

Mengod, G., Vilaro, M.T., Raurich, A., Lopez-Gimenez, J.F., Cortes, R. & Palacios J.M. (1996). 5-HT receptors in mammalian brain: receptor autoradiography and in situ hybridization studies of new ligands and newly identified receptors. *Histochemical Journal*, Vol.28, pp. 747–758.

Miller, G.M., Yatin, S.M., De La Garza, R., Goulet, M. & Madras, B.K. (2001). Cloning of dopamine, norepinephrine and serotonin transporters from monkey brain: relevance to cocaine sensitivity. *Molecular Brain Research*, Vol.87, pp. 124-143.

Moldow, R.L. & Fischman, A.J. (1987). Cocaine induced secretion of ACTH, beta-endorphin, and corticosterone. *Peptides*, Vol.8, pp. 819–822.

Molodtsova, G.F. (2008). Serotonergic mechanisms of memory trace retrieval. *Behavioural Brain Research*, Vol.195, pp. 7-16.

Morgan, D., Grant, K.A., Gage, H.D., Mach, R.H., Kaplan, J.R., Prioleau, O., Nader, S.H., Buchheimer, N., Ehrenkaufer, R.L., & Nader, M.A. (2002). Social dominance in monkeys: dopamine D2 receptors and cocaine self-administration. *Nature Neuroscience*, Vol.5, pp. 169–174.

Nader, M.A. & Barrett, J.E. (1990). Effects of chlordiazepoxide, buspirone, and serotonin receptor agonists and antagonists on responses of squirrel monkeys maintained under second-order schedules of intramuscular cocaine injection or food presentation. *Drug Development Research*, Vol.20, pp. 5-17.

Nader, M.A., Czoty, P.W., Gould, R.W. & Riddick, N.V. (2008). Positron emission tomography imaging studies of dopamine receptors in primate models of addiction. *Philosophical Transactions of the Royal Academy of Science B Biological Sciences*, Vol.363, pp. 3223-3232.

National Drug Control Budget (2011). *FY 2011 Funding Highlights*, June 2011, Available from: http://www.whitehousedrugpolicy.gov/publications/policy/11budget/fy11High light.pdf

Neisewander, J.L. & Acosta, J.I. (2007). Stimulation of 5-HT$_{2C}$ receptors attenuates cue and cocaine-primed reinstatement of cocaine-seeking behavior in rats. *Behavioural Pharmacology*, Vol.18, pp. 791–800.

Nic Dhonnchadha, B.A. & Cunningham, K.A. (2008). Serotonergic mechanisms in addiction-related memories. *Behavioural Brain Research*, Vol.195, pp. 39-53.

Nic Dhonnchadha, B.A., Fox, Sutz, S.J., R.G., Rice, K.C. & Cunningham, K.A. (2009). Blockade of the serotonin 5-HT$_{2A}$ receptor suppresses cue-evoked reinstatement of cocaine-seeking behavior in a rat self-administration model. *Behavioural Neuroscience*, Vol.123, pp. 382-396.

Nic Dhonnchadha, B.A., Ripoll, N., Clenet, F., Hascoet, M. & Bourin, M. (2005). Implication of 5-HT$_2$ receptor subtypes in the mechanism of action of antidepressants in the four plates test. *Psychopharmacology*, Vol.179, pp. 418-429.

Nilsson, S., Helou, K., Walentinsson, A., Szpirer, C., Nerman, O. & Stahl, F. (2001). Rat–Mouse and Rat–Human Comparative Maps Based on Gene Homology and High-Resolution Zoo-FISH. *Genomics*, Vol.287, pp. 287-298.

Nwaneshiudu, C.A. & Unterwald, E.M. (2010). NK-3 receptor antagonism prevents behavioral sensitization to cocaine: a role of glycogen synthase kinase-3 in the nucleus accumbens. *Journal of Neurochemistry*, Vol.115, pp. 635-642.

O'Brien, C.P. (1997). A range of research-based pharmacotherapies for addiction. *Science*, Vol.278, pp. 66–70.

O'Brien, C.P., Childress, A.R., Ehrman, R. & Robbins SJ. (1998). Conditioning factors in drug abuse: can they explain compulsion? *Journal of Psychopharmacology*, Vol.12, pp. 15–22.

Odum, A.L. & Shahan, T.A. (2004). D-amphetamine reinstates behavior previously maintained by food: importance of context. *Behavioural Pharmacology*, Vol.15, pp. 513–516.

Oeth, K.M. & Lewis, D.A. (1992). Cholecystokinin-containing and dopamine-containing mesencephalic neurons provide distinct projections to monkey prefrontal cortex. *Neuroscience Letters*, Vol.145, pp. 87-92.

Ogren, S.O., Eriksson, T.M., Elvander-Tottie, E., D'Addario, C., Ekstrom, J.C., Svenningsson, P., Meister, B., Kehr, J. & Stiedl, O. (2008). The role of 5-HT$_{1A}$ receptors in learning and memory. *Behavioural Brain Research*, Vol.195, pp. 54-77.

Owashi, T., Iritani, D., Niizato, K., Ikeda, K. & Kamijima, K. (2004). The distribution of serotonin transporter immunoreactivity in hippocampal formation in monkeys and rats. *Brain Research*, Vol.1010, pp. 166-168.

Parsons, L. H., Weiss, F., & Koob, G. F. (1998). Serotonin1B receptor stimulation enhances cocaine reinforcement. *Journal of Neuroscience*, Vol.18, pp. 10078–10089.

Paulson, P.E., Camp, D.M & Robinson, T.E. (1991). Time course of transient behavioral depression and persistent behavioral sensitization in relation to regional brain monoamine concentrations during amphetamine withdrawal in rats. *Psychopharmacology*, Vol.103, pp. 480–492.

Pearlson, G.D., Jeffery, P.J., Harris, G.J., Ross, C.A., Fischman, M.W. & Camargo, E.E. (1993). Correlation of acute cocaine-induced changes in local cerebral blood-flow with subjective effects. *American Journal of Psychiatry*, Vol.150, pp. 495-497.

Piazza, P.V. & Le Moal, M. (1998). The role of stress in drug self-administration. *Trends in Pharmacological Sciences*, Vol.19, pp. 67-74.

Pifl, C., Reither, H. & Hornykiewicz, O. (1991). Lower efficacy of the dopamine D1 agonist, SKF 38393, to stimulate adenylyl cyclase activity in primate than in rodent striatum. *European Journal of Pharmacology*, Vol.202, pp. 273-276.

Piggott, M.A., Marshall, E.F., Thomas, N., Lloyd, S., Court, J.A., Jaros, E., Costa, D., Perry, R.H. & Perry, E.K. (1999). Dopaminergic activities in the human striatum: rostrocaudal gradients of uptake sites and of D$_1$ and D$_2$ but not of D$_3$ receptor binding or dopamine. *Neuroscience*, Vol.90, pp. 433–445.

Placenza, F.M., Fletcher, P.J., Rotzinger, S. & Vaccarino FJ. (2004). Infusion of the substance P analogue, DiMe-C7, into the ventral tegmental area induces reinstatement of cocaine-seeking behaviour in rats. *Psychopharmacology*, Vol.177, pp. 111-120.

Placenza, F.M., Vaccarino, F.J., Fletcher, P.J. & Erb, S. (2005). Activation of central neurokinin-1 receptors induces reinstatement of cocaine-seeking behavior. *Neuroscience Letters*, Vol.390, pp. 42–47.

Platt, D.M., Rowlett, J.K. & Spealman, R.D. (2007). Noradrenergic mechanisms in cocaine-induced reinstatement of drug seeking in squirrel monkeys. *Journal of Pharmacology and Experimental Therapeutics*, Vol.322, pp. 894-902.

Pompeiano, M., Palacios, J.M. & Mengod, G. (1992). Distribution and cellular localization of mRNA coding for 5-HT1A receptor in the rat brain: correlation with receptor binding. *Journal of Neuroscience*, Vol.12, pp. 440–453.

Porrino, L.J. & Lyons, D. (2000). Orbital and medial prefrontal cortex and psychostimulant abuse: studies in animal models. *Cerebral Cortex*, Vol.10, pp. 326-333.

Porrino, L.J., Domer, F.R., Crane, A.M. & Sokoloff, L. (1988). Selective alterations in cerebral metabolism within the mesocorticolimbic dopaminergic system produced by acute cocaine administration in rats. *Neuropsychopharmacology*, Vol.1, pp. 109-118.

Porrino, L.J., Lyons, D., Miller, M.D., Smith, H.R., Friedman, D.P., Daunais, J.B. & Nader, M.A. (2002). Metabolic mapping of the effects of cocaine during the initial phases of self-administration in the nonhuman primate. *Journal of Neuroscience*, Vol.22, pp. 7687-7694.

Pouydebat, E., Gorce, P., Coppens, Y. & Bels, V. (2009). Biomechanical study of grasping according to the volume of the object: Human versus non-human primates. *Journal of Biomechanics*, Vol.42, pp. 266-272.

Pouydebat, E., Reghem, E., Borel, A. & Gorce, P. (2011). Diversity of grip in adults and young humans and chimpanzees (*Pan troglodytes*). *Behavioural Brain Research*, Vol.218, pp. 21-28.

Price, G.W., Roberts, C., Watson, J., Burton, M., Mulholland, K., Middlemiss, D.N. & Jones, B.J. (1996). Species differences in 5-HT autoreceptors. *Behavioural Brain Research* Vol.73, pp. 79-82.

Reader, S.M., Hager, Y. & Laland, K.N. (2011). The evolution of primate general and cultural intelligence. *Philosophical Transactions of the Royal Academy of Science B Biological Sciences*, Vol.366, pp. 1017-1027.

Ripley, T.L., Gadd, C.A., De Felipe, C., Hunt, S.P. & Stephens, D.N. (2002). Lack of self-administration and behavioural sensitisation to morphine, but not cocaine, in mice lacking NK1 receptors. *Neuropharmacology*, Vol.43, pp. 1258-1268.

Ritz, M.C., Cone, E.J. & Kuhar, M.J. (1990). Cocaine inhibition of ligand binding at dopamine, norepinephrine and serotonin transporters: a structure–activity study. *Life Sciences*, Vol.46, pp. 635–645.

Ritz, M.C., Lamb, R.J., Goldberg, S.R. & Kuhar, M.J. (1987). Cocaine receptors on dopamine transporters are related to self-administration of cocaine. *Science*, Vol.237, pp. 1219–1223.

Roberts, D.C.S., Corcoran, M.E. & Fibiger, H.C. (1977). Role of ascending catecholaminergic systems in intravenous self-administration of cocaine. *Pharmacology Biochemistry and Behavior*, Vol.6, pp. 615-620.

Roberts, D.C.S., Phelan, R., Hodges, L.M., Hodges, M.M., Bennett, B., Childers, S. & Davies, H. (1999). Self-administration of cocaine analogs by rats. *Psychopharmacology*, Vol.144, pp.389-397.

Robinson, T.E. & Berridge, K.C. (2008). The incentive sensitization theory of addiction: some current issues. *Philosophical Transactions of the Royal Society of London B: Biological Sciences*, Vol.363, pp. 3137–3146.

Roth, B.L. (2006). *The Serotonin Receptors* (1st edition), Humana Press, 1-58829-568-0, New Jersey (USA).

Sanchez-Gonzalez, M.A., Garcia-Cabezas, M.A., Rico, B. & Cavada, C. (2005). The primate thalamus is a key target for brain dopamine. *Journal of Neuroscience*, Vol.25, pp. 6076–6083.

Sanchez, M.M., Young, L.J., Plotsky, P.M. & Insel, T.R. (1999). Autoradiographic and in situ hybridization localization of corticotropin-releasing factor 1 and 2 receptors in nonhuman primate brain. *Journal of Comparative Neurology*, Vol.408, pp. 365-377.

Sanchez, M.M., Young, L.J., Plotsky, P.M. & Insel, T.R. (2000). Distribution of corticosteroid receptors in the rhesus brain: Relative absence of glucocorticoid receptors in the hippocampal formation. *Journal of Neuroscience*, Vol.20, pp. 4657-4668.

Santana, N., Bortolozzi, A., Serrats, J., Mengod, G. & Artigas, F. (2004). Expression of Serotonin(1A) and Serotonin(2A) receptors in pyramidal and GABAergic neurons of the rat prefrontal cortex. *Cerebral Cortex*, Vol.14, pp. 1100-1109.

Saphier, D., Welch, J.E., Farrar, G.E. & Goeders, N.E. (1993). Effects of intracerebroventricular and intra-hypothalamic cocaine administration on adrenocortical secretion. *Neuroendocrinology*, Vol.57, pp. 54-62.

Sarnyai, Z., Mello, N.K., Mendelson, J.H., Eros-Sarnyai, M. & Mercer, G. (1996). Effects of cocaine on pulsatile activity of the hypothalamic–pituitary–adrenal axis in male rhesus monkeys: neuroendocrine and behavioral correlates. *Journal of Pharmacology and Experimental Therapeutics*, Vol.277, pp. 225-234.

Schama, K.F., Howell, L.L. & Byrd, L.D. (1997). Serotonergic modulation of the discriminative-stimulus effects of cocaine in squirrel monkeys. *Psychopharmacology*, Vol.132, pp. 27-34.

Schmidt, K.L. & Cohn, J.F. (2001). Human facial expressions as adaptations: Evolutionary questions in facial expression research. *Yearbook of Physical Anthropology*. Vol.44, pp. 3-24.

Schmidt, M.V., Wang, X.D. & Meijer, O.C. (2011). Early life stress paradigms in rodents: potential animal models of depression? *Psychopharmacology*, Vol.214, pp. 131-140.

Schultz, W. (2004). Neural coding of basic reward terms of animal learning theory, game theory, microeconomics and behavioural ecology. *Current Opinion in Neurobiology*, Vol.14, pp.139-147.

Schultz, W. (2006). Behavioral theories and the neurophysiology of reward. *Annual Reviews in Psychology*, Vol.57, pp. 87-115.

Severini, C., Improta, G., Falconieri-Erspamer, G., Salvadori, S. & Erspamer, V. (2002). The tachykinin peptide family. *Pharmacological Reviews*, Vol.54, pp. 285-322.

Shaham, Y., Erb, S., Leung, S., Buczek, Y. & Stewart, J. (1998). CP-154,526, a selective, non-peptide antagonist of the corticotrophin-releasing factor receptor attenuates stress-induced relapse to drug seeking in cocaine and heroin-trained rats. *Psychopharmacology*, Vol.137, pp. 184-190.

Sibley, D.R. & Monsma, F.J. Jr. (1992). Molecular biology of dopamine receptors. *Trends Pharmacological Science*, Vol.13, pp. 61-69.

Sinha, R. (2001). How does stress increase risk of drug abuse and relapse? *Psychopharmacology*, Vol.158, pp. 343-359.

Smiley, J.F., Levey, A.I., Ciliax, B.J. & Goldman-Rakic, P.S. (1994). D_1 dopamine receptor immunoreactivity in human and monkey cerebral cortex: predominant and extrasynaptic localization in dendritic spines. *Proceedings of the National Academy of Sciences United States of America*, Vol.91, pp. 5720-5724.

Smith, H.R., Beveridge, T.J.R. & Porrino, L.J. (2006). Distribution of norepinephrine transporters in the non-human primate brain. *Neuroscience*, Vol.138, pp. 703-714.

Smith, Y., Kieval, J., Couceyro, P.R. & Kuhar, M.J. (1999). CART peptide-immunoreactive neurones in the nucleus accumbens in monkeys: Ultrastructural analysis, colocalization studies, and synaptic interactions with dopaminergic afferents. *Journal of Comparative Neurology*, Vol.407, pp. 491-511.

Spealman, R.D. (1995). Noradrenergic involvement in the discriminative stimulus effects of cocaine in squirrel-monkeys. *Journal of Pharmacology and Experimental Therapeutics*, Vol.275, pp. 53-62.

Spealman, R.D., Lee, B., Tiefenbacher, S., Platt, D.M., Rowlett, J.K. & Khroyan, T.V. (2004). Triggers of relapse: Nonhuman primate models of reinstated cocaine seeking. *Motivational Factors in the Etiology of Drug Abuse*, Vol.50, pp. 57-84.

Steketee, J.D. & Kalivas, P.W. (2011). Drug Wanting: Behavioral Sensitization and Relapse to Drug-Seeking Behavior. *Pharmacological Reviews*, Vol.63, pp. 348-365.

Tella, S.R. (1995). Effects of monoamine reuptake inhibitors on cocaine self-administration in rats. *Pharmacology Biochemistry and Behavior*, Vol.51, pp. 687-692.

Thompson, T. & Schuster, C.R. (1964). Morphine self-administration, food-reinforced and avoidance behaviors in rhesus monkeys. *Psychopharmacologia*, Vol.5, pp. 87-94.

Tomaz, C., Dickinsonanson, H. & McGaugh, J.L. (1992). Basolateral Amygdala lesions block diazepam-induced anterograde amnesia in an inhibitory avoidance task. *Proceedings of the National Academy of Sciences of the United States of America*, Vol.89, pp. 3615-3619.

Ukai, M., Mori, E. & Kameyama T. (1995). Effects of centrally administered neuropeptides on discriminative stimulus properties of cocaine in the rat. *Pharmacology Biochemistry and Behaviour*, Vol.51, pp. 705–708.

Van Bockstaele, E.J.V. & Pickel, V.M. (1993). Ultrastmcture of serotonin-immunoreactive terminals in the core and shell of rat nucleus accumbens: cellular substrates for interactions with catecholamine afferents. *Journal of Comparative Neurology*, Vol.344, pp. 603-617.

Vanderschuren, L. & Everitt, B.J. (2004). Drug seeking becomes compulsive after prolonged cocaine self-administration. *Science*, Vol.305, pp. 1017-1019.

Vermeulen, R.J., Jongenelen, C.A., Langeveld, C.H., Wolters, E.C., Stoof, J.C. & Drukarch, B. (1994). Dopamine D_1 receptor agonists display a different intrinsic activity in rat, monkey and human astrocytes. *European Journal of Pharmacology*, Vol.269, pp. 121–125.

Volkow, N.D., Wang G-J., Fowler, J.S., Logan, J., Gatley, S.J., Hitzemann, R., Chen, A.D., Dewey, S.L. & Pappas, N. (1997). Decreased striatal dopaminergic responsiveness in detoxified cocaine-dependent subjects. *Nature*, Vol.386, pp. 830–833.

Volkow, N.D., Wang, G.J., Fowler, J.S., Hitzemann, R., Angrist, B., Gatley, S.J., Logan, J., Ding, Y.S. & Pappas, N. (1999). Association of methylphenidate-induced craving with changes in right striato–orbitofrontal metabolism in cocaine abusers: implications in addiction. *American Journal of Psychiatry*, Vol.156, pp. 19–26.

Weed, M.R., Woolverton, W.L. & Paul, I.A. (1998). Dopamine D-1 and D-2 receptor selectivities of phenyl-benzazepines in rhesus monkey striata. *European Journal of Pharmacology*, Vol.361, pp. 129-142.

Weerts, E.M., Fantegrossi, W.E. & Goodwin, A.K. (2007). The value of nonhuman primates in drug abuse research. *Experimental and Clinical Psychopharmacology*, Vol.15, pp. 309-327.

Weinberg, MS; Johnson, DC; Bhatt, AP. & Spencer R.L. (2010). Medial prefrontal cortex activity can disrupt the expression of stress response habituation. *Neuroscience*, Vol.168, pp. 744-756.

Weiss, F., Maldonado-Vlaar, C.S., Parsons, L.H., Kerr, T.M., Smith, D.L. & Ben-Shahar, O. (2000). Control of cocaine-seeking behavior by drug-associated stimuli in rats: effects on recovery of extinguished operant-responding and extracellular dopamine levels in amygdala and nucleus accumbens. *Proceedings of the National Academy of Sciences of the United States of America*, Vol.97, pp. 4321–4326.

Wise, R.A. (1980). The dopamine synapse and the notion of 'pleasure centers' in the brain. *Trends in Neuroscience*, Vol.3, pp. 91–95.

Wise, R.A. (1996). Addictive drugs and brain stimulation reward. *Annual Review of Neuroscience*, Vol.19, pp. 319-340.

World Health Organization (2010). *World drug report 2010*, June 2010, Available from: http://www.unodc.org/unodc/en/data-and-analysis/WDR-2010.html

6

Comorbidity of a Serious Mental Illness with an Addiction to Psychoactive Substances

Krzysztof Krysta, Irena Krupka-Matuszczyk,
Małgorzata Janas-Kozik and Małgorzata Stachowicz
Medical University of Silesia, Katowice
Poland

1. Introduction

Available data from literature show that among patients suffering from serious mental illnesses it was observed that about 50% of them abused psychoactive substances during their lives (Kessler et al., 1996). And the dependence on such substances like cannabis, amphetamine, or cocaine is more common in patients suffering from schizophrenia than in other psychiatric patients (May-Majewski, 2002). It was found that in the North American population every fourth person suffering from schizophrenia abused alcohol (Helzer & Pryzbeck, 1998). The objective of this study is to analyze data from literature concerning the reasons for psychoactive substance abuse by persons suffering from psychiatric disorders and to discuss the most effective treatment strategies for them. A very important part of this analysis is the so called self-treatment hypothesis formulated by Khantzian (1985). Its definition embraces two elements. Firstly ill persons use psychoactive substances, because they decrease their psychological discomfort. On the other hand there is a great degree in psychopharmacological specificity in choosing the abused substance.

2. Definition of dual diagnosis

In the diagnostic process in psychiatry it often happens to set two or more diagnoses in the same patient. "Dual diagnosis" is a concept that doesn't appear in the official nomenclature of mental health and is not included in the ICD-10 and DSM-IV classifications. In a very general sense it concerns a patient who presents a psychopathological picture, in which we find simultaneously fulfilled criteria for two different psychiatric disorders. However, in recent years, the term "dual diagnosis" has become synonymous with the coexistence of psychiatric disorders and psychoactive substance dependence (Solomon et al., 1993) and this coexistence can consist of the following options:

1. Mental illness and drug dependence.
2. Drug dependence and personality disorders.
3. Acute psychotic disorders resulting from substance use.
4. Drug dependence, mental illness and organic disorders in different combinations (Sciacca, 1987).

Patients with a dual diagnosis can cause many problems in the diagnostic process and therapy at different stages of treatment both in the psychiatric and in the addiction treatment systems. One of the most common examples of a dual diagnosis encountered in psychiatric clinical practice is comorbodity of schizophrenia or bipolar disorder and psychoactive substance dependence.

3. Epidemiology and demographics of dual diagnosis

In recent years, there has been a gradually growing awareness that the problems associated with abuse and addiction to psychoactive substances are very common in people with various mental disorders, including schizophrenia and bipolar disorder. But, although there is an increasing number of reports from the literature that these coexisting disorders are very common, as yet few therapeutic programs based on empirical data targeted specifically at this group of patients have been developed (Lewin & Hennesy, 1994). Based on available evidence, we can try to desribe the scale of the problem. The incidence of bipolar disorder and coexisting abuse of psychoactive substances has been described inter alia in the Epidemiological Catchment Area Study (Regier et al, 1990). This study was conducted among participants from five different municipalities in the U.S.. It showed that, in comparison with with patients with other psychiatric disorders, people with bipolar disorder had the highest comorbidity of disorders associated with alcohol use (46%) and drugs (41%). In addition, rates of disorders associated with the use of alcohol and drugs in people with bipolar disorder were much higher than the associated disorders in the general population (14% and 6%). It was also observed that in bipolar I there was a higher risk of co-existence of problems associated with substance abuse in comparison with bipolar II, wich were respectively 61% and 48% (Lewin & Hennesy, 1994). These results were confirmed by further epidemiological studies. In the National Comorbidity Study (NCS) focused on the respondents with a lifetime alcohol or drug use disorder, recruited for the evaluation, it was found that 51,4% of them also met criteria for at least one lifetime mental disorder. 50.9% of the NCS respondents with a lifetime mental disorder also had a history of alcohol or drug abuse or dependence (Kessler et al., 1996). As mentioned above, one of the most common example of dual diagnosic in the coexistence of schizophrenia and addiction to substances. In the studies of Helzer and Pryzbeck (1998) it was found out that four times more alcoholic than non-alcoholic subjects suffer from schizophrenia. The abuse of stimulants four times more common in schizophrenic than non-schizophrenic subjects (Leduc & Mittleman, 1995). In New York State among each 100 patients hospitalised for their first episode of schizophrenia, 35% of them were addicted to illicit drugs. During the relapses of schizophrenia 22% of the patients use psychoactive substances (DeLisi et al., 1991).

3.1 Young age of patients with dual diagnosis
Patients with dual diagnosis are often young people. De Millo (1989) observed the prevalence of various psychiatric disorders among adolescents addicted to drugs, which was much higher that a paralell incidence among adults, but he also emphasises the fact that there is a lack of standardisation of diagnostic tools for this population. According to Lysaker et al. (1994) among schizophrenic patients with concomitant use of cocaine, the age of first hospitalisation was earlier than in patients not biased. In turn, according to Menezes (1996) patients with dual diagnosis are mainly young men. These observations confirm the evaluations from the studies of Maynard and Cox (1998), who compared the demographic structure of patients hospitalised in psychiatric hospitals in the United States. They showed that among patients with dual diagnosis there was a larger number of younger ones

(average age of 36-37 years), compared with those which had only a single psychiatric diagnosis (mean age of 42-43 years).

A study done in Swiss population, which was conducted in different groups of schizophrenic patients presented a higher average age of subjects without addiction, and also of those who were solely dependent on alcohol, in comparison with patients with a history of illicit drug abuse (Modestin et al., 2001).

Similarly, Kavanagh et al. (2004), examining patients with dual diagnosis in the population of Australia, found that the incidence of alcohol use in patients with dual diagnosis did not depend on the age group, whereas the use of other psychoactive substances was higher in younger groups. Epidemiological studies in England showed that the average age of patients with dual diagnosis is within the range of 34-38 years, but recent trends show a gradual decline of this age (Frisher et al., 2004).

3.2 Sex differences among dual diagnosis patients

When discussing issues related to the comorbidity of a seriuos maental disorder and addiction to psychoactive substances, an important factor to be considered is the sex. Lewine (1981) in his review of the literature devoted to the differences between men and women suffering from schizophrenia emphasises that men are characterized by poorer premorbid social functioning, earlier age of first hospitalisation, more severe negative symptoms, more severe disease. Better premorbid functioning of women with schizophrenia is an element often emphasised in the literature. Women at the time of onset have a better social contacts, higher education, more permanent job, most of them have already left home, got married, or have a regular partner (Kalisz et al., 2001). Girls more often than boys have a secondary education (Krupka-Matuszczyk, 1998). Research on gender differences in schizophrenia have shown that women experience a milder form of the disease than men, which is associated with better premorbid functioning. Gearon and Bellack (2000) draw attention to the gender difference in patients with dual diagnosis. In the group of outpatients with coexisting schizophrenia and psychoactive substance dependence found that women, despite a better premorbid functioning and later age of onset, experience a deterioration, when they begin to use drugs. This may indicate that women are particularly susceptible to the adverse effects of psychoactive substances. The use of these substances and related social deficits, and reduced ability to process information in them may impair the ability to recognise hazards, such as the threat of violence or rape and protect themselves against them (Bellack & Gearon, 1998). Prevalence of drug use also has a correlation with gender. As noted Sieroslawski, in studies conducted in Poland and Europe in the early 90's, the prevalence among boys was more than twice higher than in girls, though he stressed that in some other countries, like Britain or the USA differentiation based on gender was not so clear (Sierosławski, 1998). Since the age of onset of schizophrenia in men is lower than in women, and drug use among young men is more prevalent, perhaps it may result in a fact that the population of patients with dual diagnosis is dominated by young men. Numerous studies show a predominance of males among people with dual diagnosis. In 1994 DeQuardo et al. evaluated the frequency of substance use among schizophrenic patients. In a population of addicts analysed by them, there were 48% of men and 20% of women. Maynard and Cox (1998) analyzed cross-sectionally a population of patients hospitalized in the U.S. due to various psychiatric disorders, and they found that among those with a dual diagnosis, the majority were males. Swartz et al. (2000) conducted an epidemiological study including drug addicts in the U.S.. Among the people who developed a dual diagnosis, 70% were males, and most of them were in the age group of 30-40 years. Salyers and Mueser (2001), studying a group of 404 patients with schizophrenia and schizoaffective disorder, found that in the subgroup that had used alcohol or drugs, women constituted a minority. Other sources of demographic and social analyses of patients with dual diagnosis indicate that the population of such patients consists mostly of men, who often do not work and are poorly educated (Drake & Mueser, 2000). Hambrecht and Hafner (2000) conducted research among a population of a billion participants from Germany, noting that among patients with the first episode of schizophrenia, male gender is a greater risk factor when it comes to cannabis abuse. Similar observations were made by Cantor-Graae in studies conducted in Sweden (2001) in which it was found that among patients with schizophrenia who use substances were far fewer women. French researchers analysed the demographics of patients with schizophrenia and the use of psychoactive substances. It turned out that in that group only 16.7% were women (Dervaux et al., 2003). Kavanagh et al. (2004) examining the incidence of substance use psychoactive drugs in patients with psychoses of various aetiologies noted a prevalence of males in the evaluated group.

3.3 Level of education in the population of dual diagnosis patients

As stated by Chouinard et al. (2003), the first episode of a serious mental illness usually appears at the beginning of adult life, and this is the age when people take important life decisions on, inter alia, the occupation. Suffering from psychiatric disorders is often associated with failure to achieve an adequate education, which may be a consequence of reduced social and economic status. In a Polish follow-up study conducted by Krupka-Matuszczyk (1998) on a group of adolescents including 142 persons, it was observed that after the first hospitalisation 30% of young people did not continue education interrupted by illness. Patients with schizophrenia or bipolar disorder often appear to be poorer, positioned (economically and socially) in worse groups and regions. Achieving a lower educational level may be also the result of the use of psychoactive substances. Swaim et al. (1997) repeatedly observed a higher proportion of drug users in those who interrupted their education prematurely. In a study conducted in Australia it was found that weekly marijuana use in adolescents increases the risk of disruption of school before completing it (Lynskey et al., 2003). Oboth and Anthony (2000) found that among young Americans intravenous drug use causes frequent interruptions of education in high school. In further studies, Kavanagh et al., (2004) observed that having a lower educational attainment was correlated with the use of cannabis, but there was no such correlation with other drugs. In another study, devoted to patients with dual diagnosis, it was found that patients with schizophrenia addicted to alcohol or drugs achieve worse education in comparison to patients with schizophrenia without concomitant dependence (Potvin et al., 2003). Thus, the coexistence of addiction and a serious mental ilness may imply in a summation of the associated adverse factors affecting the level of education of the patients.

4. Diagnostic problems

Conducting epidemiological studies is complicated by the fact that the described problem is associated with a number of diagnostic questions. For example it is possible that some of the observed elevated rates of coexistence of bipolar disorder, or disorders of the bipolar spectrum, such as cyclothymia, and addiction may be caused by the effects of consumption of psychoactive substances. This diagnostic error is less likely in patients with chronic, severe bipolar disorder or in those patients who clearly developed symptoms of bipolar disorder before they began using substances (Lewin & Hennesy, 2004). It is also sometimes difficult to make a differential diagnosis between schizophrenia and a drug related psychosis. Some helpful observations from the patient's behaviour may suggest the clinician the possibility of substance abuse by persons treated for various mental disorders. For example, patients can often ask the nurse for painkillers, and pharmaceuticals to treat different symptoms. This behaviour often distinguishes them from patients without substance abuse problems who are reluctant to take medications because of unpleasant experiences with side effect and because of an association with a stigma of a mental illness. Another clue suggesting addiction is a behaviour of the patient in the community of patients. Patients with a co-dependency often show a better functioning in a group of mentally ill persons. They show higher social skills and they are more adequate in the field of sexual behaviour. Patients with a co-dependence more often have a tendency to intimidate others, causing fear and respect among the staff and other patients (Solomon et al., 1993).

5. Reasons for substance abuse among mentally ill people

Why are disorders related to substance use so common in patients with serious mental illnesses? One of the attempts to explain this phenomenon is the self-medication hypothesis formulated by Khantzian (1985). In defining the self-medication, he draws attention to its two aspects. 1) There is a considerable degree of specificity in the choice of a psychoactive substance. 2) People use, abuse and become addicted to psychoactive substances because they reduce the feeling of psychological discomfort. This suggests that people with psychiatric disorders use specific substances (e.g. use heroin during a manic episode or stimulants during a depressive episode) in an attempt to prevent or "self-medicate" unpleasant symptoms, which ultimately leads to the re-use of these substances. The motivation to do it is often a result of subjective profits that the patients using them experience. The patients with schizophrenia use those substances in order to handle depression, to experience more profoundly different emotions, and to reduce the side-effects of the medication they are prescribed. The data show that illicit drugs are used to reduce depression (72%), and tension (64%) to increase pleasant emotions (62%), to enhance the ability to work and to learn (17%), to decrease the side-effects of the medication.(15%), to reduce hallucinations (11%) , suspicion (4%) and other symptoms (Dixon et al., 1991). The analysis of the causes of abuse of psychoactive substances by subjects with schizphrenia was made by a Canadian team, which attempted to balance gains and losses incurred by the patients reaching for psychoactive substances. In the patients' opinion marijuana and alcohol improved their social functioning. However besides the positive outcomes, the respondents emphasised that the reduction of depressive symptoms was often only their wish, because except for achieving such effects as relaxation, pleasure, being more active etc., the psychoactive substances may happent to be an uncontrolled and unexpected reason for an increase of depressive symptoms. In addition, in spite of achieving a feeling of increased satisfaction, the patients might experience an exacerbation of existing, or develop new positive symptoms of schizophrenia (Addington & Duchak, 1997). When evaluating the attractiveness of different substances for the patients suffering from schizophrenia it is very important to distinguish between positive and negative symptoms of this disease. The positive symptoms usually implicate the abuse of tranquilisers, and the negative symptoms are most frequently a reason to develop a dependence than the positive symptoms. The incidence of negative symptoms is usually accompanied by increased suffering and the patient uses the substance to reduce it even if the relief is only transient. The study done in Australia (1995) was very important. 53 patients with comorbid diagnoses of schizophrenia and addiction to psychoactive substances were interviewed with the use of Brief Symptom Inventory and Schizophrenia/Substance Abuse Interview Schedule. Most of the patients reported that the use of substances was the reason for a development or exacerbation of their disease, 80% of them used drugs to handle their dysphoria and anxiety. The amphetamines caused their subjective improvement better than alcohol, however the choice of the substance depended mainly on what they could afford. Only cannabis exacerbated the positive symptoms and only amphetamines reduced negative symptoms (Baigent et al., 1995). In other studies it was proven that different substances have influence on different problems related to the disease. For example alcohol, cannabis and cocaine decrease depression, cannabis and alcohol decrease the level of anxiety and cocaine increases it (Coben & Levy, 1998). The analysis of subjective experiences of the patients shows that handling the positive symptoms is the most difficult for them as alcohol has here only a limited influence, cannabis increases these symptoms and the effect of cocaine may be diverse depending on the individual patients.

6. Impact of substance use on the course of psychiatric disorders

The observations of the clinicians treating the dual diagnosis patients concerning the influence of the substance abuse on the course of the mental illness are inconsistent. According to some of them the patients suffering from schizophrenia abusing substances present less positive and negative symptoms, according to others the substance abuse highly deteriorates the course of the disease. Especially the stimulants like cocaine have a negative impact on the intensity of psychiatric symptoms. According to data from literature the only result of substance abuse is the increase of frequency of hospitalizations (LeDuc & Mittleman, 1995), and according to some other studies the impact on different symptoms may be diverse, e.g. alcohol causes an increase of positive symptoms, and it is also responsible for a higher frequency of suicidal attempts (Soyka, 1994). We have available data from the literature on the relationship between substance use and severity of clinical symptoms. Lysaker et al., (1994), found that patients with schizophrenia who use cocaine have less intense negative symptoms than patients, who do not use cocaine. Serper et al. (1995) found in schizophrenic patients with a concomitant use of cocaine lower scores of negative symptoms and higher scores of depression and anxiety. Salyers and Mueser (2001) examining patients with schizophrenia who used alcohol and drugs, observed lower intensity of negative symptoms than in patients without concomitant dependence. However, Soyka et al., (2001) found that the coexistence of addiction, causes only minor differences in the scores of positive and negative symptoms. Clearer differentiation of severity was related only hallucinations among patients with dual diagnosis. Norwegian authors who analysed the relationship between substance use and severity of PANSS scores in psychotic patients who used and who did not use psychoactive substances, did not observe differences in positive negative and general symptoms (Moller & Linaker, 2004). In contrast, Canadian researchers found that patients with dual diagnosis had a higher score in

PANSS than patients with schizophrenia alone (Margolese et al., 2003). Buhler et al (2002) examined populations of nonabused patients with schizophrenia and those addicted to alcohol and drugs (mainly cannabis). They found that patients with dual diagnosis experienced more severe positive symptoms. Similar results have also resulted in a study conducted by Green et al. (2002). In the work of Addington and Addington (1997) there was no overall significant difference in symptoms measured by PANSS scale between the group using and not using psychoactive substances. The exception was the subgroup of people who used cocaine, in which a higher severity of positive symptoms was observed. In a study conducted by Pencer and Addington (2003) analysing the cognitive functions in patients with first episode of psychosis, using psychoactive substances, an assessment of PANSS at the start, after one year and two years of observation was done. There was no difference in negative symptoms between the two groups, while those who did not use drugs had less severe positive symptoms. It must be remembered that the subjects throughout the period of observation have used psychoactive substances. Substance abuse can also have a negative impact on the course of the bipolar disorder. For example, it may be associated with earlier age of onset of the disorder and cause more difficulties in the therapy of the subtypes of the disease, such as rapid cycling, dysphoria and mixed states. Salloum et al. (2002) conducted a study covering 256 patients with acute manic episode, done in a municipal psychiatric ward, in which it was found that patients with severe symptoms of disease, abusing alcohol presented a significantly higher lability of mood, impulsivity and increased incidence of aggressive behaviour than patients with an acute manic episode without accompanying alcohol abuse. Furthermore, the coexistence of bipolar disorder and substance abuse is associated with an increased number of psychiatric hospitalisations and it is more difficult to achieve remission of acute manic episodes.

7. Treatment strategies for patients with dual diagnosis

These observations lead to a conlusion that a specific approach for the treatment of comorbid mental ilness and disturbances associated with the use of psychoactive substances is necessary. Currently, clinicians must often rely on their own observations rather than on empirical data to determine which therapies are best for this group of patients.

7.1 Pharmacological treatment

In schizophrenic patients with comorbid substance abuse the treatment with second-generation antipsychotics may have beneficial effects on their symptoms. There are reports in the literature, which indicate the ability of these drugs to reduce other symptoms of the disease, as well as reducing the amount of drug used by patients treated with them.

In the studies of subjects with schizophrenia and schizoaffective disorder, previously diagnosed as drug resistant, a subgroup of patients with dual diagnosis was selected. When they were switch on clozapine from classical neuroleptics in within six months, the authors noted that patients with a coexistence and without a coexistence of drug dependence responsed equally to the treatment (Buckley et al., 1994). Similar observations were made Volavka (1999), who noted that during a 6-month treatment with clozapine it could not be determined whether the difference in the treatment response between patients with schizophrenia and schizoaffective disorder depends on the fact if they use or do not use psychoactive substances. In turn, Zimmet et al (2000) found that over 85% of patients who used psychoactive substances during their treatment with clozapine reduced the quanities of abused psychoactive substances. To similar conclusions also led the studies by Green et al., (2002) and also by Drake et al., (2000) in relation to patients who use alcohol, as well as research of Buckley et al. (1998) embracing patients with dual diagnosis abusing alcohol, cigarettes and cocaine. As it turned out, the classical neuroleptic treatment did not reduce the amount of abused substances. Probably the positive effects of clozapine treatment is due to the fact that it acts on mesocortical and mesolimbic dopaminergic neurons that are associated the reward system (Green et al., 1999). According to Noordsy et al., (2003) in patients with schizophrenia the reward system does not function properly, which increases the susceptibility to substance use. This may also underly the poorer tolerability of conventional antipsychotics in patients with dual diagnosis and the effectiveness of clozapine and, to a lesser extent, of other atypical antipsychotics in the treatment of this group of patients. According to Stip et al., (2003) and Weisman (2003) in the treatment of patients with dual diagnosis the most promising results were obtained with clozapine, and slightly worse results with olanzapine and quetiapine. Other studies have shown a reduction in the frequency of alcohol use after the change of treatment from classical neuroleptics to risperidone (Huang, 1996).

As for the effect of various drugs used to treat bipolar disorder, a summary is made here Maremmani et al (2010). According to them, for example, carbamazepine is beneficial in preventing relapse in abusers of cocaine and has a positive effect on discomfort associated with fluctuations in mood, but it has no effect on the behaviour directed to obtain the substance. Selective response to lithium is achieved in alcoholics with a coexisting depression. Oxcarbazepine has a good effect of aggressive patients, while valproic acid generally is considered the drug effective in patients with coexisting bipolar disorder and addiction, but also in people with anxiety disorders and the accompanying dependence on psychoactive substances. The authors of that study conclude that some of these medicines are safe and effective agents that can be used in the treatment of addicted persons with mood disorders.

7.2 Psychotherapy and rehabilitation

Due to the above-described specific problems associated with diagnosing and treatment of patients with dual diagnosis, specific treatment programs should be developed for them, which combine elements of both psychiatric treatment and addiction therapy. Understanding the causes of the problems described above is necessary for an effective prevention of drug abuse by people with mental illnesses. An example of therapeutic program for dual diagnosis patients with comorbid addiction to substances, with which the authors have a possibility to co-operate, is the Therapeutic Community "Famila" in Gliwice, Poland, which was founded by May-Majewski in the 80-ties. A comprehensive model of treating patients with dual diagnosis, offered by the Center for Addiction Treatment "Familia" allows them to move freely between the settings of two therapeutic models. The program is stationary, conducted in three separate buildings. They have registered 100 beds. The whole program employs three psychiatrists, 6 psychologists and 8 specialists in addiction therapy and nurses. The therapy takes place in a therapeutic community in which the average age is 23 years and in various small groups depending on the current needs of the patient. The treatment of the patient in the psychiatric ward usually follows a complex diagnostic process. Depending on the patient's current condition, which for example may be acute or chronic, the patient may continue his or her treatment in a therapeutic community. The most important rules of the program are: 1) authority, 2) clear rules and principles. The fulfillment of these conditions is essential in building a therapeutic offer for the patients with an addiction to psychoactive substances and psychiatric disorders. These standards apply in therapeutic communities, where adherence to rules and principles is possible through the common responsibilty of all members of this community, both therapists and the patients. The most important factor in a succeful therapy are: receiving feedback from others, allowing to express emotions, a sense of belonging to a group, giving feedback to others, discovering that others have similar problems, receiving support from others, giving support to others, receiving tips and ideas from others. The participant of a therapeutic program is expected to make a gradual transition from the periphery of the therapeutic communitiy to a position, when he or she takes over certain responsibilities (May-Majewski, 2002). Training of social skills is also a very important part of rehabilitation of patients with dual diagnosis. It includes skills such as: communication, interpersonal problem solving, active participation in their pharmacotherapy, learning to take care of their own health (Sawicka, 2001). A very important element that should be included in these programs is also a cognitive skills training, because, according to the the literature, patients participating in cognitive skills training significantly improve their performance on neuropsychological tests, they increase their insight. Keshavan and Hogarty (1999) developed the concept of "social cognition", which is associated with the term "emotional intelligence". The so-called "social cognition" is the central element of pathophysiology of certainn mental disorders like schizophrenia. People predisposed to the development of schizophrenia may use immature (concrete as opposed to abstract) styles which are inadequate for the more complex and abstract cognitive requirements specific to adults. In this way, they do not understand the essence of the subtleties and nuances of social interaction (Lewis, 2004). It appears that cognitive impairment is associated with various aspects of social functioning and problems in vocational activities. Data from literature suggest that they are particularly important for social functioning, quality of life, social skills, ability to benefit from learning new skills (Tamminga, 1998).

8. Conclusion

Understanding the causes of the problem described above is necessary for effective prevention of substance abuse by people with mental health problems. The results of available studies suggest that these patients have an increased risk of a relapse of both the disease and the addiction to substances. In addition to the symptoms they experience, one of the very important problem in the lives of these patients is their difficulty in social functioning. Effective therapy for these individuals should include: making it possible to create a protective environment, assisting these people in makin important changes in their lives, such as finding a good job, friends abstaining from drugs and alcohol, a group of people who can help the patient to find sense their lives. Patients directed to a therapeutic program must be motivated to make changes in their current life. This decision must be conscious and and be a free choice of the patient. It is also necessary to apply specific, individualied forms of therapy of, mental disorders and those associated with subsatnce abuse.

9. References

Addington, J. & Addington, D. (1997). Substance Abuse And Cognitive Functioning in Schizophrenia, *Journal of Psychiatry and Neuroscience*, Vol.22, No.4, (March 1997), pp. 99-104, ISSN:1180-4882

Addington J.; & Duchak V. (1997). Reasons For Substance Use in Schizophrenia. *Acta Psychiatrica Scandinavica*, Vol.96, No.5 (December 1997), pp. 329-333, ISSN:0001 - 690X

Baigent, M.; Holme, G. & Hafner, R.J. (1995). Self Reports of the Interaction Between Substance Abuse and Schizophrenia, *Australian and New Zealand Journal of Psychiatry*, Vol.29, No.1 (March 1995), pp. 69-74, ISSN 0004-8674

Bellack, A.S. & Gearon, J.S. (1998). Substance Abuse Treatment for People with Schizophrenia. *Addictive Behaviors*, Vol.23, No.6 (November-December 1998), pp.749-766, ISSN 0306-4603

Buckley, P.F. (1998). Substance Abuse in Schizophrenia: a Review. *The Journal of Clinical Psychiatry*, Vol.59, Suppl.3, pp. 26-30, ISSN 0160-6689

Buckley, P.; Thompson, P.; Way, L. & Meltzer, H.Y. (1994). Substance Abuse Among Patients with Treatment-resistant Schizophrenia: Characteristics and Implications for Clozapine Therapy. *American Journal of Psychiatry*, Vol.151, No.3 (March 1994), pp. 385-389, ISSN 0002-953X

Bühler, B.; Hambrecht, M.; Löffler; W.; an der Heiden; W. & Häfner, H. (2002). Precipitation and Determination of the Onset and Course of Schizophrenia by Substance Abuse - a Retrospective and Prospective Study of 232 Population-based First Illness Episodes. *Schizophrenia Research*, Vol.54, No.3, (April 2002), pp. 243-251, ISSN 0920-9964

Cantor-Graae, E.; Nordström, L.G. & McNeil, T.F. (2001). Substance Abuse in Schizophrenia: a Review of the Literature and a Study of Correlates in Sweden. *Schizophrenia Research*, Vol.48, No.1, (March 2001), pp. 69-82, ISSN 0920-9964

Chouinard, S.; Stip, E.; Comtois, G.; Corbière, M.; Bolé, P.; Lamontagne, L.; Lecavalier, M. & Beauregard, F. (2003). Young Patients with Severe Mental Illness Returning to School: Results of a Pilot Project Conducted in Montreal. *Santé mentale au Québec*, Vol.28, No.2, (Autumn 2003), pp. 273-290, ISSN 0383-6320

DeLisi, L.E.; Boccio, A.M.; Riordan, H.; Hoff, A.L.; Dorfman, A.; McClelland, J.; Kushner, M.; Van Eyl, O. & Oden, N. (1991). Familial Thyroid Disease and Delayed Language Development in First Admission Patients with Schizophrenia. *Psychiatry Research*, Vol.38, No.1, (July, 1991), pp. 39-50, ISSN 0165-1781

DeMilio, L. (1989). Psychiatric Syndromes in Adolescent Substance Abusers. *American Journal of Psychiatry*, Vol.146, No.9, (September 1989), pp. 1212-1214, ISSN 0002-953X

DeQuardo, J. R.; Carpenter, C. F. & Tandon, R. (1994). Patterns of Substance Abuse in Schizophrenia: Nature and Significance. *Journal of Psychiatric Research*, 1994, Vol.28, No.3, (May-June 1994), pp. 267-275, ISSN 0022-3956

Dervaux, A.; Laqueille, X.; Bourdel, M.C.; Leborgne, M.H.; Olié, J.P.; Lôo, H. & Krebs, M.O. (2003) Cannabis and Schizophrenia: Demographic and Clinical Correlates. *L'Encéphale*, 2003, Vol.29, No.1, pp. 11-17, ISSN 0013-7006

Dixon, L.; Haas, G.; Weiden, P.J.; Sweeney, J. & Frances, A.J. (1991). Drug Abuse in Schizophrenic Patients: Clinical Correlates and Reasons for Use. *American Journal of Psychiatry*, Vol.148, No.2, pp. 224-230, ISSN 0002-953X

Drake, R.E. & Mueser, K.T. (2000). Psychosocial Approaches to Dual Diagnosis. *Schizophrenia Bulletin*, Vol.26, No.1, pp. 105-118, ISSN 0586-7614

Drake, R.E.; Xie, H.; McHugo, G.J. & Green, A.I. (2000). The Effects of Clozapine on Alcohol and drug use disorders among patients with schizophrenia. *Schizophrenia Bulletin*, Vol.26, No.2, pp. 441-449, ISSN 0586-7614

Frisher, M.; Collins, J.; Millson, D.; Crome, I. & Croft P. (2004). Prevalence of Comorbid Psychiatric Illness and Substance Misuse in Primary Care in England and Wales. *Journal of Epidemiology and Community Health*, Vol.58, No.12, (December 2004), pp. 1036-1041, ISSN 0143-005X

Gearon, J.S. & Bellack, A.S. (2000). Sex differences in illness presentation, course, and level of Functioning in Substance-abusing Schizophrenia Patients. *Schizophrenia Research*, Vol.43, No1, pp. 65-70, (May 2000), ISSN 0920-9964

Green, A.I., Salomon, M.S., Brenner, M.J., Rawlins, K. (2002). Treatment of schizophrenia and comorbid substance use disorder. *Current drug targets. CNS and neurological disorders*, Vol.1, No.2, (April 2002) pp.129-139, ISSN: 1568-007X

Green, A.I., Zimmet, S.V., Strous, R.D., Schildkraut, J.J. (1999). Clozapine for comorbid substance use disorder and schizophrenia: do patients with schizophrenia have a reward-deficiency syndrome that can be ameliorated by clozapine? *Harvard review of psychiatry*, Vol.6, No.6, (March-April 1999) pp.287-296, ISSN: 1067-3229

Hambrecht, M. & Häfner, H. (2000). Cannabis, Vulnerability, and the Onset of Schizophrenia: an Epidemiological Perspective. *Australian and New Zealand Journal of Psychiatry*, Vol.34, No.3 (June 2000), pp. 468-475, ISSN 0004-8674

Helzer, J.E. & Pryzbeck, T.R. (1988). The Co-occurrence of Alcoholism with Other Psychiatric Ddisorders in the General Population and its Impact on Treatment. *Journal of Studies on Alcohol and Drugs*, Vol.49, No.3, (May 1988), pp. 219 –224, ISSN 1937-1888

Kalisz, A. & Cechnicki, A. (2001). Różnice w Czynnikach Rokowniczych Między Mężczyznami, i Kobietami Hospitalizowanymi po raz Pierwszy z Rozpoznaniem Schizofrenii. *Psychiatria Polska*, Vol.35, No.6, (November-December 2001), pp. 951-963, ISSN 0033-2674

Kavanagh, D.J.; Waghorn, G.; Jenner, L.; Chant, D.C.; Carr, V.; Evans, M.; Hemnan, H.;

Jablensky, A. & McGrath, J.J. (2004). Demographic and Clinical Correlates of Comorbid Substance Use Disorders in Psychosis: Multivariate Analyses from an Epidemiological Sample. *Schizophrenia Research*, Vol.66, No.2-3, (February 2004), pp. 115-124., ISSN 0920-9964

Keshavan, M.S. & Hogarty, G.E. (1999). Brain Maturational Processes and Delayed Onset in Schizophrenia. *Development and Psychopathology*, Vol.11, No.3, (Summer 1999), pp. 525-543, ISSN 0954-5794

Kessler, R.C.; Nelson C.B.; McGonagle, K.A.; Edlund, M.J .; Frank, R.G.; & Leaf P.L. (1996). The Epidemiology of Co-occurring Addictive and Mental Disorders: Implications for Prevention and Service Utilization, *The American Journal of Orthopsychiatry*, Vol.66, No.1, (January 1996), pp. 17–3, ISSN 0002-9432

Khantzian, E.J. (1985). The Self-medication Hypothesis of Addictive Disorders: Focus on Heroin and Cocaine dependence. *The American Journal of Psychiatry,* (November 1985), Vo.142, No.11, pp. 1259-1264, ISSN 002-953X

Leduc, P. & G. Mittleman, G. (1995). Schizophrenia and Psychostimulant Abuse: a Review and Re-analysis of Clinical Evidence. *Psychopharmacology,* Vol.21, No.4, (October 1995), pp. 407–427, ISSN 0033-3158

Levin, F.R. & Hennessy, G. (2004). Bipolar Disorder and Substance Abuse. *Biological Psychiatry,* Vol.56, No.10, (November 2004), pp. 738–748, ISSN 0006-3223

Lewine, R.R. (1981). Sex Differences in Schizophrenia: Timing or Subtypes? *Psychological Bulletin,* Vo.90, No.3, (November 1981), pp. 432-434, ISSN 0033-2909

Lynskey, M.T., Coffey, C., Degenhardt, L., Carlin, J.B., Patton, G. (2003). A longitudinal study of the effects of adolescent cannabis use on high school completion. *Addiction,* Vol.98, No.5, (May 2003), pp. 685-692, ISSN: 0965-2140

Lysaker, P.; Bell, M.; Beam-Goulet, J. & Milstein, R. (1994). Relationship of Positive and Negative Symptoms to Cocaine Abuse in Schizophrenia. *The Journal of Nervous and Mental Disease,* Vol.182, No.2, (February 1994), pp. 109-112, ISSN 0022-3018

May-Majewski, A. (2002). Normy i Zasady Leczenia Pacjentów z Podwójną Diagnozą. *Wiadomości Psychiatryczne,* Vol.5, No.1, ISSN 1505-7429

Maynard, C. & Cox, G.B. (1998).Psychiatric hospitalization of persons with dual diagnoses: estimates from two national surveys. *Psychiatric Services,* No.49, (December 1998), pp. 1615-1617, ISSN 1075-2730

Margolese, H.C.; Malchy, L.; Negrete, J.C.; Tempier, R. & Gill, K. (2004). Drug and Alcohol Use Among Patients with Schizophrenia and Related Psychoses: Levels and Consequences. *Schizophrenia Research,* Vol.67, No.2-3, (April 2004), pp. 157-166, ISSN 0920-9964

Maremmani, I.; Pacini, M.; Lamanna, F.; Pani, P.P.; Perugi, G.; Deltito, J.; Salloum, I.M.& Akiskal, H. (2010). Mood Stabilizers in the Treatment of Substance Use Disorders. *CNS Spectrums,*Vol.15, No.2, pp. 95-109, ISSN 1092-8529

Modestin, J.; Gladen, C.J. & Christen, S. (2001). A Comparative Study on Schizophrenic Patients with Dual Diagnosis. *Journal of Addictive Diseases,* Vol.20, No.4, pp.41-51, ISSN 1055-0887

Møller, T. & Linaker, O.M. (2004). Symptoms and Lifetime Treatment Experiences in Psychotic Patients with and without Substance Abuse. *Nordic Journal of Psychiatry,* Vol.58, No.3, pp. 237-242, ISSN 0803-9488

Noordsy, D.L., & Green, A.I. (2003). Pharmacotherapy for Schizophrenia and Co-occurring substance use disorders. *Current Psychiatry Reports,*Vol.5, No.5, (October 2003), pp. 340-346, ISSN 1523-3812

Obot, I.S. & Anthony, J.C. (2000). School Dropout and Injecting Drug Use in a National Sample of White Non-Hispanic American adults. *Journal of Drug Education,* Vol.30, No.2, pp.145-155, ISSN 0047-2379

Pencer, A. & Addington, J. (2003). Substance Use and Cognition in Early Psychosis. *Journalof Psychiatry and Neuroscience,* Vol.28, No.1, (January 2003), pp. 48-54, ISSN 1180-4882

Potvin, S.; Stip, E. & Roy, J.Y. (2003). Schizophrenia and Addiction: An Evaluation of the Self-medication Hypothesis. *L'Encéphale,* Vo.29, No.3 Pt 1, (May-June 2003), pp.193-203, ISSN 0013-7006

Salloum, I .M.; Cornelius, J. R.; Mezzich, J. E. & Kirisci, L. (2002). Impact of Concurrent Alcohol Misuse on Symptom Presentation of Acute Mania at Initial Evaluation. *Bipolar Disorders*, Vol.4, No.6, (December 2002), pp. 418-21, ISSN 1398-5647

Salyers M.P., Mueser K.T. (2001). Social functioning, psychopathology, and medication sideeffects in relation to substance use and abuse in schizophrenia. *Schizophrenia Research*, Vol.48, No.1, (March 2001), pp.109-123, ISSN: 0920-9964

Sawicka, M. (2005). Podobieństwa i Różnice w Stylu Radzenia Sobie ze Stresem Pomiędzy Osobami Chorymi na Schizofrenię, Uzależnionymi a Osobami z Podwójnym Rozpoznaniem. *Psychiatria Polska*, Vol.29, No.6, pp. 1199-1210, ISSN 0033-2674

Serper; M.R., Alpert, M.; Richardson, N.A.; Dickson, S.; Allen, M.H. & Werner, A. (1995). Clinical effects of recent cocaine use on patients with acute schizophrenia. *The American Journal of Psychiatry*, Vol.152, No.10, (October 1995), pp. 1464-1469, ISSN 0002-953X

Sciacca, K. (1987). Alcohol and Substance Abuse Programs at New York State PsychiatricCenters Develop and Expand. *AID Bulletin Addiction Intervention with the Disabled*, Vol.9, No.2, (Winter 1987), pp. 1-3

Sierosławski, J. (1998). Używanie Narkotyków przez Młodzież Polską na Tle Wybranych Krajów Europy. Wyniki badań ESPAD 1995. *Serwis Informacyjny Narkomania*, No.2, pp. 25-40, ISSN 1233-9318

Solomon J.; Zimberg, S. & E. Shollar (1993). *Dual Diagnosis: Evaluation, Treatment, Trainingand Program Development*, Spinger, ISBN 978-0306445439, London, UK

Soyka, M. (1994). Addiction and Schizophrenia. Nosological, Clinical and Therapeutic Questions. 2. Substance Dependence and Schizophrenia. *Fortschritte der Neurologie-Psychiatrie*, Vol.62, No.6, (June 1994), pp. 186-196, ISSN 0720-4299

Soyka, M.; Albus, M.; Immler, B.; Kathmann, N. & Hippius, H. (2001). Psychopathology inDual Diagnosis and Non-addicted Schizophrenics - are There Differences? *European Archives of Psychiatry and Clinical Neuroscience*, Vol.,251, No.5, (October 2001) pp. 232-238, ISSN 0940-1334

Stip, E.; Remington, G.J.; Dursun, S.M.; Reiss, J.P.; Rotstein, E.; MacEwan, G.W.; Chokka, P.R.; Jones, B. & Dickson, R.A.; Canadian Switch Study Group. (2003). A Canadian Multicenter Trial Assessing Memory and Executive Functions in Patients with Schizophrenia Spectrum Disorders Treated with Olanzapine. *Journal of Clinical Psychopharmacology*,Vol.23, No.4, (August 2003), pp 400-404, ISSN 0271-0749

Swaim, R.C.; Beauvais, F.; Chavez, E.L. & Oetting, E.R. (1997). The Effect of School Dropout Rates on Estimates of Adolescent Substance Use among Three Racial/Ethnic Groups. *American Journal of Public Health*, Vol.87, (January 1997), No.1, pp. 51-55, ISSN 0090-0036

Regier, D.A.; Farmer, M.E.; Rae, D.S.; Locke, B.Z.; Keith, S.J.; Judd, L.L. & Goodwin, F.K. (1990). Comorbidity of Mental Disorders with Alcohol and Other Drug Abuse. *JAMA: The Journal of the American Medical Association*, Vol.264, No.19, (November 1990), pp. 2511–2518, ISSN 0098-7484

Swartz, J.A.; Lurigio, A.J. & Goldstein, P. (2000). Severe Mental Illness and Substance Use Disorders Among Former Supplemental Security Income Beneficiaries For Drug Addiction and Alcoholism. *Archives of General Psychiatry*, Vo.57, No., (July 2000), pp. 701-707, ISSN: 0003-990X

Tamminga, C.A.; Buchanan, R.W. & Gold, J.M. (1998). The Role of Negative Symptoms and Cognitive Dysfunction in Schizophrenia Outcome. *International Clinical Psychopharmacology*, Vo.13, Suppl.3, (March 1998), pp. 21-26, ISSN 0268-1315

Volavka, J. (1999). The Effects of Clozapine on Aggression and Substance Abuse inSchizophrenic Patients. *The Journal of Clinical Psychiatry*, Vol.60, Suppl.12, pp. 43-46, ISSN 0160-6689

Weisman, R.L. (2003). Quetiapine in the Successful Treatment of Schizophrenia with Comorbid Alcohol and Drug Dependence: a Case Report. *International Journal of Psychiatry and Medicine*, Vol.33, No.1, pp. 85-89, ISSN 0091-2174

Zimmet, S.V., Strous, R.D., Burgess, E.S., Kohnstamm, S. & Green, A.I. (2000). Effects of Clozapine on Substance Use in Patients with Schizophrenia and Schizoaffective Disorder: a Retrospective Survey. *Journal of Clinical Psychopharmacology*, Vol.20, No.1, (February 2000), pp.94-98, ISSN 0271-0749

Part 2

Biological Neuropsychiatry

7

Neurotransmitter and Behaviour: Serotonin and Anxiety

André Rex and Heidrun Fink[1]

Department of Neurology, Center for Stroke Research,
Charité University Medicine, Berlin,
[1]Institute of Pharmacology and Toxicology, School of Veterinary Medicine,
Freie Universität Berlin, Berlin,
Germany

1. Introduction

There are many indications that mental disorders such as depression and anxiety disorders are directly related to mechanisms of central synaptic transmission of serotonin (5-HT).

5-HT is a peripherally and centrally occurring transmitter, which is involved in regulation of anxiety-related behaviour (Iversen 1984; Griebel 1995) and mood, but mediates also learning, appetite, food intake, sexual behaviour, sleep and influences body temperature as well as motor activity (Lucki 1998).

2. Central serotonergic system

In mammals 5-HT is distributed throughout the body. About 5% are located in the central nervous system (CNS). After 5-HT was found in the CNS (Twarog and Page 1953), detailed studies of the origin and projection areas of serotonergic neurons in the CNS began (Falck et al. 1962).

Only about 500 000 neurons in the CNS use 5-HT as a transmitter, but serotonergic neurons have connections to almost all structures of the brain and show a high degree of axonal branching. Dahlström and Fuxe (Dahlstrom and Fuxe 1964) demonstrated by histochemical methods that the raphe nuclei are the origin of almost all serotonergic neurons. Amin and colleagues (Amin et al. 1954) determined 5-HT levels in various brain areas and found the highest concentrations in hypothalamus, midbrain and area postrema.

5-HT receptors are distributed throughout the CNS, with different distribution patterns for the different receptor types. Most 5-HT postsynaptic receptors are located on the subsequent neurons. The release of 5-HT is regulated by presynaptic 5-HT receptors that are located either at the soma or at the nerve endings of the serotonergic neurons. Today, the "5-HT Receptor Nomenclature Committee of the International Union of Pharmacology (NC-IUPHAR) recognizes seven 5-HT receptor families with 16 receptor subtypes (Hoyer et al. 2002).

In the regulation of anxiety-related behaviour by serotonergic transmission, mainly 5-HT1A receptors, 5-HT2A/2C receptors and 5-HT3 receptors are involved (Griebel 1995; Rex et al. 2007). Involvement of 5-HT1B/1D receptors in the modulation of anxiety-related behaviour is discussed.

3. Anxiety and anxiety disorders

Fear or anxiety has protective functions to avoid situations that cause pain, injury or even death (Vaas 2000).

In man, fear is associated with arousal, characterized by symptoms such as restlessness, tremor, less α-waves and frequent β-waves in the electroencephalogram, tachypnea, and tachycardia, elevated systolic blood pressure, hyperemia of the skeletal muscles, decreased blood flow to the internal organs, hypermotility of the stomach, decreased salivation and mydriasis. Clinical studies however, found no uniform physiologic reaction pattern due to large individual differences (Kielholz and Battegay 1967). It was found that the decrease in the frequency of α-waves in the electroencephalogram and the increase in finger tremor and respiratory rate correlated best with the perceived anxiety of the subjects.

But what about anxiety and fear in animals? If one assumes that fear is ... "an emotional reaction to the recognition or the recognition of a perceived threat, regardless of whether that risk is also a given objective" is considered (Tembrock 2000) and that animals in an aversive environment or threatening situations show similar physiological symptoms as people, it can be expected that at least highly developed animals due to physiological and ethological homologies can feel anxiety or fear (Silverman 1978).

We are aware that anxiety and fear are human emotions. However, to ease reading also in relation to animals we speak of fear, anxious and less anxious behaviour.

A distinction between pathological and "normal" anxiety is difficult. If, however, continued intense fear without real danger and threat perception occurs, or the fear response is "unreasonable" compared to the sources of threats, they get disease value.

Anxiety disorders are among the most common mental disorders. Up to 15% of all people suffer during their life from an anxiety disorder (lifetime prevalence) (Kessler et al. 2010).

Treatment of anxiety disorders and consequences of the disease cause high costs and are connected with severe social problems (Wittchen and Jacobi 2005). One in four patients with generalized anxiety disorder is not in a position to meet its daily life requirements (Becker and Hoyer 2000). The course of anxiety disorders without adequate treatment is chronic recurrent and a spontaneous remission was found in only about 14% of the patients (Wittchen 1991).

4. Pharmacotherapy of anxiety disorders

A rational pharmacotherapy with anxiolytics is the basis for successful treatment of anxiety disorders, often combined with psychotherapy (Bandelow et al. 2005). In general, the drug therapy lasts for at least 12 months.

In the search for effective anxiolytic agents, chlordiazepoxide was synthesized in 1957 as the first benzodiazepine by Sternberg. The benzodiazepines, such as chlordiazepoxide and diazepam, were the first primary anti-anxiety agents. Until the mid-90s benzodiazepines were the most commonly prescribed anxiolytics. Despite known sedative effects and addictive potential, they are safe drugs for the short-term treatment of anxiety (Lader 2005).

During the last decade, a fundamental change has taken place in the pharmacotherapy of anxiety disorders.

Nowadays, benzodiazepines, which are still the primary acute intervention in panic disorder or drugs of second choice or for an interim treatment in generalized anxiety disorder and social phobias, are prescribed less often (Lohse et al. 2004). At present, mainly drugs that affect the serotonergic system, such as buspirone, SSRIs or NSMRI, are recommended as first choice (Bandelow, Zohar et al. 2005) (Table 1).

Anxiety Disorders	Recommended pharmacotherapy
Panic disorder	acute: benzodiazepines chronic: non-selective monoamine reuptake inhibitors (NSMRI), SSRI
Generalized anxiety disorder	SSRI, NSMRI, selective 5-HT-norepinephrine reuptake Inibitors (SSNRI), buspirone in treatment failure + start: benzodiazepines or opipramol
Social phobia	SSRI, moclobemide in treatment failure + to start: benzodiazepines
Obsessive compulsive disorder	NSMRI, SSRIs, in treatment failure: combination with neuroleptics

Table 1. Summary of drugs that are recommended for the treatment of anxiety and compulsive disorders by the Drug Commission of the German Medical Association and the German Society for Psychiatry, Psychotherapy and Neurology.

In Germany, phytotherapeutics, prescribed or self-prescribed by the patients, are used widely although there is no evidence-based proof of efficacy in anxiety disorders (Kinrys et al. 2009). A special role had preparations kava-kava herbal products (Piper methysticum). The use of kava-kava and similar "natural remedy" in the industrialized countries increased strongly. In some clinical studies, the substance proved to be similarly effective as benzodiazepines with very few adverse drug reactions (Witte et al. 2005). In higher doses, kava-kava has also sedative and hypnotic effects.

5. Neurotransmitter systems and anxiety

Since the discovery of the mode of action of benzodiazepines late 70s (Möhler and Okada 1977), γ-aminobutyric acid (GABA) is most frequently associated with anxiety disorders and their pharmacotherapy. Benzodiazepines augment the GABAergic inhibition via GABA-A receptors (Rudolph et al. 2001). Inverse agonists at the binding site for benzodiazepines, such as the beta-carboline-3-carboxylic acid N-methylamide, have anxiety-causing effects (Moriarty 1995).

In addition to GABA, 5-HT plays an important role in the development and the persistence of anxiety disorders (Griebel 1995). Studies show that patients with anxiety disorders may have genetic polymorphisms in the 5-HT transporter (Overview: (Lesch and Gutknecht 2005) or in the 5-HT2A receptor (Golimbet et al. 2004) and the 5-HT1A receptor (Gordon and Hen 2004). In patients with panic disorder the number of 5-HT1A receptors in the limbic system was shown to be reduced (Neumeister et al. 2004). Preclinical evidence also points towards an involvement of 5-HT3 receptors in the regulation of anxiety (Costall and Naylor 1992; Rex, Bert et al. 2007), but clinical efficacy is still uncertain (Adell 2010).

First indications of a link between 5-HT and anxiety-related behaviour resulted from the observation that methysergide and metergoline, later on known as 5-HT antagonists, had an anxiolytic effect in animal studies (Robichaud and Sledge 1969). The same anxiolytic effect was seen following inhibition of 5-HT synthesis by para-chlorophenylalanine in rats in the

Geller-Seifter test. This conflict-reducing effect was prevented by treatment with 5-hydxroxytryptophan (5-HTP), the precursor of 5-HT (Geller and Blum 1970). Therefore, it was expected that an increased activity of the central serotonergic system would be connected with anxiety and vice versa reduced activity with declined anxiety (Iversen 1984). Several studies have shown that an increase in 5-HT concentration in the brain increased anxiety and a reduction of 5-HT level reduces anxiety.

Other neurotransmitters that affect fear-related behaviour include the neuropeptide cholecystokinin (CCK), neuropeptide S, adenosine, excitatory amino acids and angiotensin. While the fear-producing effect of cholecystokinin is firm, the role of other neurotransmitters/-modulators for the development of anxiety, however, is not sufficiently understood.

CCK,, one of the best characterized neuropeptides, was, like 5-HT, discovered originally in the digestive tract and found later in the CNS (Vanderhaeghen et al. 1975). Two major receptor types were discovered: CCK2 and CCK1 receptors in the brain, whereas in the periphery almost exclusively CCK1 receptors occur (Beinfeld et al. 1981).

The CCK2 receptor is involved in the regulation of fear-related behaviours in humans and animals (Fink et al. 1998). In patients with a history of panic disorder and in healthy volunteers panic attacks could be triggered by a CCK-4 injection (De Montigny 1989; Bradwejn and Koszycki 2001).

Adenosine is also involved in the regulation of anxiety-related behaviour. High doses of the nonselective adenosine receptor antagonist caffeine induce fear in healthy people (Nehlig et al. 1992) and trigger panic attacks in patients with known anxiety disorder (Charney et al. 1985). Rats treated with caffeine, were more anxious in the elevated plus-maze test (X-maze) (Kayir and Uzbay 2005) and a free exploratory paradigm (Bert et al. 2011), while an adenosine-1 agonist had an anxiolytic effect in the X-maze (Florio et al. 1998).

For long the renin-angiotensin system has been considered as a classical endocrine system, with main effects in the peripheral blood pressure regulation, before an independent renin-angiotensin system in the CNS was demonstrated (Fischer-Ferraro et al. 1971). In the CNS, angiotensinII (ATII) is acting as a neurotransmitter involved in the regulation of anxiety-related behaviour. In animal studies intraventricular administration of ATII caused anxiogenic (Braszko et al. 2003), but also anxiolytic (Holy and Wisniewski 2001) effects in the X-maze test. Both, angiotensin1-receptor (AT1) antagonists (Srinivasan et al. 2003) and AT2-receptor antagonists (Braszko, Kulakowska et al. 2003) and reduced ATII levels by ACE inhibitors reduce the fear in rats (Srinivasan, Suresh et al. 2003).

Although clinical reports point to an anxiety-reducing effects of ACE inhibitors and AT-receptor antagonists, there are no valid data in man available (Gard 2004).

6. Animal models of anxiety and animal anxiety tests

Anxiety tests in the clinic have the advantage that the volunteers may self-report their experiences. To trigger anxiety, the subjects receive either fear-inducing agents (caffeine, pentylenetetrazol, lactate infusions or CO_2 inhalation), or they undergo psychological tests in an aversive environment (Graeff et al. 2003).

If animals can experience fear (Tembrock 2000), it would be possible to observe behaviour and neurochemical changes similar to changes in humans.

Animal anxiety tests are necessary for the development and characterization of novel anxiolytics. A disadvantage of animal studies is that only indirect conclusions about the emotions involved are possible by observing the behaviour and physiological side effects.

6.1 Historical developments

There are many animal tests for anxiety available (File 1985; Lister 1990). These tests may be divided roughly into three groups:

1. Tests in which anxiety is induced chemically, such as the drug discrimination test (Lal and Emmett-Oglesby 1983); 2. Tests based on conditioned fear / aversion, as the conditioned-emotional-response test (Davis 1990), the Geller-Seifter test, or the bird-punished-drinking test (Geller 1960) and last but not least 3. unconditioned tests, inducing anxiety by a new aversive environment, leading to behavioural inhibition. The unconditioned tests of anxiety include the X-maze (Handley and Mithani 1984), the black and white box test (Crawley and Goodwin 1980), the modified open field test (Rex et al. 1998), the social interaction test (Cappell and Latane 1969; File and Pope 1974) and the free exploratory paradigm (Griebel et al. 1993).

In unconditioned tests a conflict situation is created for the animals and changes in the innate behaviour in this aversive situation are observed. Examples for innate behaviour of animals and inhibiting factors used are: natural exploratory behaviour and avoidance of aversive open spaces without protection, co-existing curiosity and fear reactions to the appearance of a stranger of their own species, or vocalisations during sudden isolation.

The animal anxiety tests have to be validated pharmacologically with drugs whose anxiolytic or anxiety-inducing effects are known, and biologically by the variation of test conditions and their impact on the animals' behaviour (File 1985).

Since it is assumed that the different animal anxiety tests detect various forms of anxiety, for the determination of drug effects on behaviour also various anxiety tests should be used (Hagan et al. 2000).

In humans and animals two fundamentally different forms of anxiety can be distinguished: short-term changes in the emotional state (state anxiety) and a personality trait representing enduring anxiety (trait anxiety) (Cattell and Scheier 1958). In humans state anxiety and trait anxiety are differentiated with the "State Trait Anxiety Inventory"(Spielberger 1972).

To our knowledge only the free exploration test, in which home cage leaving behaviour in a real home environment is used to measure trait anxiety in rodents.

6.2 Recent developments and improvements

Despite the use of benzodiazepines, antidepressants and 5-HT1A agonists in the pharmacotherapy of anxiety disorders, only about 40-70% of the patients reach a symptom-free state (remission) or symptomatic improvement (response) (Kjernisted and Bleau 2004). Remission rates with SSRIs are even lower than under the conventional benzodiazepines (Pollack 2004). Therefore for the treatment of anxiety disorders, novel drugs with a rapid onset and with a constant therapeutic effect, and with fewer adverse effects are needed.

Consequently, there is still a need for improved animal tests for anxiety, which are capable to predict the anxiolytic efficacy of a drug and to mirror different facets of anxiety related disorders (Iversen 1984).

In the 80s and 90s of the last century, tests for anxiety were directed towards the discovery of drugs acting at the GABA receptors, because benzodiazepines were the gold-standard in the pharmacotherapy of anxiety disorders (Stephens and Andrews 1991). In contrast to the reliable detection of effects of GABAergic drugs on anxiety-related behaviour, it appeared that the anxiety tests available gained insufficient information regarding cholecystokininergic or serotonergic influences on anxiety-related behaviour (Griebel 1995; Rodgers and Johnson 1995). In order to assess fear-related behaviours more comprehensively, new tests for anxiety were developed or established tests changed. Examples for this progress are the elevated zero maze test (Shepherd et al. 1994) and improvements of the open field test.

6.2.1 Modified open field test and its validation

The open field has been used since about 80 years to study the locomotor and exploratory activity in laboratory rodents (Hall 1934). It could be shown that the movement pattern of animals in the brightly lit open field depends on their anxiety. The duration and frequency of the stay of animals in the central region or the amount of thigmotaxis indicate the intensity of anxiety in the animals. In assessing the behaviour of animals in the open field it has to be taken into account that a complex behaviour, which is composed of anxiety-related behaviour, neophobia, exploration, motivation, habituation and spatial learning, is analyzed.

In pre-clinical testing easy and quick tests are needed, which in the ideal case, reduce the assessment of a complex behaviour to a "yes-no decision". We modified the open field test on the basis of existing tests (Britton and Britton 1981). In our test, hungry rats were placed in a brightly lit and unfamiliar open field, with a petri dish of the usual rat chow in the middle of the open field. The hungry animals had the conflict between food supply and the fear of an unknown and aversive environment that suppresses food intake. As a parameter of an anxiety- modifying effect, we determined the percentage of rats of a group, which began to feed in the open field and could simplify the test (Rex et al. 1996; Rex, Stephens et al. 1996).

The modified open field test has been validated behaviourally and pharmacologically (Rex, Voigt et al. 1998). A shorter fasting period results in a less frequent food intake in the open field, similar to the offer of unfamiliar food.

Variations in the illumination of the test arena also changed the incidence of feeding in the open field. Increased illumination prevented the food intake entirely, while a reduction of light intensity increased the proportion of rats that fed in the aversive open field (Rex et al. 1994). These findings are consistent with other studies of rat behaviour in an open, aversive environment, showing that rats in a dimly lit open field had more social interactions than in a brightly lit open field (File and Hyde 1978; Rex et al. 2004).

We were able to show in this simple animal test not only the known anxiolytic effects of GABA agonists, such as diazepam and the β-carboline abecarnil (Rex, Stephens et al. 1996), but also the dose-related anxiety-reducing effects of 5-HT1A agonists, 5-HT2A antagonists and 5-HT3A antagonists. Hypnotics, antipsychotics such as haloperidol and stimulants such as amphetamine, without fear-reducing effect, did not increase the incidence of feeding in the open field (Rex, Voigt et al. 1998). To exclude false positive or false negative results locomotor activity and substance-related effects on food intake were also determined (Rex, Voigt et al. 1998).

6.2.2 Risk assessment in the X-maze

Often, serotonergic drugs fail to change traditional parameters of anxiety-related behaviour (De Vry 1995; Griebel 1995). However, the risk assessment behaviour of animals treated with serotonergic drugs differed from the behaviour of the controls. Therefore, in addition to developing new anxiety tests, a more detailed analysis and precise description of the behaviour in the commonly used tests was suggested. The determination of the risk behaviour of rats and mice in the X-maze is now common in the assessment of anxiety-related behaviour (Rodgers et al. 1997). We observed that guinea pigs after placement on the X-maze remained motionless in the centre of the test apparatus ("freezing"). The duration of freezing was shortened by anxiolytics such as diazepam, the 5-HT1A agonist 8-OH-DPAT or the CCK2-receptor antagonist L365, 260 and significantly prolonged by fear-inducing substances, such as CCK-4 (Rex et al. 1994). Similar findings were observed in rats. Rats of a more anxious strain showed a longer freezing-period compared with a less anxious strain (Rex et al. 1999).

6.2.3 Variation of pre-test and test procedures

The widespread use of unconditioned tests (Lister 1990) also led to varying results across different laboratories, caused by various reasons.

Variations in the construction of the experimental apparatus, for example, can affect the explorative activity of the animals. These variations include the mechanical stability of the entire experimental apparatus (Jones et al. 2002), the use of different materials of the walls of the open fields (Ohl and Keck 2003) or the use of opaque or translucent wall materials for the closed arms of X-maze (Anseloni and Brandao 1997).

Similar effects have variations in the handling and husbandry of animals before and during the test, which can alter both the spontaneous behaviour and sensitivity to anxiety-modulating drugs. Examples include: repeated "handling" (Andrews and File 1993), stress factors in the environment (also in the animal unit) (Haller and Halasz 1999), light conditions in the animal unit and in the test arena, social stress or isolation (Rodgers and Cole 1993) or test-experience of the animals (Hagan, Harper et al. 2000).

We could show that the rearing conditions in rats have an impact on the fear-related behaviour of the animals. It appears that rats that were reared either single housed or in groups, differed in anxiety-related behaviour. Animals reared in social isolation, behaved much more fearless on the X-maze (Marsden et al. 1995).

For the above reasons, a pharmacological and a behavioural validation is needed to compare own results with those in the literature. As an example for our laboratory, we established and validated the social interaction test in rats.

6.2.4 Validation of the social interaction test

The social interaction test, based on the open field test, was developed by (Cappell and Latane 1969) and validated throughout (File, 1978). When two rats, unknown to each other, are placed in a test arena, there will be contacts between the two animals. The time and frequency of individual forms of active social interaction during the tests are measured. In the aversive environment of a brightly lit open field contacts between the two animals are less frequent than in a non aversive environment (File 1985). Benzodiazepines stimulate the interaction between the two rats under aversive conditions (File and Hyde 1978). The use of non-GABAergic drugs led to conflicting results (De Vry 1995; Griebel 1995).

To assess the influence of organismic test variations on the fear-related behaviour, we tested a generally more anxious rat strain (Wistar [Wist: Shoe] Dimed Schönwalde GmbH, Germany) and a less anxious rat strain (Sprague Dawley [SD: Shoe], Dimed Schönwalde GmbH, Germany). We found that the duration of individual housing before the test and the associated social deprivation, had a significant influence on the duration and frequency of social contacts. Without a previous isolation we observed little interest in the other animal (Rex, Voigt et al. 2004).

Reduction of the aversive nature of the test arena by lower illumination or by a previous habituation to the test arena led to increased social interaction and confirmed the results of (File and Hyde 1978). Here, the change of behaviour of the more anxious Wistar rats was more pronounced. Diazepam increased social contacts only in the more anxious Wistar rats (Rex, Voigt et al. 2004). The well-known anxiogenic mCPP decreased the number and duration of mutual contacts in both rat strains (Rex, Voigt et al. 2004).

6.3 Impact of strain differences

Considering the widespread use of rodents in behavioural experiments, strain differences and their impact on the findings in the assessment and comparison of results with the available literature have to be considered. Genetic differences between individual strains or substrains in rodents may produce conflicting results and lead to misinterpretation of results (Jax 2003).

It is known that the fear-related behaviour differs between various strains of rats or mice (e.g. Trullas and Skolnick 1993; Rex, Sondern et al. 1996).

During the validation of the social interaction test, we observed that anxious Wistar rats and less anxious Sprague Dawley rats differed in the severity of behavioural changes after modifications of the test (Rex, Voigt et al. 2004). It was not known to what extend these behavioural differences were genetic determined or caused by environmental conditions during breeding and animal keeping. To determine the influence of breeding, husbandry and genetic conditions on the anxiety-related behaviour, we examined the anxiety-related behaviour of inbred and outbred rats under identical and different breeding and housing conditions.

6.3.1 Inbred laboratory rodents

We compared the fear-related behaviour of inbred Fischer 344 rats supplied by two national breeders (Charles River Laboratories Inc., Germany and Harlan-Winkelmann Ltd, Germany) and from a regional vendor (Dimed Schönwalde GmbH, Germany). Because of their extensive homocygosity inbred animals should show a small variation in behaviour. In the analysis of the anxiety-related behaviour in the X-maze, black and white box and the modified open field we found small but significant differences in anxiety-related behaviour between animals from different breeders (Bert et al. 2001).

In a second set of experiments we obtained pregnant Fischer 344 rats from the three above-mentioned vendors. The F1 generations were reared in our animal house. Interestingly, the F1 generation showed despite identical housing conditions behavioural differences between the stocks and strains (Bert, Fink et al. 2001).These differences in anxiety-related behaviour seem to be primarily innate. It is possible that a long term breeding of the rats with original genetic uniformity at different places led to the formation of substrains (Jax 2003).

6.3.2 Outbred laboratory rodents

In behavioural pharmacology experiments outbred rats, like Wistar rats or Sprague Dawley rats, are used more often. Outbred rats with their greater genetic diversity are thought to reflect the genetic diversity of the human population. We observed significant differences in anxiety-related behaviour between different outbred rat strains. These behavioural differences were detected in several unconditioned anxiety tests and are therefore not attributable to a specific test stimulus (Rex, Sondern et al. 1996). Interestingly, behavioural differences between different stocks of one strain and the behavioural differences between strains were similar (Rex, Sondern et al. 1996; Bert, Fink et al. 2001). Even when pregnant rats from different breeders were obtained and the F1 generation was raised under the same conditions, the F1 generation showed similar differences in anxiety-related behaviour.

This confirms again, that behavioural differences between the rat strains can be caused primarily by genetic differences (Rex, Sondern et al. 1996; Rex, Voigt et al. 1999; Rex et al. 2007).

In a second approach, we examined the fear-related behaviour of two lines of Sprague Dawley rats with common origin. 20 years ago the Institute of Cytology and Genetics in Novosibirsk (Russia) started breeding Sprague-Dawley (SD) rats obtained from Charles River Sulzfeld, Germany. To best knowledge, there were no further deliveries from Charles River to Novosibirsk (communication with Dr. J. Geller, CEO Charles River Germany). Examination of the anxiety-related behaviour and neurochemical experiments using both stocks revealed differences in their exploratory and anxiety-related behaviour, in habituation and learning, physical development, and serotonergic neurotransmission. Therefore, rats of the same stock but obtained from different breeders should be used with caution in research involving these measures (Rex, Kolbasenko et al. 2007).

Intentionally selectively bred sublines of rat strains have be used for more than 40 years. The selective breeding includes lines of rat strains, which differ significantly in anxiety-related behaviour, such as the HAB / LAB (high anxiety-related behaviour / low anxiety-related behaviour) rats (Liebsch et al. 1998) or the Maudsley (reactive / nonreactive) rat lines (Broadhurst 1975).

Since each of the selectively bred lines start from one common rat strain, there should be only minor genetic differences between the lines, causing the change in behaviour in anxiety tests (Landgraf 2003). Genetic and pharmacological investigations of these rat lines may contribute to the elucidation of the neurobiological basis of fear and anxiety disorders.

However, it has to be taken into account, that a complex emotion like fear has a polygenic base.

7. Combination of anxiety tests with neurochemical analysis

7.1 Brain microdialysis

The microdialysis as an in vivo sampling technique allows to gain a sterile and protein-free dialysate from one or more limited regions of the brain and subsequently to analyze changes in the levels of substances in the extracellular fluid in vivo in anesthetized and in awake animals over time.

Introduction of brain microdialysis in awake animals represented a major advance, since substance effects in anesthetized and in awake animals may differ dramatically (Boix et al. 1992; Boix et al. 1993).

Together with the group of C.A. Marsden at the University of Nottingham, U.K. we established the method of microdialysis in an awake animal during a behavioural experiment (Rex et al. 1991; Marsden, Beckett et al. 1995). This made it possible to detect changes in the release of neurotransmitters associated to drug administration and behavioural changes. Accompanying experiments in the open field (Cadogan et al. 1994) and on the X-maze (Rex et al. 2003) ensured that the implanted microdialysis probe with the attached tubings does not change the natural behaviour of animals.

The microdialysis has been used in animal anxiety tests such as the X-maze (Rex, Marsden et al. 1991; Rex et al. 1993; Voigt et al. 1999), social interaction test (Cadogan, Kendall et al. 1994), and the Vogel-test (Matsuo et al. 1996). For our studies, the microdialysis probes were implanted into brain regions involved in the regulation of anxiety-related behaviour, such as the prefrontal cortex or the hippocampus (Rex et al. 2008).

7.2 Brain serotonin concentrations

Although the relationship between anxiety and the central serotonergic transmission system is not simple, it can be assumed that changes in the activity of the serotonergic transmission system may lead to a change in the anxiety-related behaviour as well as in brain 5-HT concentration. Therefore, we investigated the relationship between anxiety-related behaviour and 5-HT concentrations in brain regions, which are involved in the regulation of anxiety-related behaviour, such as the prefrontal cortex, the ventral hippocampus and the raphe nuclei. Both, intracellular stored 5-HT and the released, extracellular located, 5-HT are measured. In general, after release into the synaptic cleft 5-HT is transported back into the presynaptic terminal by the 5-HT transporter and metabolized mainly to 5-hydroxyindole aceticacid (5-HIAA), which also can be determined. Changes in the ratio of 5-HT and 5-HIAA in the tissue indicate functional changes in central serotonergic transmission system.

8. Anxiety and serotonin

8.1 Traditional concept of anxiety and serotonin

25 years ago, the role of the central serotonergic transmission system in the regulation of anxiety-related behaviour could be summarized as follows: An increased availability of 5-HT or stimulation of postsynaptic 5-HT receptors is associated with anxiety. A reduced availability or release of 5-HT or blockade of postsynaptic 5-HT receptors triggers an anxiolysis (Iversen 1984). Earlier studies in panic disorder patients with elevated 5-HT plasma levels supported the 5-HT hypothesis of anxiety disorders (Giannini et al. 1983).

Contrary to this paradigm, in animals a local application of 5-HT into the dorsal raphe nucleus had anxiety-reducing effects. In own studies, destruction of serotonergic neurons in the raphe nuclei by the neurotoxin 5.7-DHT reduced 5-HT tissue levels without changing the anxiety-related behaviour (Rex, Thomas et al. 2003).

These results indicate that the relationship between anxiety-related behaviour and central serotonergic transmission system is not as clear as originally described by Iversen (Iversen 1984).

8.2 Strain differences in anxiety and central serotonin

If there is a connection between anxiety-related behaviour and the 5-HT concentration in the CNS, it should be possible that rat strains that differ in their anxiety-related behaviour also differ in the 5-HT concentration in the brain, too. In rats of different strains (Rex, Sondern et al. 1996), the 5-HT levels in brain tissue were determined. It could be shown that rats with a more anxious behaviour had increased 5-HT levels in projection areas of the central serotonergic transmission system (Bert, Fink et al. 2001; Rex, Voigt et al. 1999 ; Rex, Voigt et al. 2004).

8.3 Anxiogenic drugs and serotonin release
8.3.1 SSRIs
The 5-HT-releasing drug fenfluramine increases 5-HT concentration in the rat cortex substantially (Thomas et al. 2000) and leads to a more anxious behaviour on the X-maze (File and Guardiola-Lemaitre 1988).

The acute administration of NSMRIs or SSRIs, which increase 5-HT levels in the synaptic cleft leads to a more fearful behaviour in rats on the X-maze (Bagdy et al. 2001). This fear-enhancing effect of SSRIs is also observed in humans (Stahl 1998). It is particularly pronounced at the beginning of therapy (Gunnell et al. 2005) and generally it declines within two to three weeks.

8.3.2 CCK-receptor agonists
As described, CCK2-receptor ligands are also involved in the regulation of anxiety-related behaviour (Crawley and Corwin 1994; Fink, Rex et al. 1998). We have shown that the CCK2-receptor agonist CCK-4 induced in rats and guinea pigs a clear anxious behaviour on the X-maze, in the modified open field, in the black and white box and ultrasonic vocalisation test (Rex, Barth et al. 1994; Fink, Rex et al. 1998). Since both, CCK and 5-HT, affect the anxiety-related behaviour, an interaction between the two neurotransmitter systems was suggested. In the modified open field test we could show that the 5-HT1A agonist 8-OH-DPAT reduced as an anxiolytic and consequently as a "functional antagonist" dose-dependently the anxiogenic effect of CCK-4 (Rex et al. 1996).

During exposure to the X-maze, CCK-4 increased the release of 5-HT up to threefold (but not in home cage), whereas administration of the CCK1-receptor agonist A71738 and the non-selective CCK1/2-receptor agonist CCK-8s, did not affect the fear-related behaviour nor did change the 5-HT release compared to control animals (Rex and Fink 1998). The anxiogenic effect of CCK-4 in tests for anxiety could be antagonized by the selective CCK2-receptor antagonist L365,260 (Rex et al. 1993; Rex and Fink 1998). We could show an anxiolytic-like effect of L365,260 that abolished not only the effects of CCK2-receptor agonists, but had even own anxiety-reducing effects in animal anxiety tests (Hughes et al. 1990; Fink, Rex et al. 1998).

Our results can be summarized as follows: CCK-4 affected the function of central serotonergic transmission system only slightly or not at rest, but stimulated during acute fear the release of 5-HT in the cortex and hippocampus.

8.4 Arousal and serotonin release
There is general agreement that aversion, based on animal models of anxiety in animals leads to activation in the limbic system and cortex (arousal reaction). So far, it is uncertain whether the increased release of 5-HT during the test for anxiety is caused by anxiety or by the arousal reaction.

Besides the results of various in vivo microdialysis experiments that confirm our hypothesis of an involvement of central serotonergic system in anxiety-related behaviour (Wright et al. 1992; Rex, Marsden et al. 1993; Matsuo, Kataoka et al. 1996; Rex, Voigt et al. 1999; Rex, Voigt et al. 2004), other studies suggested a link between stress-related hyperactivity of rats and the increased release of 5-HT in projection areas (Linthorst et al. 2002).

We could show that the mild stressor "white noise" (Buller et al. 2003), did not increase hippocampal 5-HT release in anxious rats, although the rats were highly active during exposure to white noise (Rex et al. 2005). Comparing our results with other findings in which increased 5-HT release was found during a forced stay in an inescapable stressful situation, like the forced swim test, we think that these situations most likely cause fear in this animals. This is supported by the results of Linthorst and colleagues who interpret an extremely increased 5-HT release in some animals as an anxiety / panic-stimulated release (Linthorst, Penalva et al. 2002).

It was also assumed by others that the increased release of 5-HT during the stay on the X-maze (Rex, Marsden et al. 1993), in the aversive open field (Cadogan, Kendall et al. 1994) or during the forced swim test (Linthorst, Penalva et al. 2002) is caused not by fear but just by exposure to a new unfamiliar environment per se. To check whether a new, but not aversive environment also causes an increased release of 5-HT, we performed microdialysis studies with anxious rats in a non-aversive version of the X-maze. By closing the open arms the remaining arms represented with their high walls rather a protective environment for the animals. The initial stay of the animals in the modified X-maze did not increase 5-HT release, although the animals actively explored the new environment (Rex, Voigt et al. 2005).

Another argument for an anxiety-related increased 5-HT release in hippocampus and cortex emerged from studies in which behavioural strain differences have been analyzed. In several microdialysis studies, we could measure an increased release of 5-HT during the stay on the X-maze only in anxious rat strains. In rats with a non-anxious behaviour, the release of 5-HT in the X-maze test under the same conditions was not increased as much (Rex, Voigt et al. 1999; Rex, Voigt et al. 2004).

Together, our results suggest that acute fear increases the extracellular 5-HT concentration in the serotonergic projection areas and there is a connection between the amount of released 5-HT and the anxiety of the animals.

9. Anxiolysis and serotonin

9.1 Role of 5-HT1A, 5-HT1B/1D receptors

The release of 5-HT is regulated by presynaptic somatodendritic 5-HT1A receptors and presynaptic 5-HT1B/1D receptors at the nerve endings of serotonergic neurons (De Vry 1995).

The functional significance of postsynaptic 5-HT1A receptors and 5-HT1B/1D receptors is still not completely clarified (Göthert and Schlicker 1997). Differentiation of effects mediated by pre-or postsynaptic receptors with the existing substances is difficult. While a stimulation of presynaptic 5-HT1A receptors and 5-HT1D receptors by agonists reduces 5-HT release in the projection areas (Rex, Fink et al. 1993; De Vry 1995; Rex et al. 1997) antagonists at the 5-HT1A and 5-HT1D receptors do not always induce an increase of 5-HT release (Roberts et al. 1999), as 5-HT is released tonically only to a small extent.

Also own microdialysis studies showed that blockade of autoreceptors without previous stimulation of 5-HT release had no measurable effect. If guinea pigs stayed in the familiar cage, neither the selective 5-HT1A antagonist WAY 100635 nor the 5-HT1B/1D-Antagonist GR 127 935, changed release of 5-HT in the ventral hippocampus and the prefrontal cortex (Rex et al. 1996; Rex, Voigt et al. 2008).

Whereas in the resting state the tonic 5-HT release and therefore the effects of antagonists on 5-HT1A and 5-HT1B/D receptors are small, in an aversive environment, such as the X-maze the release of 5-HT was stimulated. Treatment with the 5-HT1B/1D-antagonist GR 127935 led to a quicker but short-lasting increase in extracellular 5-HT concentration in the cortex, compared to treatment with saline (Rex, Fink et al. 1996).

In other studies in which a drug-induced increased extracellular 5-HT concentration was examined, the regulatory function of 5-HT1A and 5-HT1D receptors could be shown more clearly. If pre-treatment with a SSRI increased the 5-HT concentration in the synaptic cleft, both, 5-HT1A antagonists(Hughes et al. 2005), as well 5-HT1B/1D-antagonists had a potentiating effect on 5-HT release in the CNS. These results suggest that control of the firing rate of serotonergic neurons and thus of transmitter release by presynaptic 5-HT1A- and 5-HT1B/1D-receptors is pronounced when 5-HT release is stimulated.

5-HT1A agonists such as buspirone and tandospirone are used in the treatment of anxiety disorders. Their anxiety-reducing effect is explained by stimulation of presynaptic 5-HT1A receptors and the subsequent reduction in 5-HT release (Stahl 1998).

However, the role of postsynaptic 5-HT1A receptors for an anxiolytic effect is still not clear. So we used a neurobiochemical approach to try to discriminate the function of presynaptic and postsynaptic 5-HT1A receptors in vivo.

9.2 5-HT1A receptors and brain metabolic activity

It is known that the energy metabolism in the CNS is linked closely to the activity of the cells. Determination of the redox status of cells allows conclusions about the functional state of these cells (Ames 2000). Complementary to established methods, the laser-induced fluorescence spectroscopy offers the possibility of "on line" - measurements of the metabolic state of intact tissues.

After verification that in vivo laser-induced fluorescence spectroscopy detects changes in mitochondrial/metabolic activity in the CNS, we determined the mitochondrial activity in the ventral hippocampus after administration of the 5-HT1A agonist 8-OH-DPAT (Rex and Fink 2006).

Systemic administration of 8-OH-DPAT induced dose-dependent changes in mitochondrial activity of hippocampal neurons. In the highest dose 8-OH-DPAT significantly increased the NADH fluorescence, while the middle dose had no effect on NADH fluorescence and the lowest dose resulted in a slight but not significant increase in NADH fluorescence.

We interpret the results as follows: The highest dose of 8-OH-DPAT stimulates postsynaptic 5-HT1A receptors in the ventral hippocampus and thus inhibiting the activity of the following neurons, leading to an increase in NADH fluorescence. Our conclusions are sustained by electrophysiological studies, in which higher doses of 8-OH-DPAT lowered activity in the hippocampus and cortex (Tada et al. 1999).

Since 8-OH-DPAT has in behavioural tests an anxiety-reducing effect in doses that affect the postsynaptic 5-HT1A receptors it cannot be excluded that the postsynaptic 5-HT1A receptors play a role in the regulation of anxiety-related behaviour.

10. Anxiolytic drugs and serotonin

It was shown that aversive stimuli and substances with an anxiety-enhancing effect increase the 5-HT release in some serotonergic projection areas, such as the ventral hippocampus and the prefrontal cortex. Therefore, we investigated whether anxiolytics of different drug classes inhibit 5-HT release in general.

10.1 Different classes of anxiolytic drugs and serotonin release

Benzodiazepines and 5-HT1A agonists are therapeutically used anxiolytics. CCK2 antagonists were effective in various animal anxiety models, such as the X-maze (Rex, Barth et al. 1994), the modified open field (Rex, Voigt et al. 1998), social interaction and the elevated zero maze (Revel et al. 1998). Therefore, we investigated the effects of diazepam (Rex, Marsden et al. 1993; Rex et al. 1993a), 8-OH-DPAT (Rex et al. 1993) and the CCK2 antagonist L 365.260 (Rex, Fink et al. 1994) on 5-HT release in the prefrontal cortex using microdialysis during the X-maze test.

As shown before, exposure to the X-maze resulted always in a marked increased 5-HT release (Rex, Marsden et al. 1991; Marsden, Beckett et al. 1995). Pretreatment with diazepam or 8-OH-DPAT or L 365.260 reduced this aversion induced increase in 5-HT release in the prefrontal cortex and caused a less anxious behaviour of the animals on the X-maze.

Under non-aversive conditions, like before and after exposure to the X-maze, diazepam, 8-OH-DPAT and L 365.260 decreased basal 5-HT release in the prefrontal cortex.

Both the reduction in the aversion induced 5-HT release and the anxiolytic effects of diazepam, 8-OH-DPAT and L 365.260 were antagonized by pretreatment with the benzodiazepine antagonist flumazenil, the non-selective 5-HT1 antagonist methiothepine and the selective CCK2-receptor agonist CCK-4, respectively (Rex, Fink et al. 1993; Rex, Marsden et al. 1993; Rex, Marsden et al. 1993).

Our results indicate a receptor mediation of the observed effects and they are consistent with the hypothesis that an acute stay in an aversive environment is associated with increased 5-HT release and an anxiolytic effect with a decreased release of 5-HT. The results are supported by in vitro studies showing that both, diazepam and the 5-HT1A agonist buspirone as well as the CCK2 antagonist GV 150 013, decreased the electrically stimulated release of 5-HT from cortical slices significantly (Siniscalchi et al. 2001).

10.2 Benzodiazepines and serotonin concentrations

Already in the 70s it has been shown that benzodiazepines reduce 5-HT synthesis (Dominic et al. 1975) and the 5-HT turnover (Wise et al. 1972).

After systemic administration chlordiazepoxide inhibited the firing rate of serotonergic neurons in the dorsal raphe nucleus (Trulson et al. 1982) and after injection into the dorsal raphe chlordiazepoxide reduced anxious behaviour in the conditioned-emotional-response test (Thiebot et al. 1980).

The dorsal and median raphe nuclei have a high density of GABA receptors. Microinjections of GABA in the dorsal raphe nucleus and in serotonergic projection areas, such as the amygdala and the hippocampus, reduced the firing rate of serotonergic neurons. This reduced firing rate was reduced even further by administration of benzodiazepines (Gallager 1978). On the other hand, the anxiety-reducing effect of benzodiazepines in a conflict test was abolished by the intraventricular administration of 5-HT (Wise, Berger et al. 1972).

We have seen "antiserotonergic" effects of diazepam on both the tissue concentration as well as the 5-HT release (Rex, Marsden et al. 1993; Bert, Fink et al. 2001). In the rat brain diazepam reduced tissue concentrations of 5-HT in serotonergic projection areas, such as cortex and hippocampus which confirmed the results of Pei and colleagues (Pei et al. 1989). Interestingly, diazepam had a greater effect in animals with high tissue concentrations of 5-HT, while the effect was smaller in animals with low 5-HT levels.

In a Wistar rat strain (HsdCpb: WU, Harlan, Germany), which showed a non-anxious behaviour in different anxiety tests, diazepam reduced the already low 5-HT levels in hippocampus and cortex only marginally and did not change the anxiety-related behaviour. In these non-anxious rats exposure to the X-maze did not increase 5-HT release in the hippocampus (Rex, Voigt et al. 1999).

In the more anxious Wistar rats (Han: Wist (SYN WI), Institute for Risk Assessment, Germany) and Fischer rats (F344/NHsd, Harlan, Germany) with higher 5-HT concentrations in the tissue and aversion-induced release of 5-HT on the X-maze (Rex, Voigt et al. 1999), diazepam induced an anxiolytic-like behaviour on the X-maze and reduced the concentration of 5-HT in the hippocampus and frontal cortex significantly (Bert, Fink et al. 2001).

Since similar doses of diazepam in rat strains with different 5-HT concentrations in the brain have different effects on anxiety-related behaviour (Bert, Fink et al. 2001), it can be assumed that the effect of benzodiazepines depends of the activity of the serotonergic neurotransmission system and the GABAergic system interacts with the central serotonergic transmission system.

To further test the hypothesis of a close link between anxiolytic effects and a decreased release of 5-HT, we examined an anxiolytic effective herbal product.

10.3 Herbal anxiolytic kava-kava

The herbal product kava-kava had been widely used as an anxiolytic. Although kava pyrones have been identified as the pharmacologically active ingredients of kava-kava (Singh and Blumenthal 1997), the mechanism of action has not been clarified (Smith et al. 2001). The kava-kava pyrones bind probably not to the GABA-A receptors (Garrett et al. 2003). We examined the effects of kava-kava in the X-maze and the social interaction test. In both tests a standardized kava-kava preparation caused dose-dependent anxiety-reducing effect in rats, similar to the effect of diazepam (Rex et al. 2002). Our results were later confirmed in mice (Garrett, Basmadjian et al. 2003).

In a second experiment we determined the concentration of 5-HT in a tissue sample (punch), containing the dorsal and the medial raphe nucleus and in tissue samples of the ventral hippocampus and the prefrontal cortex. Kava-kava led to a reduction in 5-HT concentration in the cortex and hippocampus.

Since the tissue concentration is not related strongly to the release of 5-HT, we investigated the release of 5-HT in the ventral hippocampus following administration of kava-kava. Using in vivo microdialysis we showed for the first time that kava-kava, like 8-OH-DPAT and diazepam, decreased the 5-HT release in the projection areas.

11. Long term reduction of serotonin and anxiolysis

Under the premise that a correlation between the amount of tissue concentration of 5-HT and the expression of anxiety-related behaviour exists, it could be assumed that a reduction of 5-HT concentration in the CNS would be associated with anxiolysis. The 5-HT concentration in the brain can be reduced by destruction of serotonergic neurons for a long time.

Systemic para-chloroamphetamine reduced the 5-HT content in the CNS of rats and these animals showed an anxiolytic-like behaviour in the Geller-Seifter test (Geller and Blum 1970).

Intracerebral administration of the neurotoxin 5.7-DHT, causing destruction of serotonergic neurons, reduced the 5-HT content in the CNS and induced anxiolytic-like effects in conditioned anxiety tests (Iversen 1984; Soderpalm and Engel 1992; Thiebot, Jobert et al. 1980). These studies confirmed seemingly a simple relation between 5-HT and anxiety.

However, studies in which unconditioned tests were used and/or individual nuclei in the raphe region were lesioned, showed contradictory results. While 5.7-DHT reduces anxiety after intraventricular application (Griebel 1995), administration of the neurotoxin into either the median or the dorsal raphe nucleus had no effect on behaviour in several anxiety tests (Griebel 1995, Thomas et al 2000). Only in the social interaction test (File et al. 1979) a lesion of the dorsal raphe nucleus caused a less anxious behaviour of the animals.

In our studies, neither the lesion of the median raphe nucleus (Thomas, Fink et al. 2000) nor of the dorsal raphe nucleus (Rex, Thomas et al. 2003) alone changed the fear-related behaviour of the rats. The 5-HT levels in the projection areas, such as cortex and hippocampus were decreased significantly (Thomas, Fink et al. 2000; Rex, Thomas et al. 2003) and comparable to the effects of 5.7-DHT lesion on 5-HT concentrations in the CNS described in the literature (Tabatabaie and Dryhurst 1998).

For the first time not only the 5-HT levels in the tissue, but also the release of 5-HT in lesioned and non-lesioned rats in the familiar cage and during exposure to the X-maze were determined. Rats in which either the dorsal or the median raphe nucleus was lesioned by 5.7-DHT, differed in the tissue concentrations of 5-HT, but not in anxiety-related behaviour and in the aversion induced 5-HT release, compared to untreated control animals (Rex, Thomas et al. 2003).A reason, that the lesion of only one of the two major raphe nuclei did not relate to the aversion induced 5-HT release and the behaviour of animals, could lie in the overlapping innervations' of the hippocampus and the cortex by the dorsal raphe nucleus and the median raphe nucleus. The lesion of one of the raphe nuclei can be compensated by the innervations' of the other raphe nuclei, at least in part.

A lesion of almost all serotonergic neurons by intraventricular administration of 5.7-DHT (Griebel 1995) or simultaneous lesions of the dorsal and of the median raphe nuclei (Thomas, Fink et al. 2000), however, interrupt all serotonergic projections to the hippocampus. The 5-HT concentrations were reduced much more and there was no increased release of 5-HT observed during the exposure to the X-maze and the rats behaved "anxiety-free" on the X-maze. The destruction of serotonergic neurons in the raphe nuclei prevents storage of 5-HT in the nerve endings in the projection areas. Consequently, 5-HT is not released due to aversion and thus no anxious behaviour was induced.

The findings presented so far support the hypothesis that there is a relationship between decreased release of 5-HT and less anxious behaviour of animals.

We could also show that reduced 5-HT release does not necessarily change the anxiety-related behaviour. The non-selective 5-HT1 agonist 5-carboxamidotryptamine (5-CT) reduced the basal release of 5-HT and prevented the increased 5-HT release on the X-maze, similar to the 5-HT1A agonist 8-OH-DPAT. Nevertheless, we observed no change in anxiety-related behaviour compared to control animals after treatment with 5-CT (Rex, Fink et al. 1996).

At the present it can be generalized that anxiolytics reduce the release of 5-HT in the brain. However, a reduced concentration of 5-HT and reduced 5-HT release under resting conditions does not automatically lead to an anxiety-free behaviour of animals.

12. Conclusions

Similar to humans, anxiety-related behaviour in animals appears to be influenced by genetic factors and environmental conditions. Changes in housing and breeding conditions and/or variations in experimental conditions and the experimental procedure may change the behaviour of the animals profoundly. Strain differences have a strong influence on the anxiety-related behaviour in the animals. Additionally, separate maintaining and breeding of rodents over several generations may lead to the development of sublines with different anxiety-related behaviour.

Further developments of animal anxiety tests, the knowledge of their limits and the evaluation of additional ethological behavioural parameters can be used to detect changes in anxiety-related behaviour more accurately.

A correlation between the level of 5-HT concentration in the CNS and the anxiety of rat strains, but not general activation, could be proved experimentally. Anxious rats have higher tissue levels of 5-HT in projection areas of neurons originating in the median and the dorsal raphe nuclei as rat strains with "fearless" behaviour. Anxiolytics decrease extracellular 5-HT levels in the projection areas of the serotonergic neurons in the CNS, especially in more anxious rat strains.

Studies using in vivo microdialysis while performing tests for anxiety in awake and freely moving animals with permanently reduced 5-HT concentrations in specific brain regions showed that not only the absolute level of 5-HT concentration in the CNS, but also the amount of 5-HT released during an aversive situation, can be related to the behaviour of the animals.

Anxiolytics of different drug classes reduce the serotonin release during an aversive situation, whereas anxiety-causing substances increase the serotonin release under the same conditions significantly. However, a reduced release of serotonin does not always lead to fearless behaviour in rodents.

The central serotonergic transmission is also influenced by other neurotransmission systems, e. g. GABA and CCK systems..

In summary our results demonstrate the major role of the serotonergic neurotransmission in the regulation of anxiety-related behaviour. Studies on the role of the serotonergic system under aversive and non-aversive conditions may lead to a better understanding of the mechanisms involved in the development of anxiety disorders and the possible development of novel therapeutic approaches in the treatment of anxiety disorders, too.

13. References

Adell, A. (2010). Lu-AA21004, a multimodal serotonergic agent, for the potential treatment of depression and anxiety. IDrugs 13(12): 900-10.

Ames, A., 3rd (2000). CNS energy metabolism as related to function. Brain Res Brain Res Rev 34(1-2): 42-68.

Amin, A. H., Crawford, T. B.&Gaddum, J. H. (1954). The distribution of substance P and 5-hydroxytryptamine in the central nervous system of the dog. J Physiol 126(3): 596-618.

Andreatini, R.&Bacellar, L. F. (1999). The relationship between anxiety and depression in animal models: a study using the forced swimming test and elevated plus-maze. Braz J Med Biol Res 32(9): 1121-6.

Andrews, N.&File, S. E. (1993). Handling history of rats modifies behavioural effects of drugs in the elevated plus-maze test of anxiety. Eur J Pharmacol 235(1): 109-12.

Anseloni, V. Z.&Brandao, M. L. (1997). Ethopharmacological analysis of behaviour of rats using variations of the elevated plus-maze. Behav Pharmacol 8(6-7): 533-40.

Bagdy, G., Graf, M., Anheuer, Z. E., Modos, E. A.&Kantor, S. (2001). Anxiety-like effects induced by acute fluoxetine, sertraline or m-CPP treatment are reversed by pretreatment with the 5-HT2C receptor antagonist SB-242084 but not the 5-HT1A receptor antagonist WAY-100635. Int J Neuropsychopharmacol 4(4): 399-408.

Bandelow, B., Zohar, J.&Hollander, E. (2005). Medikamentöse Behandlung von Angst- und Zwangs- und posttraumatischen Belastungsstörungen. Frankfurt, Wissenschaftliche Verlagsgesellschaft.

Becker, E.&Hoyer, E. J. (2000). Das Generalisierte Angstsyndrom - Häufig nicht erkannt. DNP: 36-39.

Beinfeld, M. C., Meyer, D. K.&Brownstein, M. J. (1981). Cholecystokinin in the central nervous system. Peptides 2 Suppl.2: 77-79.

Bert, B., Fink, H., Sohr, R.&Rex, A. (2001). Different effects of diazepam in Fischer rats and two stocks of Wistar rats in tests of anxiety. Pharmacol Biochem Behav 70(2-3): 411-20.

Bert, B., Schmidt, N., Voigt, J. P., Fink, H.&Rex, A. (2011). Evaluation of cage leaving behaviour as a free choice paradigm Journal of Pharmacological and Toxicological Methods under revision.

Boix, F., Huston, J. P.&Schwarting, R. K. (1992). The C-terminal fragment of substance P enhances dopamine release in nucleus accumbens but not in neostriatum in freely moving rats. Brain Res 592(1-2): 181-6.

Boix, F., Mattioli, R., Adams, F., Huston, J. P.&Schwarting, R. K. (1993). Peripherally administered substance P affects extracellular dopamine concentrations in the neostriatum but not in the nucleus accumbens under anesthesia. Brain Res Bull 31(6): 655-60.

Bradwejn, J.&Koszycki, D. (2001). Cholecystokinin and panic disorder: past and future clinical research strategies. Scand J Clin Lab Invest Suppl 234: 19-27.

Braszko, J. J., Kulakowska, A.&Winnicka, M. M. (2003). Effects of angiotensin II and its receptor antagonists on motor activity and anxiety in rats. J Physiol Pharmacol 54(2): 271-81.

Britton, D. R.&Thatcher Britton, K. (1981). A sensitive openfield measure of anxiolytic drug activity. Pharmacol.Biochem.Behav. 15: 577-582.

Broadhurst, P. L. (1975). The Maudsley reactive and nonreactive strains of rats: a survey. Behav Genet 5(4): 299-319.

Buller, K. M., Crane, J. W., Spencer, S. J.&Day, T. A. (2003). Systemic apomorphine alters HPA axis responses to interleukin-1 beta administration but not sound stress. Psychoneuroendocrinology 28(6): 715-32.

Cadogan, A. K., Kendall, D. A., Fink, H.&Marsden, C. A. (1994). Social interaction increases 5-HT release and cAMP efflux in the rat ventral hippocampus in vivo. Behav Pharmacol 5(3): 299-305.

Cappell, H.&Latane, B. (1969). Effects of alcohol and caffeine on the social and emotional behavior of the rat. Q J Stud Alcohol 30(2): 345-56.

Cattell, R. B.&Scheier, I. H. (1958). The nature of anxiety: a review of thirteen multi-variate analyses comprising 814 variables. Psychol Rep 4(4): 351-388.

Charney, D. S., Heninger, G. R.&Jatlow, P. I. (1985). Increased anxiogenic effects of caffeine in panic disorders. Arch Gen Psychiatry 42(3): 233-43.

Costall, B.&Naylor, R. J. (1992). Astra Award Lecture. The psychopharmacology of 5-HT3 receptors. Pharmacol Toxicol 71(6): 401-15.

Crawley, J.&Goodwin, F. K. (1980). Preliminary report of a simple animal behavior model for the anxiolytic effects of benzodiazepines. Pharmacol Biochem Behav 13(2): 167-70.

Crawley, J. N.&Corwin, R. L. (1994). Biological actions of cholecystokinin. 15: 731-755.

Cryan, J. F.&Kaupmann, K. (2005). Don't worry 'B' happy!: a role for GABA(B) receptors in anxiety and depression. Trends Pharmacol Sci 26(1): 36-43.

Dahlstrom, A.&Fuxe, K. (1964). Localization of monoamines in the lower brain stem. Experientia 20(7): 398-9.

Davis, M. (1990). Animal models of anxiety based on classical conditioning: the conditioned emotional response (CER) and the fear-potentiated startle effect. Pharmacol Ther 47(2): 147-65.

De Montigny, C. (1989). Cholecystokinin tetrapeptide induces panic-like attacks in healthy volunteers. Archives of General Psychiatry 46: 511-517.

De Vry, J. (1995). 5-HT1A receptor agonists: recent developments and controversial issues. Psychopharmacology (Berl) 121(1): 1-26.

Dominic, J. A., Sinha, A. K.&Barchas, J. D. (1975). Effect of benzodiazepine compounds on brain amine metabolism. European Journal of Pharmacology 32: 124-127.

Falck, B., Hillarp, N. A., Thieme, G.&Torp, A. (1962). Fluorescence of catechol amines and related compounds condensed with formaldehyde. J Histochem Cytochem 10: 348-354.

File, S. E. (1985). Models of anxiety. Br.J.Clin.Pract.Symp.Suppl. 38: 15-20.

File, S. E.&Guardiola-Lemaitre, B. J. (1988). l-fenfluramine in tests of dominance and anxiety in the rat. Neuropsychobiology 20(4): 205-11.

File, S. E.&Hyde, J. R. (1978). Can social interaction be used to measure anxiety? British Journal of Pharmacology 62: 19-24.

File, S. E.&Pope, J. H. (1974). The action of chlorpromazine on exploration in pairs of rats. Psychopharmacologia 37(3): 249-54.

Fink, H., Rex, A., Voits, M.&Voigt, J. P. (1998). Major biological actions of CCK--a critical evaluation of research findings. Exp Brain Res 123(1-2): 77-83.

Fischer-Ferraro, C., Nahmod, V. E., Goldstein, D. J.&Finkielman, S. (1971). Angiotensin and renin in rat and dog brain. J Exp Med 133(2): 353-61.

Florio, C., Prezioso, A., Papaioannou, A.&Vertua, R. (1998). Adenosine A1 receptors modulate anxiety in CD1 mice. Psychopharmacology (Berl) 136(4): 311-9.

Gallager, D. W. (1978). Benzodiazepines: potentiation of a GABA inhibitory response in the dorsal raphe nucleus. European Journal of Pharmacology 49: 133-143.

Gard, P. R. (2004). Angiotensin as a target for the treatment of Alzheimer's disease, anxiety and depression. Expert Opin Ther Targets 8(1): 7-14.

Garrett, K. M., Basmadjian, G., Khan, I. A., Schaneberg, B. T.&Seale, T. W. (2003). Extracts of kava (Piper methysticum) induce acute anxiolytic-like behavioral changes in mice. Psychopharmacology (Berl) 170(1): 33-41.

Geller, I. (1960). The acquisition and extinction of conditioned suppression as a function of the base-line reinforcer. J Exp Anal Behav 3: 235-40.

Geller, I.&Blum, K. (1970). The effects of 5-HTP on para-Chlorophenylalanine (p-CPA) attenuation of conflict behavior. Eur J Pharmacol 9(3): 319-24.

Giannini, A. J., Castellani, S.&Dvoredsky, A. E. (1983). Anxiety states: relationship to atmospheric cations and serotonin. J Clin Psychiatry 44(7): 262-4.

Golimbet, V. E., Alfimova, M. V.&Mitiushina, N. G. (2004). Polymorphism of the serotonin 2A receptor gene (5HTR2A) and personality traits. Mol Biol 38(3): 404-12.

Gordon, J. A.&Hen, R. (2004). Genetic approaches to the study of anxiety. Annu Rev Neurosci 27: 193-222.

Göthert, M.&Schlicker, E. (1997). Regulation of 5-HT release in the CNS by presynaptic 5-HT autoreceptors and by 5-HT heteroreceptors. Serotoninergic Neurons and 5-HT Receptors in the CNS. H. G. Baumgarten &M. Göthert. Berlin Heidelberg New York, Springer. 129: 307-350.

Graeff, F. G., Parente, A., Del-Ben, C. M.&Guimaraes, F. S. (2003). Pharmacology of human experimental anxiety. Braz J Med Biol Res 36(4): 421-32.

Green, E. (1981). Genetics and Probability in Animal Breeding Experiments. New York, Oxford University Press.

Griebel, G. (1995). 5-Hydroxytryptamine-interacting drugs in animal models of anxiety disorders: more than 30 years of research. Pharmacol Ther 65(3): 319-95.

Griebel, G., Belzung, C., Misslin, R.&Vogel, E. (1993). The free-exploratory paradigm: an effective method for measuring neophobic behaviour in mice and testing potential neophobia-reducing drugs. Behav Pharmacol 4(6): 637-644.

Gunnell, D., Saperia, J.&Ashby, D. (2005). Selective serotonin reuptake inhibitors (SSRIs) and suicide in adults: meta-analysis of drug company data from placebo controlled, randomised controlled trials submitted to the MHRA's safety review. BMJ 330(7488): 385.

Hagan, J. J., Harper, A. J., Elliott, H., Jones, D. N.&Rogers, D. C. (2000). Practical and theoretical issues in gene-targeting studies and their application to behaviour. Rev Neurosci 11(1): 3-13.

Hall, C. S. (1934). Emotional behavior in the rat. I. Defecation and urination as measures of individual differences in emotionality. J. Comp. Psychol. 18: 385– 403.

Haller, J.&Halasz, J. (1999). Mild social stress abolishes the effects of isolation on anxiety and chlordiazepoxide reactivity. Psychopharmacology (Berl) 144(4): 311-5.

Handley, S. L.&Mithani, S. (1984). Effects of alpha-adrenoceptor agonists and antagonists in a maze- exploration model of 'fear'-motivated behaviour. Naunyn Schmiedebergs Archive of Pharmacology 327: 1-5.

Holy, Z.&Wisniewski, K. (2001). Examination of the influence of 3,5-DHPG on behavioral activity of angiotensin II. Pol J Pharmacol 53(3): 235-43.

Hughes, J., Boden, P., Costall, B., Domeney, A., Kelly, E., Horwell, D. C., Hunter, J. C., Pinnock, R. D.&Woodruff, G. N. (1990). Development of a class of selective cholecystokinin type B receptor antagonists having potent anxiolytic activity. Proc.Natl.Acad.Sci.U.S A. 87: 6728-6732.

Hughes, Z. A., Starr, K. R., Langmead, C. J., Hill, M., Bartoszyk, G. D., Hagan, J. J., Middlemiss, D. N.&Dawson, L. A. (2005). Neurochemical evaluation of the novel 5-HT1A receptor partial agonist/serotonin reuptake inhibitor, vilazodone. Eur J Pharmacol 510(1-2): 49-57.

Iversen, S. D. (1984). 5-HT and anxiety. Neuropharmacology 23(12B): 1553-60.

Jax (2003). The importance of understanding substrains in the genomic age. JAX Notes(491): 1-3.

Jones, N., Duxon, M. S.&King, S. M. (2002). Ethopharmacological analysis of the unstable elevated exposed plus maze, a novel model of extreme anxiety: predictive validity and sensitivity to anxiogenic agents. Psychopharmacology (Berl) 161(3): 314-23.

Kayir, H.&Uzbay, I. T. (2005). Nicotine antagonizes caffeine- but not pentylenetetrazole-induced anxiogenic effect in mice. Psychopharmacology (Berl): 1-6.

Kessler, R. C., Ruscio, A. M., Shear, K.&Wittchen, H. U. (2010). Epidemiology of anxiety disorders. Curr Top Behav Neurosci 2: 21-35.

Kielholz, P.&Battegay, R. (1967). Angst: Psychische und somatische Aspekte. Bern, Hans Huber.

Kinrys, G., Coleman, E.&Rothstein, E. (2009). Natural remedies for anxiety disorders: potential use and clinical applications. Depress Anxiety 26(3): 259-65.

Kjernisted, K. D.&Bleau, P. (2004). Long-term goals in the management of acute and chronic anxiety disorders. Can J Psychiatry 49(3 Suppl 1): 51S-63S.

Lader, M. (2005). Management of panic disorder. Expert Rev Neurother 5(2): 259-66.

Lal, H.&Emmett-Oglesby, M. W. (1983). Behavioral analogues of anxiety. Animal models. Neuropharmacology 22: 1423-1441.

Landgraf, R. (2003). Neurobiologie und Genetik der Angst im Tiermodell. Nervenarzt 74(3): 274-8.

Lesch, K. P.&Gutknecht, L. (2005). Pharmacogenetics of the serotonin transporter. Prog Neuropsychopharmacol Biol Psychiatry 29(6): 1062-73.

Liebsch, G., Montkowski, A., Holsboer, F.&Landgraf, R. (1998). Behavioural profiles of two Wistar rat lines selectively bred for high or low anxiety-related behaviour. Behav Brain Res 94(2): 301-10.

Linthorst, A. C., Penalva, R. G., Flachskamm, C., Holsboer, F.&Reul, J. M. (2002). Forced swim stress activates rat hippocampal serotonergic neurotransmission involving a corticotropin-releasing hormone receptor-dependent mechanism. Eur J Neurosci 16(12): 2441-52.

Lister, R. G. (1990). Ethologically-based animal models of anxiety disorders. Pharmac.Ther. 46: 321-340.

Lohse, J. L., Lorenzen, A.&Mueller-Oerlinghausen, B. (2004). Psychopharmaka. Arzneiverordnungsreport 2004. U. Schwabe &D. Paffrath. Berlin, Heidelberg, New York, Springer Verlag: 769-810.

Lucki, I. (1998). The spectrum of behaviors influenced by serotonin. Biol Psychiatry 44(3): 151-62.

Marsden, C. A., Beckett, S. R. G., Wilson, W., Bickerdike, M., Fink, H., Rex, A.&Cadogan, A. K. (1995). Serotonin involvement in animal models of anxiety and panic. Serotonin in the central nervous system and periphery. E. Takada &G. Curzon. Amsterdam, Elsevier: 135-143.

Matsuo, M., Kataoka, Y., Mataki, S., Kato, Y.&Oi, K. (1996). Conflict situation increases serotonin release in rat dorsal hippocampus: in vivo study with microdialysis and Vogel test. Neurosci Lett 215(3): 197-200.

Möhler, H.&Okada, T. (1977). Benzodiazepine receptor: demonstration in the central nervous system. Science 198(4319): 849-51.

Moriarty, D. D. (1995). Anxiogenic effects of a beta-carboline on tonic immobility and open field behavior in chickens (Gallus gallus). Pharmacol Biochem Behav 51(4): 795-8.

Nehlig, A., Daval, J. L.&Debry, G. (1992). Caffeine and the central nervous system: mechanisms of action, biochemical, metabolic and psychostimulant effects. Brain Res Brain Res Rev 17(2): 139-70.

Neumeister, A., Young, T.&Stastny, J. (2004). Implications of genetic research on the role of the serotonin in depression: emphasis on the serotonin type 1A receptor and the serotonin transporter. Psychopharmacology (Berl) 174(4): 512-24.

Ohl, F.&Keck, M. E. (2003). Behavioural screening in mutagenised mice--in search for novel animal models of psychiatric disorders. Eur J Pharmacol 480(1-3): 219-28.

Pei, Q., Zetterstrom, T.&Fillenz, M. (1989). Both systemic and local administration of benzodiazepine agonists inhibit the in vivo release of 5-HT from ventral hippocampus. Neuropharmacology 28: 1061-1066.

Pollack, M. H. (2004). Unmet needs in the treatment of anxiety disorders. Psychopharmacol Bull 38(1): 31-7.

Rex, A. (1996). Verhaltenspharmakologische und neurochemische Untersuchungen zu Interaktionen zwischen dem Neuropeptid Cholezystokinin und dem Neurotransmitter Serotonin. Medizinische Fakultät. Berlin, Humboldt-Universität.

Rex, A., Barth, T., Voigt, J. P., Domeney, A. M.&Fink, H. (1994). Effects of cholecystokinin tetrapeptide and sulfated cholecystokinin octapeptide in rat models of anxiety. Neurosci Lett 172(1-2): 139-42.

Rex, A., Bert, B.&Fink, H. (2007). [History and new developments. The pharmacology of 5-ht3 antagonists]. Pharm Unserer Zeit 36(5): 342-53.

Rex, A.&Fink, H. (1998). Effects of cholecystokinin-receptor agonists on cortical 5-HT release in guinea pigs on the X-maze. Peptides 19(3): 519-26.

Rex, A.&Fink, H. (2006). Effects of 8-OH-DPAT on hippocampal NADH fluorescence in vivo in anaesthetized rats. J Neurosci Res 83(4): 551-6.

Rex, A., Fink, H.&Marsden, C. A. (1993). The effect of CCK-4 and L 365.260 on cortical extracellular 5-HT release on exposure to the elevated plus maze. Anxiety: Neurobiology, Clinic and Therapeutic Perspectives. M. Hamon, H. Ollat &M. H. Thiébot. London

Paris, Colloque INSERM/John Libbey Eurotext: 207-208.

Rex, A., Fink, H.&Marsden, C. A. (1994). Effects of BOC-CCK-4 and L 365.260 on cortical 5-HT release in guinea-pigs on exposure to the elevated plus maze. Neuropharmacology 33(3-4): 559-65.

Rex, A., Fink, H., Skingle, M.&Marsden, C. A. (1996). Involvement of 5-HT1D receptors in cortical extracellular 5-HT release in guinea-pigs on exposure to the elevated plus maze. J Psychopharmacol 10: 219-224.

Rex, A., Kolbasenko, A., Bert, B.&Fink, H. (2007). Choosing the right wild type: behavioral and neurochemical differences between 2 populations of Sprague-Dawley rats from the same source but maintained at different sites. J Am Assoc Lab Anim Sci 46(5): 13-20.

Rex, A., Marsden, C. A.&Fink, H. (1991). Increased 5-HT release in the guinea-pig frontal cortex on exposure to the X-Maze. Monitoring molecules in neuroscience. H. Rollema, B. Westerink &W. J. Drijfhout. Groningen, University Centre for Pharmacy. 5: 250-252.

Rex, A., Marsden, C. A.&Fink, H. (1993). 5-HT 1A receptors and changes in extracellular 5-HT in the guinea-pig prefrontal cortex: involvement in aversive behaviour. J Psychopharmacol 7: 338-345.

Rex, A., Marsden, C. A.&Fink, H. (1993). Effect of diazepam on cortical 5-HT release and behaviour in the guinea-pig on exposure to the elevated plus maze. Psychopharmacology (Berl) 110(4): 490-6.

Rex, A., Marsden, C. A.&Fink, H. (1997). Cortical 5-HT-CCK interactions and anxiety-related behaviour of guinea-pigs: a microdialysis study. Neurosci Lett 228(2): 79-82.

Rex, A., Morgenstern, E.&Fink, H. (2002). Anxiolytic-like effects of kava-kava in the elevated plus maze test--a comparison with diazepam. Prog Neuropsychopharmacol Biol Psychiatry 26(5): 855-60.

Rex, A., Sondern, U., Voigt, J. P., Franck, S.&Fink, H. (1996). Strain differences in fear-motivated behavior of rats. Pharmacol Biochem Behav 54(1): 107-11.

Rex, A., Stephens, D. N.&Fink, H. (1996). Anxiolytic action of diazepam and abecarnil in a modified open field test. Pharmacol Biochem Behav 53(4): 1005-11.

Rex, A., Thomas, H., Hortnagl, H., Voits, M.&Fink, H. (2003). Behavioural and microdialysis study after neurotoxic lesion of the dorsal raphe nucleus in rats. Pharmacol Biochem Behav 74(3): 587-93.

Rex, A., Voigt, J. P.&Fink, H. (1999). Behavioral and neurochemical differences between Fischer 344 and Harlan-Wistar rats raised identically. Behav Genet 29(3): 187-92.

Rex, A., Voigt, J. P.&Fink, H. (2005). Anxiety but not arousal increases 5-hydroxytryptamine release in the rat ventral hippocampus in vivo. Eur J Neurosci 22(5): 1185-9.

Rex, A., Voigt, J. P., Gustedt, C., Beckett, S.&Fink, H. (2004). Anxiolytic-like profile in Wistar, but not Sprague-Dawley rats in the social interaction test. Psychopharmacology (Berl) 177(1-2): 23-34.

Rex, A., Voigt, J. P., Voits, M.&Fink, H. (1998). Pharmacological evaluation of a modified open-field test sensitive to anxiolytic drugs. Pharmacol Biochem Behav 59(3): 677-83.

Rex, A., Voigt, J. P., Wicke, K. M.&Fink, H. (2008). In vivo/ex vivo and behavioural study on central effects of 5-HT1B/1D and 5-HT1A antagonists in guinea pigs. Pharmacol Biochem Behav 88(3): 196-204.

Roberts, C., Boyd, D. F., Middlemiss, D. N.&Routledge, C. (1999). Enhancement of 5-HT1B and 5-HT1D receptor antagonist effects on extracellular 5-HT levels in the guinea-pig brain following concurrent 5-HT1A or 5-HT re-uptake site blockade. Neuropharmacology 38(9): 1409-19.

Robichaud, R. C.&Sledge, K. L. (1969). The effects of p-chlorophenylalanine on experimentally induced conflict in the rat. Life Sci 8(17): 965-9.

Rodgers, R. J., Cao, B. J., Dalvi, A.&Holmes, A. (1997). Animal models of anxiety: an ethological perspective. Braz J Med Biol Res 30(3): 289-304.

Rodgers, R. J.&Cole, J. C. (1993). Anxiety enhancement in the murine elevated plus maze by immediate prior exposure to social stressors. Physiol Behav 53(2): 383-8.

Rodgers, R. J.&Johnson, N. J. (1995). Cholecystokinin and anxiety: promises and pitfalls. Crit Rev Neurobiol 9(4): 345-69.

Rudolph, U., Crestani, F.&Mohler, H. (2001). GABA(A) receptor subtypes: dissecting their pharmacological functions. Trends Pharmacol Sci 22(4): 188-94.

Shepherd, J. K., Grewal, S. S., Fletcher, A., Bill, D. J.&Dourish, C. T. (1994). Behavioural and pharmacological characterisation of the elevated zero-maze as an animal model of anxiety. Psychopharmacology 116: 56-64.

Silverman, P. (1978). Animal behaviour in the laboratory. London, Chapman and Hall.

Singh, Y. N.&Blumenthal, M. (1997). Kava: An Overview. Distribution, mythology, botany, culture, chemistry, and pharmacology of the South Pacific's most revered herb. HerbalGram 39: 33-55.

Siniscalchi, A., Rodi, D., Cavallini, S., Marino, S., Beani, L.&Bianchi, C. (2001). Effects of cholecystokinin tetrapeptide (CCK(4)) and anxiolytic drugs on the electrically evoked [(3)H]5-hydroxytryptamine outflow from rat cortical slices. Brain Res 922(1): 104-11.

Smith, K. K., Dharmaratne, H. R., Feltenstein, M. W., Broom, S. L., Roach, J. T., Nanayakkara, N. P., Khan, I. A.&Sufka, K. J. (2001). Anxiolytic effects of kava extract and kavalactones in the chick social separation-stress paradigm. Psychopharmacology (Berl) 155(1): 86-90.

Soderpalm, B.&Engel, J. A. (1992). The 5,7-DHT-induced anticonflict effect is dependent on intact adrenocortical function. Life Sci 51(5): 315-26.

Spielberger, C. D. (1972). Anxiety: current trends in theory and research. New York, Academic Press.

Srinivasan, J., Suresh, B.&Ramanathan, M. (2003). Differential anxiolytic effect of enalapril and losartan in normotensive and renal hypertensive rats. Physiol Behav 78(4-5): 585-91.

Stahl, S. M. (1998). Mechanism of action of serotonin selective reuptake inhibitors. Serotonin receptors and pathways mediate therapeutic effects and side effects. J Affect Disord 51(3): 215-35.

Stephens, D. N.&Andrews, J. S. (1991). Screening for anxiolytic drugs. Behavioural models in psychopharmacology: Theoretical, industrial and clinical perspectives. P. Willner. Cambridge, University Press: 50-75.

Tabatabaie, T.&Dryhurst, G. (1998). Molecular mechanisms of action of 5,6- and 5,7-dihydroxytryptamine. Highly Selective Neurotoxins: Basic and Clinical Applications. R. M. Kostrzewa. Totowa, Humana Press: 269 – 291.

Tada, K., Kasamo, K., Ueda, N., Suzuki, T., Kojima, T.&Ishikawa, K. (1999). Anxiolytic 5-hydroxytryptamine1A agonists suppress firing activity of dorsal hippocampus CA1 pyramidal neurons through a postsynaptic mechanism: single-unit study in unanesthetized, unrestrained rats. J Pharmacol Exp Ther 288(2): 843-8.

Tembrock, G. (2000). Angst. Darmstadt, Wissensch. Buchges.

Thiebot, M. H., Jobert, A.&Soubrie, P. (1980). Conditioned suppression of behavior: its reversal by intra raphe microinjection of chlordiazepoxide and GABA. Neurosci Lett 16(2): 213-7.

Thomas, H., Fink, H., Sohr, R.&Voits, M. (2000). Lesion of the median raphe nucleus: a combined behavioral and microdialysis study in rats. Pharmacol Biochem Behav 65(1): 15-21.

Trullas, R.&Skolnick, P. (1993). Differences in fear motivated behaviors among inbred mouse strains. Psychopharmacology (Berl) 111(3): 323-31.

Trulson, M. E., Preussler, D. W., Howell, G. A.&Frederickson, C. J. (1982). Raphe unit activity in freely moving cats: effects of benzodiazepines. Neuropharmacology 21(10): 1045-50.

Twarog, B. M.&Page, I. H. (1953). Serotonin content of some mammalian tissues and urine and a method for its determination. Am J Physiol 175(1): 157-61.

Ungerstedt, U.&Hallstrom, A. (1987). In vivo microdialysis--a new approach to the analysis of neurotransmitters in the brain. Life Sciences 41: 861-864.

Ungerstedt, U.&Rostami, E. (2004). Microdialysis in neurointensive care. Curr Pharm Des 10(18): 2145-52.

Vaas (2000). Emotionen. Lexikon der Neurowissenschaft. Heidelberg, Berlin, Spektrum Akademischer Verlag. 1: 386-397.

Vanderhaeghen, J. J., Signeau, J. C.&Gepts, W. (1975). New peptide in the vertebrate CNS reacting with antigastrin antibodies. Nature 257(5527): 604-5.

Voigt, J. P., Rex, A., Sohr, R.&Fink, H. (1999). Hippocampal 5-HT and NE release in the transgenic rat TGR(mREN2)27 related to behavior on the elevated plus maze. Eur Neuropsychopharmacol 9(4): 279-85.

Wise, C. D., Berger, B. D.&Stein, L. (1972). Benzodiazepines: anxiety-reducing activity by reduction of serotonin turnover in the brain. Science 177(44): 180-3.

Wittchen, H. U. (1991). Der Langzeitverlauf unbehandelter Angststörungen: Wie häufig sind Spontanremissionen? Verhaltenstherapie 1: 273-282.

Wittchen, H. U.&Jacobi, F. (2005). Size and burden of mental disorders in Europe--a critical review and appraisal of 27 studies. Eur Neuropsychopharmacol 15(4): 357-76.

Witte, S., Loew, D.&Gaus, W. (2005). Meta-analysis of the efficacy of the acetonic kava-kava extract WS1490 in patients with non-psychotic anxiety disorders. Phytother Res 19(3): 183-8.

Wright, I. K., Upton, N.&Marsden, C. A. (1992). Effect of established and putative anxiolytics on extracellular 5-HT and 5-HIAA in the ventral hippocampus of rats during behaviour on the elevated X-maze. Psychopharmacology (Berl) 109(3): 338-46.

8

Molecular Mechanism of the Involvement of the Susceptibility Genes, *DISC1, PACAP, TRAP1* and *Dysbindin* in Major Psychiatric Disorders Such as Schizophrenia, Depression and Bipolar Disease

Taiichi Katayama[1], Shinsuke Matsuzaki[1,2],
Tsuyosi Hattori[3] and Masaya Tohyama[1,2]
*[1]United Graduate School of Child Development, Osaka University,
Kanazawa University and Hamamatsu University School of Medicine,
[2]Department of Anatomy and Neuroscience,
Graduate school of Medicine, Osaka University
[3]Department of Molecular Neuropharmacology, Graduate School of Medicine, Osaka
University,
Japan*

1. Introduction

No effective drugs are currently available for the treatment of mental diseases, primarily because the underlying mechanism of mental diseases have not been adequately explored at the molecular level. However, recent studies have examined several molecular cascades whose disturbances are associated with mental diseases such as schizophrenia, bipolar disease and major depression. The most common characteristics of these cascades us that they are all associated with neural circuit formation, suggesting that neurodevelopmental factors play a key role in the pathogenesis of mental diseases. The present review summarizes the available information on these molecular cascades and their association with mental disease.

2. Molecular mechanism of PACAP-stathmin1 dependent psychiatric disorders (Yamada et al., 2010)

Pituitary adenylate cyclase polypeptide (PACAP) is involved in multiple brain function such as neurotransmission and neural plasticity (Hashimoto et al., 2001; Vaudry et al., 2000). It also has a neurotrophic effect via three heptahekical G protein coupled receptors, one of which is specific for PACAP (PAC$_1$ receptor) and two others that are shared with vasoactive intestinal polypeptide (VPAC$_1$ and VPAC$_2$) (Hashimoto et al., 1993). Recently, mice that lack *Adcyap 1*, the gene encoding PACAP, (*Adcyap 1$^{-/-}$* mice) were developed (Hashimoto et al., 2001, Shintani et al., 2002). *Adcyap 1$^{-/-}$* mice display remarkable behavioral abnormalities providing evidence that PACAP plays a previously uncharacterized role in the regulation of psychomotor behavior. In addition, previous association study reported that several single nucleotide polymorphism (SNPs) in the vicinity of the PACAP gene locus were associated with schizophrenia (Hashimoto, R. et al., 2007). However, although nothing was known about the mechanism of PACAP deficiency-induced psychiatric illness, we have clarified these mechanisms.

2.1 Down-regulation of PACAP expression induces up-regulation of stathmin1 expression in the dentate gyrus both *in vivo* and *in vitro*

Real-time PCR showed that stathmin1 mRNA was markedly increased in the dentate gyrus of *Adcyap 1-/-* mice. An increased in stathmin1 protein levels in the dentate gyrus of *Adcyap 1-/-* mice was confirmed by western blot analysis. These findings were confirmed also *in vitro* using PC12 cells. PACAP stimulation of PC12 cells caused a decrease in stathmin1 mRNA levels after 3 h, and expression continued to decrease over the next 24 h (Fig. 1A). Stathmin1 protein levels also decreased in response to PACAP, which caused a dose-dependent decrease of stathmin1 mRNA levels. The decrease of stathmin1 expression caused by PACAP stimulation was slightly, but statistically significantly, inhibited by pretreatment with a $PAC_1/VPAC_2$ receptor antagonist (PACAP6-38). In addition, pretreatment with a p38 antagonist (SB202190) or an ERK antagonist (PD98059) also inhibited the PACAP-induced decrease of stathmin1 expression. Co-administration of SB202190 and PD98059 strongly inhibited the effect of PACAP, reflecting the key roles played by p38 and ERK in the PACAP signaling pathway. On the other hand, VIP did not decrease stathmin1 expression. These results indicate that PACAP regulates stathmin1 expression via the PAC_1 receptor in neurons of the dentate gyrus.

2.2 Up-regulation of stathmin1 induces abnormal axonal arborization in neurons of the dentate gyrus subgranular zone

In wild-type mice, cells expressing stathmin1 were preferentially located in the innermost part of the granular cell layer, the so-called subgranular zone (SGZ), where neurogenesis of granular cells occurs in adults. Two types of stathmin1 containing processes were found, namely; dendrites and axons. Immunoreactivity for stathmin1 was significantly increased in the SGZ neurons of *Adcyap 1-/-* mice, although the actual number of immunoreactive cells was similar in mutant and wild-type mice. . The number of dot-like immunoreactive fibers belonging to axons was significantly increased in the polymorphic layer of *Adcyap 1-/-* mice, compared with wild-type mice. In support of the *in vivo* datas, over-expression of stathmin1 in the hippocampal primary culture neurons caused dramatic changes of axon fibers. Arborization of axon fibers was markedly increased by stathmin1 over-expression compared with that in normal primary cultured neurons. The number of secondary neurites on axons was also increased following over-expression of stathmin1. These findings indicated that an increase in stathmin1 expression in SGZ neurons leads to abnormal axon arborization.

If PACAP directly regulates stathmin1 expression in vivo, SGZ neurons should express PAC_1. In fact, strong expression of PAC_1 mRNA was identified throughout the entire granular cell layer, including the SGZ. Furthermore, SGZ neurons expressed both stathmin1 protein and PAC_1 mRNA. These results show that PACAP inhibits stathmin1 expression via the PAC_1 receptor.

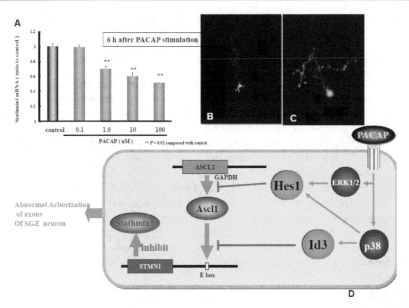

Fig. 1. PACAP-stathmin1 cascade

A: PACAP regulated stathmin1 expression via PAC1 in PC12 cells. Alteration of stathmin1 mRNA levels 24 h after PACAP treatment, at the indicated concentrations were quantified by real-time PRC. Data are expressed as mean ±SEM relative to control values (n=3, PACAP 1nM **P=0.0044, 10nM **P=0.0033, 100nM ***P=0.0003 compared with control. B,C; Stathmin1 over-expression in neurons caused abnormally pronounced arborization of axon fibers. Morphology of hippocampal primary neurons transfected with stathmin1. Over-expression of GFP (B) and GFP-stathmin1 (C). The neurons over-expressing stathmin1 have abnormally pronounced sprouting of axon fibers. D: Schematic drawing of the molecular pathway underlying PACAP regulation of stathmin1 expression. The schematic representation shows the pathway by which PACAP regulates the expression of stathmin1 by suppressing the function and expression of Ascl1 after increasing the expression of Hes1 and Id3 by activating ERK and p38.

2.2.1 Stathmin1 gene promoter activity is regulated by basic helix loop helix (bHLH) proteins via the E10 box

A BLAST search identified the genomic sequence of rat stathmin1 in a chromosome 5 contig. PCR amplification of a 1885bp genomic DNA fragment that consisted of 1561 nt upstream of the stathmin1 transcription start site (+1), exon1, and part of intron 1 (+325) was then performed. This fragment was sequenced and subcloned into a pGL3 luciferase reporter vector. This fragment was also analyzed for transcription factor-binding sites using the DNAsis program. The 1.8kbp rat stathmin1 5' genomic sequence contained 12 (E1-E12) putative E boxes (CANNTG), which are potential binding sites for bHLH proteins, including neuronal transcription activators. To investigate the promoter activity of stathmin1, we constructed several expression plasmids for the luciferase assay after transient transfection in PC12 cells. Constructs containing E10 (such as STMN1-1, STMN1-2 and STMN 1-3) showed a high level of luciferase activity compared with control cells, but constructs containing a stathmin promoter lacking the E10 box (such as STMN1-4) did not show luciferase activity. Therefore, the E10 box was found to be a key motif that regulates stathmin1 expression through bHLH factors.

2.2.2 An activating bHLH protein, Ascl1, activates the stathmin promoter

Among activating bHLH proteins, Ascl1was found to activate the stathmin1 promoter. Co-transfection of PC12 cells with the stathmin1-promoter plasmid and the Ascl1 expression plasmid induced a dose-dependent increase in luciferase activity compared with cells transfected with the stathmin1 promoter plasmid alone. To examine whether endogenous Ascl1 protein could bind to the stathmin1 promoter sequence in PC12 cells, sheared chromatin was immunoprecipitated with an anti-Ascl1 antibody or with control IgG, followed by PCR amplification of the corresponding DNA regions using stathmin1 promoter specific primers. Analysis of amplified DNA showed that more sequences were amplified by primers flanking the E10 box than by primers flanking the E10-E11 boxes. In addition, co-localization of Ascl1 and stathmin1 in SGZ neurons was demonstrated by immunohistochemistry. These results established that endogenous Ascl1 protein binds to stathmin1 promoter and act as a major regulator of stathmin1 promoter activity.

2.2.3 The inhibitory bHLH proteins, Hes1 and Id3, showed increased expression after PACAP stimulation

As described above, PACAP inhibits stathmin1 expression. In addition, PACAP stimulation of PC12 cells caused an increase in the expression of the inhibitory HLH proteins, Hes1 and Id3 expression which belong to inhibitory HLH proteins. Inhibition of the PACAP signaling pathway, as through the inhibition of p38 and ERK, suppresses the effect of PACAP on stathmin1 expression. Moreover, the increase of Id3 mRNA levels in response to PACAP stimulation was inhibited by a p38 inhibitor (SB202190), but not by an ERK inhibitor (PD98059), while induction of Hes1 mRNA by PACAP stimulation was inhibited by both an ERK inhibitor and a p38 inhibitor. Co-administration of p38 and ERK inhibitors strongly inhibited thePACAP-induced induction of Hes1 mRNA. These findings showed that Hes1 expression is regulated by both the PACAP-ERK and PACAP-p38 pathways, whereas Id3 expression is mainly controlled by the PACAP-p38 pathway.

2.2.4 Hes1 and Id3 suppress stathmin1 promoter activity via Ascl1 inhibition

PC12 cells were co-transfected with a stathmin1 promoter plasmid and a Hes1 expression plasmid or an Id3 expression plasmid with or without an Ascl1 expression plasmid. Even without exogenous Ascl1 expression, a high level of luciferase activity was detected, owing to the action of the stathmin1 promoter. Expression of Hes1 or Id3 in these cells inhibited luciferase activity related to the stathmin1 promoter activity through endogenous Ascl1. In PC12 cells transfected with the stathmin1 promoter plasmid and the Ascl1 expression plasmid, luciferase activity was higher than that in PC12 cells without the Ascl1 expression plasmid. Id3 expression in these cells inhibited the up-regulation of stathmin1 promoter luciferase activity, while Hes1 expression failed to reduce the luciferase activity induced by exogenous Ascl1.These findings suggested that Id3 inhibits activation of the stathmin1 promoter by both exogenous and endogenous Ascl1, while Hes1 only blocked the effect of endogenous Ascl1. Thus, it is likely that Id3 regulates Ascl1 at the protein level, while Hes1 regulates Ascl1 transcription. If so, inhibition of Hes1 expression should increase the transcription of Ascl1. In fact, the up-regulation of Hes1 in PC12 cells by PACAP stimulation led to inhibition of Ascl1 expression. In addition, a reduction of Hes1 expression also resulted in an elevation of Ascl1 expression to 1.2 fold the control level. These results indicate that Ascl1, which controls stathmin1 expression, was functionally regulated by Id3 and quantitatively regulated by Hes1, in response to PACAP signaling.

2.3 Role of the PACAP-stathmin1 cascade in psychiatric disorders

As described above, PACAP inhibits stathmin1 expression. In addition, over-expression of stathmin1 causes abnormal axonal arborization (Fig. 1B,C), indicating that stathmin1 regulates the maturation of neurons and neural circuit formation. Furtehrmore, *Adcyap 1-/-* mice are known to show behavioral abnormalities, some of which might have potential relevance to mental disorders such as schizophrenia (Hashimoto et al.,2001; Shintani et al., 2002), and several SNPs in the vicinity of the *PACAP* gene locus are associated with schizophrenia (Hashimoto et al., 2007). If so, stathmin1 expression should be altered in the brain of patients with schizophrenia. Our RT-PCR study showed that stathmin1 mRNA levels were significantly increased in schizophrenic patients compared with age-matched controls. In contrast, stathmin1 was not significantly increased in the brains of patients with bipolar disorder.

3. Mechanism of PACAP-DBZ/DISC1 dependent psychiatric disorders (Hattori et al.,2007; Katayama et al., 2009)

DBZ (DISC1-binding zinc finger protein) was found as a DISC1(disrupted-in schizophrenia 1)-interacting molecules by yeast-2-hybrid screening of a complementary DNA (cDNA) library. Subsequent co-immunoprecipitation studies and yeast-2 hybrid assays showed that amino acids 348-597 of DISC1 act as the DBZ binding region, which indicates that the regions of DISC1 near the translocation breakpoint (amino acid 598) participate in the interaction with DBZ. DISC1 and DBZ co-localize diffusely in the cytoplasm and centrosome, and are involved in neurite extension. PACAP regulates the association between DISC1 and DBZ (for details on DISC1, see the chapter 6).

3.1 DISC1-DBZ interaction inhibits the neurite outgrowth (Fig.2)

DBZ mRNA was expressed exclusively in the brain, but was not expressed in peripheral tissues. To examine the functional role of the DISC1-DBZ interaction, PC12 cells stably expressing DISC1-HA and mock-transfected cells were infected with Adv-DBZ-GFP or Adv-GFP for 24 h. Immunoprecipitation and western blot analysis confirmed the over-expression of DBZ-GFP and DISC1-HA as well as the association between these 2 molecules. Over-expression of both proteins in PC12 cells caused a significant reduction in the number of neurite bearing PC12 cells after PACAP stimulation. However, over-expression of either DBZ or DISC1 alone had no effect. The region of DBZ encompassing amino acids 152-301 interacts with DISC1. PC12 cells were transiently transfected with DBZ (152-301)-IRES-GFP or with GFP alone and treated with PACAP (100nM) for 48 h. The cells expressing DBZ (152-301) had a shorter neurite length than cells expressing GFP alone. Under these conditions, no significant change of apoptosis was detected and the number of transfected cells was similar. The effect of DBZ (152-301) on neurite growth was also confirmed in primary cultured hippocampal neurons.

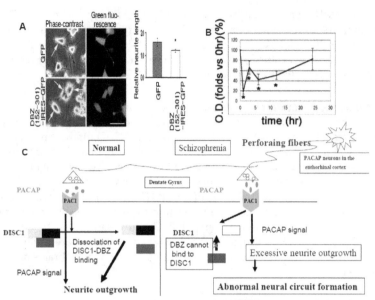

Fig. 2. A: Neurite outgrowth was inhibited by the DISC1-binding domain of DBZ [DBZ(152-301)-IRES-GFP]. PC12 cells were transfected with DBZ (152-301)-IRES-GFP or GFP alone at 2 days after plating. After 24 h , cells were starved of serum for 4h and treated with 100nM PACAP for 48h. Phase-contrast and fluorescence microscopy images are shown. Diagrams display neurite length relative to cell body diameter of transfected PC12 cells. B: PACAP-induced transient inhibition of the endogenous DISC1-DBZ interaction in PC12 cells. Immunoprecipitation and western blot analysis (with anti-DISC1 or anti-DBZ antibodies) of PC12 cells lysates collected at the indicated times after stimulation with 100nM PACAP. Immunoprecipitaes obtained with an anti-DBZ antibody incubated with 5% of each lysates (5% input), were subjected to western blot analysis with the same antibody. Quantitation of relative band densities for DISC1 co-immunoprecipitated with DBZ, as well as for total DISC1 or DBZ protein, was performed by scanning densitometry. Data were expressed as the mean ±SEM. of at least 3 independent experiments. *$P<0.05$ vs control (Student's t-test). C: A possible PACAP-DISC1/DBZ pathway . In the normal brain, PACAP leads to the temporal dissociation of the binding between DISC1 and DBZ , which in turn leads to normal neurite outgrowth. In the brain of schizophrenia patients, DBZ cannot bind to DISC1, and the PACAP pathway may proceed without inhibition, resulting in the formation of an abnormal neural circuit.

3.2 PACAP regulates DISC1-DBZ binding (Fig. 2)

Exposure to PACAP (100nM) increased the expression of endogenous DISC1 in PC12 cells by about 50% after 24 h, whereas it had no effect on DBZ expression. PACAP has a marked influence on the interaction between DBZ and DISC1. The co-immunoprecipitation of DISC1 and DBZ from PC12 cell lysates was reduced by approximately 80% 1h after treatment of cells with PACAP (100nM). However, this reduction was transient and there was a gradual return to control level by 24 h after treatment. Addition of an ERK inhibitor 24 h after PACAP treatment inhibited the rebinding of DBZ to DISC1, while an inhibitor of adenyl cyclase failed to influence the DISC1-DBZ interaction, showing that PACAP regulates DISC1-DBZ binding through the ERK cascade but not through the cAMP cascade.

3.3 Role of the PACAP-DBZ cascade with regard to PACAP-DBZ/DISC1 dependent psychiatric disorders (Fig.2)

The findings described above show that the DISC1-DBZ interaction inhibits neurite out growth, and PACAP dissociates this interaction, resulting in neurite outgrowth. The involvement of the DISC1-DBZ interaction and PACAP in neurite outgrowth suggests that these molecules should be expressed in the early ontogenetical stages. In fact, a marked elevation of both DBZ and PAC_1 (PACAP receptor) expression was observed during the perinatal stage (Hattori et al. in preparation). DISC1 shows a high level of expression in the developing cortex and hippocampus (Honda et al.,2004). In addition, down-regulation of DBZ caused a delay in the migration of cortical neurons (Sato et al., personal communication) and disturbance of cilia formation (Kumamoto et al., in preparation). The DISC1-DBZ interaction which is regulated by PACAP has therefore been shown to be involved in neurite out growth and the migration of neurons. In the brain of patients with PACAP-dependent psychiatric disorders, dissociation of the binding between DISC1 and DBZ does not occur and neurite extension may be inhibited. On the other hand, in brains in which translocation of DISC1 occurs, DBZ is unable bind to DISC1 and the dissociation of DISC1 from DBZ may not be induced, which results in an immature neural circuit.

4. Molecular mechanism of Dysbindin-MARCKS cascade dependent psychiatric disorders (Okuda et al., 2010)

Studies of postmortem brain tissue showed decreased Dysbindin (dystrobrevin binding protein 1; DTNBP1) protein and mRNA levels in patients with schizophrenia compared with controls (Bray et al., 2005; Talbot et al., 2004; Weickert et al., 2004). Chronic treatment of mice with antipsychotics did not affect the levels of Dysbindin protein and mRNA expression in their brains (Chiba et al., 2006; Talbot et al., 2004), suggesting the lower levels of Dysbindin protein and mRNA found in the postmortem brains of schizophrenia patients is not likely to be a simple artifact of antemortem drug treatment. In addition, several studies suggested that diverse high-risk SNPs and haplotypes could influence Dysbindin mRNA expression (Bray et al., 2005; Talbot et al., 2004; Weickert et al., 2004). These data indicate that the *Dysbindin* gene may confer susceptibility to schizophrenia through reduced Dysbindin expression. However, the molecular mechanisms underlying the effect of decreased Dysbindin expression on vulnerability to schizophrenia remain unknown.

4.1 Dysbindin- myristoylated alanin-rich protein kinase C substrate (MARCKS) cascade (Okuda et al., 2010)

4.1.1 Dysbindin exists within the nucleus in addition to the cytoplasm

Cell fractionation experiments using Dysbindin-FLAG-overexpressing HEK293 cells showed that Dysbindin exists mainly in the cytosol while a small amount is present in the nucleus. Immunohistochemical analysis also revealed that Dysbindin is localized mainly in the cytoplasm with a perinuclear high density region. However, a faint immunoreaction was seen within the nucleus. Furthermore, pretreatment with leptomycine-B(LPB), which inhibits the export of proteins from the nucleus to the cytoplasm, caused a slight increase of

Dysbindin and its nuclear localization. These findings show that the Dysbindin protein is shuttled between the nucleus and the cytoplasm.

4.1.2 Dysbindin binds to the transcription factor NF-YB

Using yeast 2-hybrid screening, several transcriptional factors including nuclear transcription factor Y beta (NF-YB), were identified as candidates for interaction with Dysbindin. NF-YB belong to a family of CCAAT-binding transcription factors that are important for the basal transcription of a class of regulatory genes and are involved in cellular reactions. HEK293T cells which express NF-YB endogenously were transfected with expression vectors for Dysbindin-V5 and subjected to immunoprecipitation to confirm the Dysbindin-NF-YB interaction. In addition, the Dysbindin-NF-YB interaction was shown in lysates from SH-SY5Y cells, which express both Dysbindin and NF-YB endogenously, as well as adult mouse brain lysates.

4.1.3 Downregulation of Dysbindin causes up-regulation of the expression level of MARCKS

The interaction between Dysbindin and NF-YB suggests that Dysbindin may be functionally involved in the transcription of genes regulated by NF-YB. We therefore screened for genes displaying altered expression by means of a DNA chip, using RNA extracts from the Dysbindin or NF-YB knockdown human neural cell line, SH-SY5Y. Among them identified, we focused on MARCKS, because protein kinase C has been involved in psychiatric diseases and because the promoter region of the MARCKS gene has the CCAAT binding motif specific for NF-YB.

The effect of Dysbindin on MARCKS in vitro was confirmed in vivo by examining the expression of the MARCKS protein product in the hippocampus of Dysbindin knockout mice with advanced age and comparing the levels with those of wild-type mice. In wild-type mice, a peak in MARCKS protein expression in the hippocampus was detected on postnatal days 15 and 20, and with a marked decrease in expression levels over time. However, this decrease was not observed in Dysbindin knockout mice, suggesting that down-regulation of Dysbindin may enhance the transcription of the MARCKS protein.

Chromatin immunoprecipitation analysis using SH-SY5Y cells over-expressing Dysbindin-Flag, was performed to explore the possibility that the Dysbindin-NF-YB complex could affect the transcription of MARCKS via interaction with the promoter region of MARCKS. PCR products from the chromatin immunoprecipitates suggested that Dysbindin and NF-YB simultaneously interact with the promoter region of MARCKS. These results indicate that the Dysbindin-NF-YB complex interacts with the promoter region of the MARCKS gene resulting in inhibition of MARCKS transcription.

4.1.4 The transcriptional level of the MARCKS gene is regulated by Dysbindin via the NF-YB binding motif, CCAAT-2

The 5'-UTR region of the MARCKS gene has 2 kinds of CCAAT sequences, namely; one CCAAT motif located between residues -1152 and -700 (CCAAT-1) and one located between UTR -700 and -614 (CCAAT-2). Because NF-YB binds to the CCAAT motif to regulate the transcription of target genes ˒ the role of the CCAAT motifs in the regulation of MARCKS transcription was examined by luciferase assay with 5 vectors containing shorter RNA probes (Fig. 3A); These vectors were UTR(1152)-Luc, UTR (953)-Luc, UTR (700)-Luc, UTR

(614)-Luc, and UTR (462)-Luc. The luciferase activity detected in SH-SY5Y cells expressing the UTR (1152)-Luc after retinoic acid stimulation was used as a baseline. In the cells transfected with UTR (953)-Luc containing both CCAAT sequence and UTR (700)-Luc containing CCAAT-1 sequence but lacking the CCAAT-2 sequence, luciferase activity remained at baseline level after stimulation with retinoic acid. However luciferase activity was markedly increased in cells expressing UTR (614)-Luc after retinoic acid stimulation. These results suggest that the CCAAT-2 motif plays an important role in the inhibition of MARCKS transcription. Furthermore, SH-SY5Y cells transfected with UTR (462)-Luc lacking CCAAT-1, CCAAT-2 and SP1 region showed very low luciferase activity, indicating that the SP1 is indispensable for MARCKS transcription.

To confirm that the CCAAT-2 region is important for the regulation of MARCKS transcription, several probes were designed for the luciferase assay (Fig. 3 B), namely; D1-UTR (1152)-Luc which lacks the CCAAT-2 motif and its downstream region including Sp1 from UTR (1152)-Luc, D2-UTR (1152)-Luc which lacks the SP1 region and the downstream sequence from UTR (1152)-Luc, D3-UTR (1152)-Luc which lacks only the sequence downstream of the SP1 region, D4-UTR (1152)-Luc which lacks only the CCAAT motif from UTR (1152)-Luc, and M-UTR(1152)-Luc, which has a point mutation in the CCAAT-2 motif. Luciferase activity was detected in SH-SY5Y cells transfected with each probe, using the activity in cells transfected with UTR (1152)-Luc as the baseline value. Cells transfected with M-UTR (1152)-Luc and those transfected with D4-UTR (1152)-Luc exhibited marked increases in luciferase activity, showing that the CCAAT-2 motif plays a key role in the inhibition of MARCKS transcription. Furthermore, cells expressing D1-UTR (1152)-Luc, D2-UTR (1152)-Luc or D3-UTR (1152)-Luc exhibited no luciferase activity. These findings suggest that the sequence downstream of the Sp1 region, and the Sp1 region itself, areindispensable for MARCKS transcription.

To confirm the involvement of Dysbindin in the altered MARCKS transcription levels via the CCAAT-2 motif, we compared the luciferase activity of UTR (1152)-Luc detected in Dysbindin knockdown cells with that of control cells. Knockdown of Dysbindin resulted in the up-regulation of luciferase activity in the UTR (1152)-Luc transfected cells. However, the effect of knockdown of Dysbindin knockdown on luciferase activity was not observed in D1-UTR (1152)-Luc transfected cells. These results suggest that Dysbindin regulates MARCKS transcription via the NF-YB binding motif CCAAT-2. On the other hand, the negligible levels of luciferase activity observed in cells transfected with probes lacking the sequence downstream of the Sp1 region, suggest that this this sequence is essential for MARCKS transcription. In fact, knockdown of Dysbindin caused the up-regulation of MARCKS expression (Fig. 3C).

4.2 Role of the Dysbindin-MARCKS cascade in psychiatric disorders (Fig. 3D)

SNPs in Dysbindin have been associated with intermediate cognitive phenotypes related to schizophrenia such as IQ and working and episodic memory, and a Dysbindin haplotype has been associated with higher educational attainment (Corvin et al., 2008; Donohoe et al., 2007). In addition, several papers show evidence of the involvement of Dysbindin in cognitive functions (Burdick et al., 2006; Zinkstok et al., 2007).

Furthermore, accumulating evidence suggests the involvement of Dysbindin in neurotransmission. At the cellular level, Dysbindin is located at both pre- and post-synaptic terminals., and is thought to be involved in postsynaptic density function and the

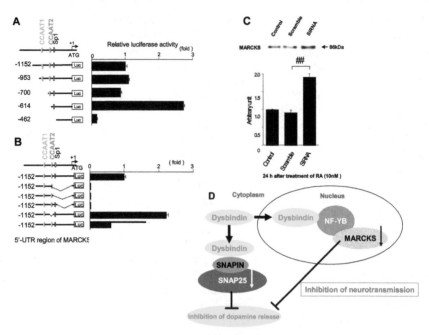

Fig. 3. A,B: Dysbindin regulates the transcription of MARCKSvia the CCAAT-2 sequence. A: The following 5 vectors contaiing shorter DNA probes were used for the luciferase assay; UTR(1152)-Luc, UTR (953)-Luc, UTR (700)-Luc, UTR (614)-Luc, and UTR (462)-Luc. Vectors were transfected into SH-SY5Y cells and luciferase activity was measured. The luciferase activity of UTR (1152) was used as the control. Columns and vertical bars denote the means ±SEM (triplicate independent experiments). B: The UTR (1152)-Luc vector and deletion or point mutations of the UTR (1152)-Luc vectors, [D10UTR(1152)-Luc], [D2-UTR (1152)-Luc], [D3-UTR (1152)-Luc], [D4-UTR(1152)-Luc] and [M-UTR (1152)-Luc], were transfected into SH-SY5Y cells and luciferase activity was measured. [D4-UTR(1152)-Luc], which lacks CCAAT-2, and [M-UTR (1152)-Luc], which has a point mutation in the CCAAT-2 sequence, showed increased luciferase activity. The luciferase activity of UTR (1152) was used as the control. Columns and vertical bars denote the means ±SEM(triplicate independent experiments). C: Dysbindin knockdown results in the up-regulation of MARCKS. SH-SY5Y cells were transfected with scrambled RNAi or siRNA for Dysbindin. Cell lysate of un-treated cells (cont.), scrambled RNAi-transfected cells (Scr.) and RNAi for Dysbindin-transfected cells (siRNA) were subjected to western blotting with an anti-MARCKS antibody. Columns and vertical bars denote the means ±SEM(triplicate independent experiments). Dysbindin knockdown cells exhibited significant up-regulation of MARCKS expression compared with control cells (P<0.001, Student's t-test). D: A possible Dysbindin pathway related to the regulation of dopamine release. In the cytoplasm of the nigrostriatal dopamine neurons, Dysbindin binds to Snapin. This binding inhibits the expression of SNAP25, which may suppress dopamine release. In the nuclei of these neurons, Dysbindin inhibits MARCKS expression via the binding to NF-YB. Reduction of MARCKS expression in dopaminergic neurons may causes the down-regulation of dopamine transport from the soma to the terminal. Thus Dysbindin inhibits dopamine release by 2 pathway.

trafficking of receptors (NMDA,GABAergic and nicotinic) (Sillitoe et al., 2003; Talbot et al., 2004). Over-expression of Dysbindin increases glutamate release from pyramidal neurons in cell culture, possibly because of its role in vesicular trafficking (Numakawa et al., 2004). Decreases in Dysbindin mRNA and protein levels have been reported in regions previously implicated in schizophrenia such as the prefrontal; cortex, midbrain and hippocampus (Talbot et al., 2004; Weickert et al., 2004). On the other hand, abnormal activation of nigrostriatal and mesolimbic dopaminergic systems is thought to be one of the most important etiologies for schizophrenia (Angrist & van Kammen, 1984; Creese et al., 1976; Lieberman et al., 1987; Seeman &Lee, 1975), suggesting a functional relationship between dopamine and Dysbindin. In support of this, midbrain dopamine neurons also contain Dysbindin (Kumamoto et al., 2006). Suppression of Dysbindin expression in PC12 cells resulted in an increase of the expression of SNAP25 which plays an important role in neurotransmitter release, and increased the release of dopamine. On the other hand, up-regulation of Dysbindin expression in PC12 cells showed a tendency to decrease the expression of SNAP25 and the release of dopamine. These findings show that Dysbindin inhibits dopamine release via down-regulation of SNAP25 expression (Kumamoto et al., 2006).

Thus, Dysbindin inhibits MARCKS expression and decreased expression of Dysbindin is characteristic of the schizophrenic brain. In addition, a decrease in Dysbindin levels up-regulates dopamine release. MARCKS influences neurotransmission *via* F-actin and vesicular transport *via* synaptic vesicles. The enhanced dopaminergic transmission produced by the lower expression level of Dysbindin may be partially attributed to activation of MARCKS. Thus, the impairment of neuronal transmission in the schizophrenic brain may be caused by alterations of MARCKS expression levels *via* changes in Dysbindin.

Sandy (*sdy*) mice that express no Dysbindin, showed behavioral abnormalities, which could be endophenotypes of schizophrenia (Feng et al., 2008). These mutant mice reportedly exhibit defective synaptic structure and function of CA_1 neurons (Chen et al., 2008), though the mechanism by which the loss of Dysbindin induces schizophrenia-like behaviors, remains unclear. Recently, we revealed that Dysbindin is involved in neural development through the regulation of the actin skeleton organization (Kubota et al., 2008). This study showed that knockdown of Dysbindin resulted in the aberrant organization of the actin cytoskeleton in SH-SY5Y cells. Furthermore, morphological abnormalities of the actin cytoskeleton were similarly observed in growth cones of cultured hippocampal neurons derived from sdy mice. In addition, a significant correlation was found between Dysbindin expression levels and the phosphorylation level of c-Jun N-terminal kinase (JNK), which is implicated in the regulation of cytoskeletal organization. These findings revealed that Dysbindin plays a key role in coordinating JNK signaling and actin cytoskeleton organization, which are required for neuronal development.

5. Mechanism of tumor necrosis factor receptor (TNFR) associated protein 1 (TRAP1)-N-cadherin alteration-induced psychiatric disorders

An increase in serum tumor necrosis factor-α (TNF-α) level is closely related to the pathogenesis of major depression (Irwin & Miller, 2007). The tumor necrosis factor receptor assoicated protein (TRAP1) was detected in whole brain lysates (Song et al., 1995). TRAP1 is a member of the heat shock protein 90 (HSP90) family and possesses ATPase activity, but lacks chaperone activity (Felts et al., 2000). However, the function and molecular mechanism of the TNF-TRAP system remain unclear. In the following section, we will describe the evidence that TRAP1 regulates the expression of adhesion molecule (Kubota et al., 2009).

5.1 TRAP1 is widely expressed in neurons through the brain, including in regions known to be affected in patients with major depression

In situ hybridization histochemistry and immunocytochemistry revealed that TRAP1 mRNA and protein are broadly expressed in neurons throughout the gray matter of the brain and the spinal cord, including in regions known to be affected in patients with major depression patients, such as the medial prefrontal cortex, hippocampus and nuclei producing monoamine: the substantia nigra pars compacta, dorsal raphe nucleus and locus ceruleus (Nestler et al., 2002; Berton and Nestler, 2006). However, glial cells such as astrocytes and oligodendrocytes are devoid of TRAP1. In addition, punctate immunostaining of TRAP1 was detected in the cytoplasm, which is consistent with previously reported mitochondrial localization of TRAP1 in a cell culture (Felts et al., 2000).

5.2 TRAP1 regulates cell adhesion

A striking cell-scattering phenotype was observed in TRAP1 knockdown SH-SY5Y cells. Cells transfected with siTRAP1 were dispersed throughout the dish, compared to cells transfected with control siRNA, which grew in aggregates resembling untransfected SH-SY5Y cells (Fig. 4A,B). This phenomenon was detectable as early as 24 h after transfection and became more prominent by 72 h after transfection. Immunostaining of actin filaments in siRNA-treated cells showed no difference in cytoskeletal structure. Quantification of the percentage of cells with no inter-cellular contacts after staining for actin detected a 6.2-fold increase in cells transfected with siTRAP1(36%) compared to cells transfected with control siRNA (5.8%). The cell aggregation assay revealed that TRAP1 knockdown cells were characterized by decreased efficacy of cell-cell adhesion compared with control cells, suggesting an alteration in calcium-dependent cell adhesion is affected. These results strongly indicate that TRAP1 regulates downstream molecules crucial for cell adhesion.

5.3 N-cadherin is transcriptionally down-regulated in TRAP1 knockdown cells

Expression levels of cell adhesion molecules, including N-cadherin, are directly related to the cell-scattering phenomenon (Hayashida et al., 2006; Yasuda et al., 2007) and N-cadherin mediates calcium-dependent cell adhesion in neuronal cells (Takeuchi and Nakagawa, 2007) Our findings showed that N-cadherin levels were remarkably decreased throughout the cytoplasm of TRAP1 knockdown cells, including around the membrane where cell-adhesion takes place, compared to control cells (Fig. 4C,D). Immunoblotting experiments confirmed this finding, showing a significant decrease in N-cadherin expression in TRAP1 knockdown cells from as early as 24 h until at least 2 h after transfection. However, the expression level of β-catenin, which is involved in the regulation of cell-adhesion, was unaffected. These results suggest that the cell scattering phenotype detected in TRAP1 knockdown cell is at least partially mediated by a reduction of N-cadherin expression in those cells.

To exclude the possibility that cell viability or migration may contributes to the cell-scattering phenotype in TRAP1 knockdown cells, we examined cell viability by the 3-(4,5-dimethylthiazol2-yl)-2,5-diphenyltetrazolium bromide (MTT) assay and migration by the wound-healing assay. Although a slight decrease in cell viability was observed in TRAP1 knockdown cells compared to control cells 48 h after transfection or later, no changes were detected 24 h after transfection, when the cell-scattering phenotype of TRAP1 was already observed. No significant changes in the rate of cell migration were observed.

To determine if down-regulation of N-cadherin induced by siTRAP1 occurs at the transcriptional level, N-cadherin mRNA levels were measured by real-time RT-PCR analysis 48 h after siRNA transfection, which showed that N-cadherin mRNA levels in TRAP1 knockdown cells were approximately 45% lower than in control cells. These results indicate that TRAP1 knockdown induces transcriptional down-regulation of N-cadherin.

5.4 E2F1, a putative transcription factor of N-cadherin, is down-regulated in TRAP1 knockdown cells

To determine the possible involvement of a transcription factor in down-regulation of N-cadherin in TRAP1 knockdown cells, a search DBTSS (Database of Transcriptional Start Sites) and TRANSFAC (The Transcription Factor Database) database was conducted. This search revealed a putative binding site for E2F1 in the promoter region of the N-cadherin gene. Immunoblot analysis and real-time PCR showed that E2F1 mRNA and protein levels were significantly decreased in TRAP1 knockdown cells (Fig. 4E), although the mRNA level of c-Myc, another representative transcription factor, was not affected, In addition, SH-SY5Y cells transfected with the N-cadherin-luciferase plasmid showed strong activity of the reporter, and this activity was suppressed in TRAP1 knockdown cells, mimicking the signaling cascade detected *in vitro*. Furthermore, exogenously transfected E2F1 showed a 7.5-fold induction of luciferase reporter activity relative to the control vector. These results indicate that E2F1 plays a regulatory role upstream of N-cadherin in TRAP1 knockdown cells.

5.5 Reduced phosphorylation of STAT causes down-regulation of E2F1 in TRAP1 knockdown cells

A recognition sequence for STAT3 is located 89bp upstream of the transcription initiation site of the *E2F1* gene. Upon activation, STAT3 proteins are tyrosine-phosphorylated, dimerize and translocate to the nucleus where the nuclear phospho-STAT binds to STAT recognition sites located in the promoter region of downstream genes to promote the transcription of those genes. In TRAP1 knockdown cells, the amount of tyrosine-phosphorylated STAT3, but not the total amount of tyrosine-phosphorylated STAT3, was significantly reduced. In addition, the promoter activity of the *E2F1* gene was significantly reduced if the STAT3 recognition site was deleted and if TRAP1 was knocked down. These data indicate that TRAP1 regulates the tyrosine phopsphorylation status of STAT3, which controls the expression of E2F1, and thus modulates the transcription of N-cadherin.

5.6 Role of the TRAP1-N-cadherin cascade in psychiatric disorders (Fig. 4G)

Because N-cadherin is involved in the morphogenesis of synapses (Okamura et al., 2004; Togashi et al., 2002), the regulation of the morphology of dendritic spines by TRAP1 via N-cadherin was analyzed in cultured hippocampal neurons. Spines are divided into 2 types based on morphology, namely: pedunculated and sessile with the former possessing a substantial stalk construction that is absent in the latter (Greg et al., 1999). In TRAP1 knockdown neurons, spines were predominantly sessile. Only 20.8% of spines displayed a pedunculate morphology compared with 66.7% in control neurons. Functionally, N-cadherin regulates synaptic plasticity; The activity dependent accumulation of N-cadherin

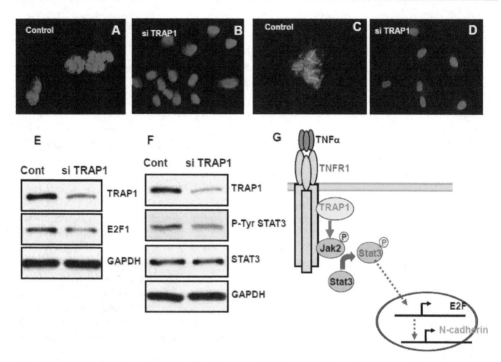

Fig. 4. TRAP1 is involved in cell-cell adhesion. A,B: Immunohistochemistry of TRAP1
knockdown and control cells stained with an anti-TRAP1 antibody (red) and DAPI(blue).
TRAP1 protein levels are markedly reduced in B. In addition, cells transfected with siTRAP1
were dispersed throughout   the dish (B), compared withcells transfected with control
siRNAthat grew in aggregates resembling untransfected SH-SY5Y cells. C,D: TRAP1
knockdown results in the down-regulation of N-cadherin. Immunohistochemistry of TRAP1
knockdown cells (D) compared with that of control cells (C) stained with an anti-N-cadherin
antibody (green) and DAPI (blue). In the TRAP1 knockdown cells (D), N-cadherin is
remarkably decreased throughout the cytoplasm, including around the membrane where
cell-adhesion takes place. C: Immunobloting of TRAP1 knockdown cells at 48 h after
transfection with anti-TRAP1, E2F1 and GAPDH antibodies.E2F1 expression was
significantly decreased in the TRAP1 knockdown cells, showing that TRAP1 knockdown
decreases the transcription activity of the N-cadherin promoter. D: Immunoblotting of
TRAP1 knockdown cells with anti-TRAP1, phosphorylated STAT3 (Tyr705) (p-Tyr STAT3),
STAT3 and GAPDH antibodies 48h after transfection. The level of tyrosine-phosphorylated
STAT was significantly reduced in the TRAP1 knockdown cells. D: Molecular pathway of
the TRAP1-N-cadherin cascade. TRAP1 regulates the tyrosine phosphorylation of STAT3,
which controls the expression of E2F, and thus, subsequently modulates the transcription of
N-cadherin. As TRAP1 mutations are deeply involved in major depression, the disturbance
of cell adhesion by the reduction of N-cadherin which causes abnormal neural circuit
formation, may be important in the pathogenesis of major depression.

at synapse is essential for spine remodeling and long term potentiation, suggesting that N-
cadherin plays important roles in higher brain function such as learning and memory. It is

therefore likely that altered expression of N-cadherin may be associated with the pathogenesis of mental disorders.

In support of this, we showed that 4 SNPs in the TRAP1 gene may be associated with the pathogenesis of mental disorders, particularly major depression, including 2 SNPs that cause an amino acid change in the TRAP1 protein:R07G (rs1 3926) and D395E (rs1 136948). Moreover, these 2 non-synonymous SNPs are located in the region critical for the binding of TRAP1 to TNFR1, suggesting that the binding affinity of TRAP1 to TNFR1 or the downstream signaling of TRAP1 might be altered in these disorders.

6. Involvement of DISC1 in psychiatric disorders (Fig. 5)

DISC1 has been identified as a potential susceptibility gene for major psychiatric disorders. Disruption of this gene by a balanced translocation (1:11,q42.1;q14.3) results in a predicted C-terminal truncation of the open reading frame. Furthermore, this anomaly is segregated with schizophrenia and affective disorders in a large Scottish family (Millar et al., 2000,2001). A frameshift mutation of DISC1 has been identified in an American family with schizophrenia and schizoaffective disorder (Sach et al., 2005), and the association of the SNPs of DISC1 with schizophrenia, schizoaffetive disorder and bipolar disorder has also been suggested (Hodgkinson et al., 2004).

6.1 Interacting partners bind to the area close to the translocation breakpoint of DISC1

DISC1 has been proposed to be a multifunctional protein that interacts with multifunctional protein that interact with multiple proteins of the centrosome and cytoskeletal system at a distinct domain (Morris et al., 2003; Ozaki et al., 2003). The function of DISC1 could therefore be regulated by DISC1 binding proteins. The DISC1 binding partners, fasciculation and elongation protein zeta-1 (Fez1), DBZ and kendrin were identified using yeast 2-hybrid analysis. The interaction between DISC1 and Fez1, DISC1 and DBZ, and DISC1 and Kendrin were confirmed by immunoprecipitation assays (Matsuzaki & Tohyama, 2007, Miyoshi et al., 2003, Hattori et al., 2007).

6.2 Role of DISC1-Fez1 interaction in psychiatric disorders (Miyoshi et al.,2003)

The DISC1-Fez1 interaction identified *in vitro* was confirmed *in vivo* by showing the co-localization of DISC1 and Fez1 in neurons of the hippocampus, cerebral cortex and olfactory bulb. Analysis of the intracellular localization of DISC1 revealed that DISC1 and Fez1 co-localize in growth cones in cultured hippocampal neurons. The interactions of these proteins are associated with F-actin. The finding that a molecular complex composed of DISC1, Fez1 and actin is located in the growth cone of neurite suggests the involvement of the DISC1-Fez1 interaction in neurite extension. In support of this, both DISC1 and Fez1 were found to be expressed in the brain during an early ontogenetical stage Honda et al., 2004). The physiological role of the DISC1-Fez1 interaction in neuronal cells, especially at the stage of neurite outgrowth, was examined using PC12 cells. After stimulation with nerve growth factor (NGF), PC12 cells cease proliferation and begin to extend neuritis. The interaction between FLAG-tagged DISC1 and endogenous Fez1 was examined over the course of neuronal differentiation. The amount of Fez1 in immunoprecipitates obtained using an anti-FLAG antibody was drastically increased upon NGF stimulation, suggesting that the DISC1-

Fez1 interaction is up-regulated by NGF stimulation.. Furthermore, when treated with NGF, DISC1-stable lines exhibited enhanced neurite extension compared to mock-stable cells. These findings established that DISC1 participates in neurite outgrowth through its interaction with Fez1. In schizophrenia with DISC1 translocation carriers, in which Fez1 cannot bind to DISC1 owing to its translocation, neuronal circuit formation may remain immature. In addition, an association between the SNPs of the *Fez1* gene and schizophrenia has also been suggested in a Japanese population (Yamada et al., 2004).

6.3 Role of the DISC1-Kendrin interaction in psychiatric disorders (Miyoshi et al., 2004; Shimizu et al. 2008)
6.3.1 The carboxy-terminal region of DISC1 is essential for the DISC1-Kendrin interaction

Kendrin, also referred to as pericentrin-B, is a calmodulin-binding protein localized specifically on centrosomes. Through the presence of the PACT domain, Kendrin is targeted to the centrosome. Co-localization of DISC1 and Kendrin was demonstrated in SH-SY5Y neuroblastoma cells transfected. In addition, co-localization of DISC1 and Kendrin at the centrosome was confirmed by immunohisotchemistry. DISC1 lacking the putative Kendrin binding region (amino acid 446-553) (KBR) is unable to target to the centrosome and distributes diffusely throughout the cytoplasm, showing that interaction of DISC1 with Kendrinis essential for its centrosomal localization. A direct yeast 2-hybrid interaction assay suggested that a short fragment of amino acids 446-533 of DISC1 constituting the binding region (KBR) was essential for the interaction with Kendrin. A subsequent study using immunoprecipitation assays in HEK293 cells in which Kendrin was endogenously expressed confirmed that KBR is critical for the interaction with Kendrin as described below. Cells were transiently transfected with expression vectors for HA-tagged full-length DISC1 (DISC1-HA) and the HA-tagged DISC1 deletion muctant lacking the KBR (DSC1ΔKBR-HA). Endogenous Kendrin was coimmunoprecipitated with DISC1-HA, but not with DISC1ΔKBR-HA. These findings indicate that KBR is the binding region of DISC1 to Kendrin. To examine whether KBR itself could bind to Kendrin, several DISC1 deletion mutants were prepared: GDBP (amino acids 348-597−FLAG, BPC (amino acids 598-854)-FLAG, BR (amino acids 446-633)-FLAG, KBR-FLAG and KBRC (amino acids 446-854)-FLAG. Surprisingly, endogenous Kendrin was detected in immunoprecipitates from cells transfected with KBRC-FLAG, but it was barely detected in immunoprecipitates from cells transfected with GDBP-FLAG, BPC-FLAG, BR-FRAG or KBR-FLAG. These findings confirm KBR as the Kendrin binding region for DISC1 to Kendrin, but also show that the binding to Kendrin is enhanced remarkably in the presence of the carboxy-terminal region downstream of KBR. Thus, KBR is required but not sufficient for the interaction, and the carboxy-terminal region of DISC1 is also indispensable for the binding to Kendrin.

6.3.2 The carboxy-terminal region of DISC1 is required for the localization of DISC1 to the centrosome

Next, we determined which part of DISC1 is indispensable for co-localization of DISC1 with Kendrin at the centrosome. KBRC-FLAG showed a diffuse pattern in the cytoplasm but clearly revealed a strong 'dot' pattern in the perinuclear area. The merged image of KBRC-FLAG and Kendrin showed that they were colocalized at the centrosome. On the other hand, localization of KBR-FLAG showed a diffuse distribution pattern in the nucleus and cytoplasm without strong staining at the centrosome. Staining of BR-FLAG and GDBP-FLAG was characterized by a small punctate distribution pattern, while BPC-FLAG exhibited a diffuse distribution in the cytoplasm. However, BPC-FLAG was not detected at the centrosome. Taken together, these findings demonstrate that the carboxy-terminal half of the DISC1 protein containing KBR and the downstream region of KBR are necessary and sufficient to target the DISC1 protein to the centrosome.

6.3.4 Inhibition of the DISC1-Kendrin interaction perturbs the microtubule network formation

The interaction of DISC1 with Kendrin at the centrosome and the key role of Kendrin in microtubule nucleation at the centrosome suggest that the interaction between DISC1 and Kendrin may affect microtubule network formation. The DISC1-binding region of Kendrin (DBR) (amino acids 2918-305) was first identified. To inhibit the DISC1-Kendrin interaction specifically at the centrosome, a FLAG-tagged DRB-PACT (DBR-PACT-FLAG) construct was prepared including DBR and PACT (a conserved centrosomal targeting motif in CG-NAP and pericentrin). Microtubule aster formation was then observed in COS cells transfected with either the DBZ-PACT-FLAG or PACT-FLAG expression vector. Mock-transfected cells showed microtubule aster formation at the centrosome. However, over-expression of DBR-PACT-FLAG resulted in a significant decrease in the percentages of cells containing the microtubule aster compared with cells expressing PACT-FLAG. In addition, over-expression of DISC1 ΔKBR-FLAG resulted in a significant decrease in the percentage of cells containing the microtubule aster compared with mock-transfected cells. These results show that the DISC1-Kendrin interaction is involved in brain maturation through the regulation of microtubule organization.

6.3.5 Role of the DISC1-Kendrin interaction in mental disorders

Over-expression of the DISC1-binding region of Kendrin perturbed the normal distribution of the stabilized microtubule network. The over-expression of DISC1 lacking the Kendrin binding site caused an impairment in microtubule aster formation. Carriers of the chromosomal translocation that segregates with mental diseases are expected to produce the truncated mutant DISC1 protein that lacks the carboxy-terminal region, or to have a reduced expression of the DISC1 protein. In the case of truncated mutant protein expression, this protein would not be able to target to the centrosome and interact with Kendrin, which might induce dysfunction of the microtubule network formation. Loss of DISC1 protein expression could lead to the dysfunction of microtubules by disrupting the DISC1-Kendrin interaction. In addition, involvement of Kendrin in olfactory cilia assembly was also reported (Miyoshi et al., 2009). Thus, the DISC1-Kendrin interaction plays a role in neuronal development by regulating microtubule organization, showing that mental diseases derived from DISC1 dysfunction are neurodevelopmental disease. In addition, our recent analysis showed an association between SNPs of the Kendrin gene and bipolar diseases (Anitha et al., 2005).

6.4 Role of DISC1 and its binding proteins with special reference to psychiatric disorders

The present review summarize results showing that DISC1 functions in neural network formation by interacting with several binding partners, including Fez1, DBZ, and

Kendrin, which binds to the area near the translocation site of DISC1. DISC1 interactions, including DISC1-Fez1, DISC1-DBZ and DISC1-Kendrin, all play a key role in neuronal development. Other groups have identified additional DISC1 interaction partner such as NudE-like (NUDEL) (Morris et al., 200; Ozeki et al., 2003), lissenchphaly-1 (LIS1) (Brandron et al., 2004), phosphodiesterase 4B (PDE4B) (Millar et al., 2005), glycogen synthase kinase 3 (GSK3) (Mao et al., 2009), the motor protein dynein and growth factor receptor bound protein 2 (Grb2) (Shinoda et al., 2007;Taya et al., 2007), and these binding partners suggested the functional involvement of DISC1 in neural development. DISC1 therefore plays crucial roles in brain development by affecting neuronal migration, neurite outgrowth and neural maturation through its interaction with several cytoskeletal proteins.

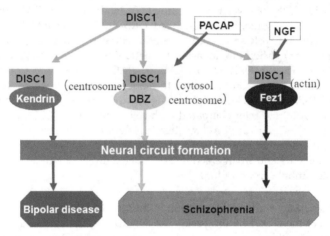

Fig. 5. DISC1 binding proteins that bind to an area near the translocation and their function. The binding between DISC1 and these molecules play a role in neurodevelopment. Accordingly mental disorders in which these molecules are implicated could be considered neurodevelopmental diseases.

7. Conclusion

The results summarized in this review indicate that the TRAP1 cascade, PACAP-stathmin1 cascade, PACAP-DBZ/DISC1 cascade, Dysbindin-MARCKS cascade, DISC1-Fez1 interaction and DISC1-Kendrin interaction are all involved in neural development. In addition, the molecules mentioned above are associated with schizophrenia or bipolar disease, showing that the neural development that is associated with these systems is disturbed in the brains of patients with either of these disease.

8. Acknowledgment

This research was partly supported by Ministry of Education, Culture, Sports, Science and Technology of Japan and by a grant from Dainippon Sumitomo Pharma Co. Ltd.
We thank Mrs. Etsuko Moriya for preparing this manuscript.

9. References

Angrist, B. & van Kammen, D.P., (1984). CNS stimulants as tools in the study of schizophrenia. *Trend Neurosci.* Vol.7, pp. 388-390

Anitha, A., Nakamura, K., Yamada, K. et al. (2008). Gene and expression analyses reveal enhanced expression of pericentrin2 (PCNT2) in bipolar disorder. *Biol. Psychiatry* Vol. 63, pp. 678-685

Berton, O. & Nestler, E.J. (2006). New approaches to antidepressant drug discovery: beyond monoamines. *Nat. Rev. Neurosc*i. Vol. 7, pp. 372−377

Brandron, N.J., Handford, E.J., Schurov, I. et al. (2004). Disrupted in Schizophrenia 1 and Nudel form a neurodevelopmentally regulated protein complex: implication for schizophrenia and other major neurological disorders. *Mol. Cell Neurosci.* Vol. 25, pp. 42-55

Bray, N.J., Preece, A., Williams, N.M., et al. (2005). Haplotypes at the dystrobrevin binding protein 1 (DTNBP1) gene locus mediate risk for schizophrenia through reduced DTNBP1 expression. *Hum. Mol. Genet.* Vol. 14, pp. 1947-1954

Burdick, K.E., Lencz, T., Funke, B. et al. (2006). Genetic variation in DTNBP1 influences general cognitive ability. Hum. Mol. Genet. Vo. 15, No.10, pp.1563-1568

Chen, X.W., Feng, Y.Q., Hao,C.J. et al. (2008). DTNBP1, a schizophrenia susceptibility gene, affects kinetics of transmitter release. J. Cell Biol. Vol. 181, 791-801

Chiba, S., Hashimoto, R., Hattori, S. et al. (2006). Effect of antipsychotic drugs on DISC1 and dysbindin expression in mouse frontal cortex and hippocampus. J. Neural Transm. Vol.113, No.9, pp. 1337-1346

Corvin, A., Donohoe, G., Nangle, J.M. et al. (2008). A dysbindin risk haplotype associated with less severe mani-type symptoms in psychosis. *Neurosci. Lett.* Vol. 431, No.2, 146-149

Creese, I., Burt, D.R. & Snyder, S.H. (1976). Dopamine receptor binding predicts clinical and pharmacological potencies of antischizophrenic drugs. *Science* Vol. 192, pp. 481-483

Donohoe, G., Morris, D.W., Nangle, J.M. et al. (2007). Variance in neurocognitive performance is associated with dysbindin-1 in schizophrenia: a preliminary study. *Neuropsychologia* Vol. 45, No. 2, pp. 454-458

Felts, S.J., Owen, B.A., Nguyen, P. et al. (2000). The hsp90-related protein TRAP1 is a mitochondrial protein with distinct functional properties. *J. Biol. Chem.* Vol. 275, pp. 3305-3312

Feng, Y.Q., Zhou, Z.Y., He, X. et al. (2008). Dysbindin deficiency in sandy mice causes reduction of snapin and displays behabiors related to schizophrenia. *Schizophr. Res.* Vol. 106, pp. 218-227

Hashimoto, H., Ishiharas, T., Shigemoto, R. et al., (1993). Molecular cloning and tissue distribution of a receptor for pituitary adenylate cyclase activating polypeptide. *Neuron* Vol. 11. pp. 333-342

Greg, S., Nelson, S. &Michael, H. (1999). Dendrites. Oxford University Press, New York

Hashimoto, H., Shintani, N., Tanaka, K. et al. (2001). Altered psychomotor behaviors in mice lacking pituitary adenylate cyclase-activating polypeptide (PACAP). *Proc. Natl. Acad. Sci. USA* . Vol. 98, pp.13355-13360

Hashimoto, R., Hashimoto, H., Shintani, N. et al. (2007). Pituitary adenylate cyclase-activating polypeptide is asociated with schizophrenia. *Mol. Psychiatry* Vol. 12, pp. 1026-1032

Hattori, S., Murotani, T., Matsuzaki, S. et al., Behavioral abnormalities and dopamine reductions in sdy mice with a deletion in Dtnbp1, susceptibility gene for schizophrenia. *Biochem. Biophys. Res. Commun.* Vol. 373, pp. 298-302

Hattori, T., Baba, K., Matsuzaki, S., et al. (2007). A novel DISC1-interacting partner DISC1-binding Zinc finger protein: implication in the modulation of DISC1-dependent neurite outgroath. *Mol. Psychiatry* Vol. 12, pp. 398-407

Hayashida, Y., Urata, Y., Muroi, E. et al. (2006). Calreticulin represses E-cadherin gene expression in Madin-Darby canine kidney cells via Slug. *J. Biol. Chem.* Vol. 281, pp. 32469-32484

Hodgkinson, C..A., Goldman, D., Jaeger, J. et al. (2004). Disrupted in schizophrenia 1 (DISC1): association with schizophrenia, schizoaffective disorder,and bipolar disorder. *Am. J. Hum. Genet.* Vol. 75, pp. 862-872

Honda, A., Miyoshi, K., Baba, K., et al. (2004). Expression of fasciculation and elongation protein zeta-1 (Fesz1) in the developing rat brain. *Mol. Brain Res.* Vol. 122, pp. 89-92

Irwin, M.R. & Miller, A.H. (2007). Depressive disorders and immunity: 20 years of progress and discovery. *Brain Behav. Immun.* Vol. 21,pp. 374-383

Katayama,T., Hattori, T., Yamada,K. et al., Role of the PACAP-PAC1-DISC1 and PACAP-PAC1-stathmin1 systems in schizophrenia and bipolar disorder; novel treatment mechanisms? *Pharmacogenomics* Vol. 10, No. 12, pp. 1967-1978, ISSN1462-2416

Kubota, K., Inoue, K., Hashimoto, R. et al. (2009). Tumor necros i s factor receptor-associated protein 1 regulates cell adhesion and synaptic morphoogy via modulation of N-cadherin expression. *J. Neurochem.* Vol. 110, pp.496-508

Kubota, K., Kumamoto, N., Matsuzaki, S. et al. (2009). Dysbindin engages in c-Jun N-terminal kinase activity and cytoskeletal organization. *Biochem. Biophy. Res. Commun.* Vol. 73, pp. 191-195

Kumamoto N., Matsuzaki, S., Inoue, K. et al. (2006). Hyperactivation of midbrain dopaminergic system in schizophrenia could be attributed to the down-regulation of dysbindin. *Biochem. Biophy. Res. Comm.* Vol. 345, pp. 904-909.

Lieberman, J.A., Kane, J.M. & Alvir, J. (1987). Provocative tests with psychostimulant drugs in schizophrenia. *Psychopharmacol. (Berl)* Vol. 91, pp. 415-433

Mao, Y., Ge, X., Franki, C.L. et al. (2009). Disrupted in schizophrenia 1 regulates neuronal progenitor proliferation via modulation of GSK3 β / β-catenin signaling. *Cell* Vol. 136, pp. 1017-1031

Matsuzaki, S. & Tohyama, M. (2007). Molecular mechanism of schizophrenia with reference to disrupted-in-schizophrenia 1 (DISC1). *Neurochem. Int.* Vol. 51, pp. 165-172

Millar, J.K., Wilson-Annan, J.C., Anderson, S. et al. (2000). Distribution of tw novel genes by a translocation co-segregating with schizophrenia. *Hum. Mol. Genet.* Vol. 9, pp. 1415-1423

Millar, J.K., Christie, A., Anderson, S. et al. (2001). Genomic structure and localization within a linkage hotspot of distrupted in schizophrenia 1, a gene disrupted by a translocation segregating withschizophrenia. *Mol. Psychaitry* Vol. 6, pp. 173-178

Millar, J.K., Pickard, B.S., Mackie, S. et al. (2005). DISC1 and PDE4B are interacting genetic factors in schizophrenia that regulate cAMP signaling. *Science* Vol. 310, pp. 1187-1191

Miyoshi, K., Asanuma, I., Miyazaki, F.J. et al. (2004). DISC1 localizes to the centrosome by binding to kendrin. *Biochem. Biophys. Res. Commun.* Vol. 317, pp. 1195-1199.

Miyoshi, K., Kasahara, K., Miyazaki, I. et al. (2009). Pericentrin, a centrosomal protein related to microcephalic primordial dwarfism, is required for olfactory cilia assembly in mice. *FASEB J.* Vol. 10, pp. 3289-3297

Miyoshi, K., Honda, A., Baba, K. et al. (2003). Disrupted-In-Schizophrenia 1, a candidate gene for schizophrenia, participates in neurite outgrowth. *Mol. Psychiatry* Vol. 8, pp. 685-684

Morris, J.A., Kandpal,G., Ma, L. et al. (2003). DISC1 (disrupted-in-schizophrenia 1) is a centrosome-associated protein that interacts with MAP1A, MIPT3,ATF4/5 and Nudel: regulation and loss of interaction with mutation. *Hum. Mol. Genet.* Vol. 12, 1591-1608

Nestler, E.J., Barrot, M., DiLeone, R.J. et al. (2002). Neurobiology of depression. *Neuron*, Vol. 34, pp. 13-25.

Numakawa, T., Yagasaki, Y., Ishimoto, T. et al. (2004). Evidence of novel neuronal functions of dysbindin, a susceptibility gene for schizophrenia. *Hum. Mol. Genet.* Vol. 13,2699-2708

Okuda, H., Kuwahara, R., Matsuzaki, S. et al. (2010). Dysbindin regulates the transcriptional level of   myristoylated alanine-rich protein kinase C substrate via the interaction with NF-YBin mice brain. *PLoS one* Vol. 5, Issue1 pp.e8773

Okumura, K., Tanaka, H., Yagita, Y. et al. (2004). Cadherin activity is required for activity-induced spine remodeling. *J. Cell Biol.* Vol. 167, pp. 961-972

Ozeki, Y., Tomoda, T., Kleiderlein, J. et al. (2003). Disrupted-in-schizophrenia-1 (DISC-1): mutant truncation prevents binding to NudE-like (NUDEL) and inhibits neurite outgrowth. *Proc. Natl. Acad. Sc. USA.* Vol. 100, pp.289-294

Sachs, N.A., Sawa, A., Holmes, S.E. et al. (2005). A frameshift mutation in disrupted in schizophrenia 1 in an American family with schizophrenia, schizoaffective disorder. *Mol. Psychiatry* Vol. 10, pp. 758-764

Seeman, P. & Lee,T. (1975). Antipsychotic drugs; direct correlation between clinical potency and presynaptic action on dopamine neurons. *Science* Vol. 188, pp. 1217-1219

Shimizu, S., Matsuzaki, S., Hattori, T. et al. (2008). DISC1-kendrin interaction is involved in centrosomal microtubule network formation. *Biochem. Biophys. Res. Commun.* Vol. 377, pp. 1051-1056

Shintani, N., Mori, W., Hashimoto, H., et al. (2992). Defects in reproductive functions in PACAP-deficient femal mice. *Regul. Pep.* Vol. 109, pp. 45-48

Shinoda, T., Taya, S., Tsuboi, D et al. (2007). DISC1 regulates neurortophion-induced axon elongation via interaction with Grb2. *J. Neurosci.* Vol. 27, pp.4-14

Sillitoe, R.V., Benson, M.A., Blake, D.J. et al. (2003). Abnormal dysbindin expression in cerebellar mossy fiber synapses in the mdx mouse model of Duchenne muscular dystrophy. *J. Neurosci.* Vol. 23, No. 16, pp. 6576-6585

Song, H.Y., Dunbar, Y., Zhang, J.D. et al. (1995). Identification of a protein with homology to hsp90 that binds the type 1 tumor necrosis factor receptor. *J. Biol. Chem.* Vol. 270, pp. 3574-3581.

Takeuchi, M. & Nakagawa, S. (2001). Cadherin-dependent cell-cell adhesion. *Curr. Protoc. Cell Biol.* Chapter9, Unit 9.3

Talbot, K., Eidem, W.L., Tinsley, M.A. et al. (2004). Dysbindin-1 is reduced in intrinsic, glutamatergic terminals of the hippocampal formation in schizophrenia. *J. Clin. Invest.* Vol. 113, pp. 1353-1363

Taya, S., Shinoda, T., Tsuboi, D. et al. (2007). DISC1 regulates the transport of the NUDEL/LIS1/14silon complex through kinesin-1. *J. Neurosci. Vol.* 27, pp. 15-26

Togashi, H., Abe, K., Mizoguchi, A. et al. (2002). Cadhelin regulates dendritic spine morphogenesis. *Neuron*, Vol. 35, pp. 77-89

Vaudry, D., Gonzalez, BJ, Basille, M. et al. (2000). Pituitary adenylate cyclase-activating polypeptide and its receptors: from structure to function. *Pharmacol. Rev. Vol.* 52, pp. 269-234

Weicker, C.S., Straub, R.E., McClintock, B.W., Matsumoto, M. et al. (2004). Human dysbindin (DTNBP1) gene expression in normal brain and in schizophrenic prefrontal cortex and midbrain. *Arch. Gen. Psychiatry* Vol. 61, pp. 544-555

Yamada, K., Matsuzaki,S., Hattori, T. et al. (2010). Increased stathmin1 expression in the dentate gyrus of mice causes abnormal axonal arborizations. *PLoS one* Vol.5, Issue1, e8596

Yamada,K., Nakamura, K., Minabe, Y. et al. (2004). Association analysis of FEZ1 variants with schizophrenia in Japanese cohorts. *Biol.Psychiatry* Vol. 56, pp. 683-690

Yasuda, S., Tanaka, H., Sugiura, H. et al. (2007). Activity-induced procadherin arcadlin regulates dendritic spine number by triggering N-cadherin endocytosis via TAO2beta and p38 MAP kinases. *Neuron* Vol. 56, pp. 456-471

Zinkstok, J.R., de Wilde, O., van Amelsvoort, T.A. et al. (2007). Association between the DTNBP1 gene and intelligence: a case-control study in young patients with schizophrenia and related disorders and unaffected siblings. Behav, Brain Func. Vol., 3, pp.19

9

Psychogenic Movement Disorders

Carlo Dallocchio

Department of Medical Specialities, Division of Neurology, Ospedale Civile
Voghera (Pavia)
Italy

1. Introduction

Abnormal movements and postures resulting from primary psychiatric disease are a diagnostic dilemma because all types of movement disorders may be mimicked by a psychogenic disease, including akinetic-rigid and hyperkinetic disorders, with the latter more frequent, particularly tremor, myoclonus, and dystonia (Williams et al., 2005; Reich, 2006).

Psychogenic movement disorders (PMDs), are a valuable model for all medically unexplained symptoms and raise arduous challenges for diagnosis and treatment indicating our restricted understanding of the true pathogenesis that causes them. A multiplicity of terms such as "hysterical conversion", "functional", "psychosomatic", "neuropsychiatric", "dissociative motor disorders",and so on, have been applied to describe neurological symptoms that cannot be attribute to any known organic disease (Mace & Trimble, 1991; Lang, 2006). The term "psychogenic" is the commonest in the movement disorder literature, but there is no unanimity whether it reflects the precise nature of a syndrome containing both neurologic and psychiatric components.

By the late-19th century, psychoanalytic theory ruled medical reasoning about these symptoms. Originally referring to these disorders as hysteria, neuropsychiatrists began illustrating the various clinical phenomenological aspects of such disorders. Paralysis, tremors, convulsions and sensory alterations were identified as sometimes being due to hysteria. Subsequently, different etiologies of dystonia, tremor, myoclonus and other movement disorders were recognized. Over the years, newer clinical criteria, laboratory investigations, particularly neurophysiological findings, and improved neuroimaging have provided significant insights about the psychogenicity of the diagnosis. However, a misdiagnosis is possible either on patients originally believed to have a conversion disorder or because PMD was never considered on differential diagnosis (Rosebush & Mazurek, 2006; Lang & Gupta, 2009).

The pathophysiology of PMDs are not yet well known, but functional brain imaging studies combined with other neurophysiologic techniques are starting to help understand them (Stone & Carson, 2011). These studies promise an understanding of these symptoms in parallel neurologic and psychiatric ways.

The diagnosis of a psychogenic movement disorder is often difficult and the level of diagnostics that the clinician has for PMD varies remarkably, depending on the clinical feature of the movement disorders and the accompanying signs and symptoms. PMDs are classified by the Diagnostic and Statistical Manual of Mental Disorders (DSM-IV) of the American Psychiatric Association as conversion disorder of motor subtype and must be differentiated from factitious disorder and malingering, in which the abnormal movements are purposefully forged. Since most patients with conversion symptoms are found to have "no psychiatric disease" by the psychiatric and "no neurologic disease" by the neurologist, a multidisciplinary treatment approach, including the movement disorders neurologist, the consulting psychiatrist, and frequently a physical therapist, is crucial in obtaining symptom remission in many subjects (Williams et al., 2005; Stone et al., 2010).

Although evidence for treatment of PMDs are lacking and is mainly based on case control, retrospective, or case report studies, the therapeutic process starts with the diagnosis and the explanation of the symptoms to the patient. To date, the treatment for each patient with PMDs is individualized and may include psychotherapeutic interventions, behavioral therapy, hypnosis, pharmachotherapy, physical therapy, and other approach.

Physicians should not underestimate the importance of distress and disability that subjects with these symptoms suffer. Failure to diagnose a PMDs inevitably delays treatment and may perpetuate a patient's situation of disability (Williams et al., 2005). In addiction, patients with somatisation had approximately twice the medical care utilisation and twice the annual medical care costs of non-somatizing patients and spend 1.3 to 3.9 days in bed per month compared to an average of one day or less for patients with major medical problems (Smith et al., 1986; Barsky et al., 2005). The current chapter reviews empirical evidence concerning clinical manifestations of PMDs and summarizes how PMDs are currently diagnosed, investigated and treated.

2. Epidemiology and risk factors

Although psychogenic neurological symptoms are common and account for 1–9% of neurological symptoms observed in the general population (Lempert et al., 1990; Factor et al., 1995), the following caveats should be borne in mind: (i) available reports result from tertiary movement disorders centers, and therefore it is difficult to valuate how common these disorders are in the general population or even what is the prevalence respect to all conversion disorders, (ii) the insufficiency of confirmatory diagnostic testing prejudices case definition even when clinical satisfactory criteria are applied and (iii) several clinical settings and situations (e.g., neurology or psychiatry in- or outpatient service, emergency room or general practitioner cases, chronic or refractory cases, etc.) may confound case ascertainment (Lang, 2006). In the only series dividing medically unexplained motor symptoms into "absence of motor function" and "presence of abnormal motor activity", 48% of the patients had index symptoms in the former category, while 52% had symptoms, such as tremor, dystonia or ataxia (Crimlisk et al., 1998).

PMDs also can occur over a wide range of ages from teenage to the mid seventies (Deuschl et al.,1998; Feinstein et al., 2001). The mean age at onset described in several case series on these disorders ranges between 37 years and 50 years and women are predominantly affected with a range of 61–87% (Hinson et al., 2005; Factor et al., 1995).

There are no data on racial distribution in the published research, however a trans-cultural comparison between patients with these disorders in the USA, in Spain, and in Brazil showed essentially similar demographic and clinical characteristics by ethnic origin (Cubo et al., 2005; Munhoz et al., 2010). Nearly 15% of patients with a psychogenic movement disorder have also an underlying organic movement disorder (Ranawaya el al., 1990).

Curiously, PMDs are frequently seen in subjects employed in health care professions or allied health care professionals possibly due to the exposure to disease and those who have witnessed the organic form of the movement disorder (e.g. Parkinson's disease) in other relatives (Miyasaki et al., 2003;)

More frequently, PMDs are encountered in the context of a second coexisting psychiatric illness. Feinstein and colleagues followed 88 patients suffering from psychogenic movement disorders, over an average of 3 years. 42 patients agreed to undergo a structured psychiatric interview. The most common life time prevalence rates were found for depression (42%), anxiety disorders (62%), a combination of depression and anxiety (29%) and conversion disorder (95%). Personality disorder (antisocial, borderline, dependent, avoidant or a mixture of those) was diagnosed in 42% of patients tested (Feinstein et al., 2001). Among the a series of 127 patients with psychogenic tremor, depression (51%) and anxiety (31%) were the most common psychiatric co-morbidities (Jankovic & Thomas, 2006).

Risk factors for these disorders include: history of sexual abuse or rape, physical trauma, previous surgery, major stressful life experiences (Williams et al., 2005; Feinstein et al., 2001). Many patients with functional neurologic symptoms report just as much physical disability and are more distressed than patients with neurologic disease. Furthermore, subjects with these symptoms are more likely to be out of work because of ill health than the general population (Stone et al., 2011).

3. Pathophysiology

In reviewing the history of psychogenic neurologic disorders, hysterical paralisis and sensory loss have been known presumably back in antiquity (Ng BY, 1999) and have been debated before the late 19th century, when Charcot, Janet, Breuer, and Freud gave a systematic psychological account of these phenomena. (Charcot, 1889; Janet, 1907; Freud, 1910). From then on, there has been a large body of literature regarding the possible psychogenic, psychoanalytical, cultural and biological mechanisms underlying PMDs.

According to Janet, traumatic events can cause a functional separation (dissociation) of structures of memory, identity, insight, and perception of the environment from conscious awareness. As a result, unexplained symptoms emerge from the activation of these dissociated structures (Janet, 1889). Patients suffering from non-organic motor symptoms are singularly susceptible to hypnosis, an inducible state of dissociation.

This theory was later developed by Breuer and Freud, who considered dissociation a psychological defence mechanism rather than a disorganizing phenomenon: the mental conflict is partially or completely resolved by the expression of physical symptoms, which is called primary gain. According to this psychodynamic model, dissociation preserves the subject from the invalidating affect associated with remembrances of trauma by its "conversion" in to somatic symptoms and once these latter have developed, may confer further advantages to the patient (attention, solicitude, social interaction, etc.) or "secondary gains"(Breuer & Freud, 1895).

In contemporary psychiatry, dissociative symptoms and dissociation as a mechanism are taken to point to a role traumatic events in pathogenesis. Various factors may provide to the pathway to conversion disorder, perhaps comprehending, concurrent somatic illness in adolescence or adulthood, parental illness in the subject childhood, and early illness. In particular physical or sexual abuse in childhood have considered key factors in the generation of vulnerability to unexplained somatic symptoms (Ovsiew, 2006).

The definite nature of emotional disorders responsible of psychogenic disorders, and their functional consequences on neural systems in the brain, still remain largely unknown.

In the closing decades of the 19th century, researchers have progressively been looking for organic correlates of PMDs and the neural mechanism perspective became more approved with the advent of novel functional neuroimaging methods. These new approaches have now allowed to detect in vivo regionally specific changes in cerebral blood flow and task-related changes in the attempt to identify specific neural correlates associated with conversion symptoms, that is the "dynamic lesion" that Charcot considered responsible for the neurological signs he observed in patients affected by "hysteric movement disorders".

PMDs evoke notable interest because, as protean disorders of willed action or intention, the underlying mechanism are supposed to be the result of unconscious processes, a sort of impairment to the volition system, once any demonstrative organic or feigning dysfunctions has been excluded (Fink, 2006). Psychogenic movements may be voluntary or involuntary. Factitious disorder and malingering describe when the disorder is voluntary, and the patients are lying. On the other hand, most patients with PMDs have a conversion aetiology and manifest movements that look voluntary, even if patients declare that the movements are involuntary. By a physiological point of view we can not tell the difference between voluntary and involuntary, but we know (most of time) that both are preceded by a normal "readiness potential" or so called Bereitschaftspotential, a manifestation of cortical contribution to the pre-motor planning of volitional movement (Shibasaki & Hallet, 2006) and share cortical structures that are involved in movement planning and execution.

In a go-nogo task, while a patient underwent functional magnetic resonance imaging (fMRI), Cojan et al. demonstrated that distinct inhibitory mechanism are implicated in simulation and conversion disorders and that conversion symptoms do not act through cognitive inhibitory circuits, but involve selective activations in midline brain regions associated with self-related representations and emotion regulation (Cojan, 2009). Other neuroimaging results have shown increase activation in limbic regions, such as orbitofrontal or cingulated cortex during conversion symptoms affecting different motor or sensory modalities (Vuilleumier, 2005, Nowak, 2009). A recent single photon emission computed tomography (SPECT) study by Czarnecki et al. suggested that the prominent hypoperfusion of the prefrontal and anterior cingulate cortex in patients with psychogenic tremor likely indicates deactivation of the anterior portion of the default mode network (the baseline state of the brain that deactivates during goal-directed activity), which could prove to be a peculiar marker of PMDs. Moreover, this study reported resting hyperperfusion in left insula and left inferior frontal gyrus in psychogenic tremor that may also prove to be a disease characteristic (Czarnecki et al. 2011).

Voon and colleagues used functional magnetic resonance imaging (fMRI) to study patients with psychogenic tremor who could voluntarily mimic their tremor and showed hypoperfusion of the right temporal parietal junction only during involuntary movements. The authors speculate that this hypoactivity may reflect the lack of an appropriate sensory prediction signal, being the right temporal parietal junction implicated as a general comparator of internal predictions with actual events. This suggests a loss of self-agency o awareness that made the movements feel involuntary (Voon et al., 2010).

There may be a pathologic unconscious influence on movement production associated with a disconnection between movement production and sense of volition (Hallet, 2010). Besides, earliest affective or stress-related factors, neuropsychological and psychosocial processes, perhaps involved primitive reflexive mechanisms of protection and alertness that are not fully independent of conscious control (Vuilleumier, 2005). This prominent evidence in favour of multi causes of PMDs requires a multifaceted approach integrating innovative neuroimaging and neurophysiological techniques with social, psychological and psychodynamic theories.

4. Clinical manifestations and diagnostic clues

The diagnosis of PMDs remains a fascinating and challenging dilemma in both clinical neurology and psychiatry. It should not be considered as a diagnosis of exclusion but should be established on positive clinical criteria to determine whether abnormal movements are produced by organic disease, psychiatric disorder, or both (Jankovic & Thomas, 2006). Taking into account that unnecessary investigations should be prevented, more notable evidence is required before a diagnosis of psychogenic disorder can be confirmed. Some studies, including exhaustive neurologic assessments and modern diagnostic techniques, have shown that a misdiagnosis is possible on long-term follow-up of patients initially diagnosed with a conversion disorder and later identified as having an organic disorder (Moene et al., 2000; Lang, 2006; Lang & Gupta, 2009). Otherwise, failure to make the diagnosis arises because PMDs were seldom contemplated in the differential diagnosis, especially in patients who have a coexistent neurologic disease, such as neurodegenerative or demyelinating disorder or epilepsy. Coexistent organic neurologic disease was present in 37% of patients with psychogenic tremor followed for over 3 years (Jankovic et al., 2004). Additionally, the problem is exacerbated by a tendency among physicians to be concerned about missing an "organic" diagnosis in order to relieve the patient from a "functional" one, even if the latter is treatable and the former is not (Rosebush & Mazurek, 2006). Another troubling side of these disorders is the reluctance of many physicians to put their judgments and conclusions into a transparent discussion with the patient. So an ambivalent communication wanes to deliver the presumed diagnosis in real terms and running the risk that patients continue to explore for months or years further opinion through "doctor shopping". (Friedman & LaFrance WC, 2010).

Because many patients or family members of patients with PMDs are strongly reluctant to the diagnosis not explained organically and may resistant to a psychiatric referral, a multidisciplinary approach, including the general or movement disorders neurologist and the consulting psychiatrist is essential. The role of the neurologist is primary in determining whether there is an underline neurologic disorder and whether it could explain the clinical picture. Hardly mental health professionals undertake a treatment of such patients without the neurologic diagnosis has been either established or dismissed (Feinstein et al., 2001; Williams et al., 2005).

Fahn and Williams developed four degrees of certainty for the diagnosis (Tab. 1) of psychogenic dystonia, which are commonly applied in clinical practice and research to all PMDs (Fahn & Williams, 1988). Shill and Gerber formulated further criteria with a denomination of "clinically proven PMDs" which requires remission when the patient is unobserved or with psychotherapy or when there is a Bereitschaftspotential on electroencephalography (for myoclonus only). Moreover, they added further criteria of PMDs to include excessive pain or fatigue and previous disease exposure (Shill & Gerber, 2006). Developing this idea, Hallett proposed that a new designation of "laboratory proven PMDs" could be considered (Peckham & Hallett, 2009). A recent study demonstrated that the finger tapping test may provide an objective tool to aid the clinical diagnostic criteria set by Fahn and Williams for identifying patients with PMDs (Criswell et al., 2010).

Documented psychogenic
Movements are persistently relieved by psychotherapy or psychological suggestion or with the administration of placebos. If the patient is observed to be symptom free when left alone, this may also be documented as psychogenic; however, this feature is usually indicative of malingering or factitious disorder.
Clinically Established Psychogenic
Inconsistent or incongruent with classical dystonia (on examination, the patient is unable to move the limbs but is able to dress herself in daily life). In addition, one or all of the following is highly suggestive: other neurologic signs present that are psychogenic (self-inflicted injuries, false weakness, false sensory findings), an obvious psychiatric disturbance is present, and multiple somatizations are present.
Probable Psychogenic
Movements are inconsistent or incongruent, but there are no other features (as above) to further support the diagnosis. Movements are consistent with organic dystonia, but there are other features on examination to suggest psychogenicity (self-inflicted injuries, false weakness, false sensory findings). Multiple somatizations are present, but movements are consistent with organic dystonia.
Possible Psychogenic
An obvious emotional disturbance is present, but movements are consistent with organic dystonia.

Table 1. The classification of psychogenic movement disorders (Williams & Fahn, 1995)

An additional support, that seems appropriate to capture the complexity of PMDs and that can be used to assess PMDs and test the efficacy of intervention strategies is the Psychogenic Movement Disorder Rating Scale (PMDRS). This clinimetric assessment describes and quantifies the complicated phenomenology of PMDs, and provides the following six types of information: movement phenomenology, anatomic distribution and severity of abnormal movements, duration of abnormal movements, assessment of two functions (gait and speech), impairment-based incapacitation by abnormal movement or function, and total severity score (Hinson et al., 2005).

It should be emphasized that observation and examination are the most important tools for the physician looking for inconsistency of movements. The first trace of psychogenicity in a patient presenting with such abnormal motor activity can be obtained by history (Table 2.A). This may comprise psychiatric history, childhood history, personality factors, drug experience, recent personal and family life events, stressful situations or work-related injury, litigation or compensation pending, personal encounter or knowledge of similar disorders serving as a "model" and possible secondary gain (Bhatia & Schneider, 2007; Nowak & Fink, 2009).

In general, the manner of onset characterizes the clinical presentation of PMDs (Table 2.B): symptoms appear abruptly, frequently in the context of precipitating factors and, the highest disability and severity are reached quickly (Feinstein et al., 2001). Important specifics of PMDs are an inconsistent character of movement (unusual presentation in amplitude, frequency, distribution), and they may increase with attention or decrease with distraction (Miyasaki, 2003). A deliberate slowness of movement is incongruent with an organic movement disorders, as well as simultaneous occurrence of variegated abnormal movements and disfunctions, and peculiarly, patients may seem to struggle and put in more effort than needed to complete the task (Hinson & Blacke Haren 2006; Bhatia & Schneider 2007). Often, this is manifest by sighing, grimacing, and using their whole body to do a movement. The movements themselves may appear bizarre and should be incongruous with a known movement disorder.

There are controversial points of view whether there is a place for placebo in management of PMDs, as it reflects ethical evaluations and can infringe the relationship between physician and patient. Although a response to placebo of a movement disorder is seriously supportive of a diagnosis of PMDs (Espay et al., 2009). Equally, spontaneous resolution and improvement of unexplained symptoms with psychiatric evaluation or psychotherapy are highly suggestive of psychogenic aetiology of them (Fahn, 1994).

Diagnostic testing should be used primarily to give further support to the underlying clinical suspicion that it is psychogenic. Routine blood test including haematology, thyroid function, renal and liver function, and evaluation for Wilson's disease may be helpful. Magnetic resonance imaging can be helpful for excluding an underlying structural, vascular or demyelinating lesion, particularly if the abnormal movement is unilateral or asymmetrical. Neurophysiology studies to evaluate tremor and myoclonus can aid in the diagnosis of PMDs. Dopamine transporter (DAT) SPECT and Fluorodopa (18F-dopa) PET scans have been proven quite helpful in distinguishing psychogenic parkinsonism from Parkinson's disease or essential tremor (Kagi et al., 2010; Czarnecki et al. 2011).

The role of the consulting psychiatrist is to interpret the psychopathology present, ascertain its relevance to the presenting PMDs symptoms and establish a positive rapport with the patient. If this appears feasible, the psychiatrist will then begin the treatment course, with adequate collaborative support from neurologist (Williams et al., 2005).

However, psychiatric aspects and categorical differentiations, which are discussed in detail elsewhere in this book, also apply to PMDs. In brief, the psychiatric examination includes research of individual psychodynamics and significant environmental events as well as a complete multiaxial delineation of specific psychopathology according to the official psychiatric classification system such as the Diagnostic and Statistical Manual of Mental Disorders, fourth Edition (DSM-IV). The primary psychopathology underlying PMDs can be divided into two categoric diagnostic subgroups: somatoform disorders on the one hand, and factitious disorders and malingering on the other. The first category includes conversion disorder and somatization disorder. Conversion disorder is likely the most common mechanism of PMDs and is defined by the DSM-IV criteria as a disorder including one or more symptoms, that are not the result of a neurological disorder, affecting voluntary motor or sensory function that suggest a medical condition and is associated with psychological factors.

The primary psychiatric diagnosis varies: most cases are considered to be conversion disorders, in which the problem is generated by an unconscious mechanism, but infrequently some are factitious disorders or malingering, in which the abnormal movements are purposefully forged. Factitious disorders include intentional production of physical or psychological symptoms, where the goal is to assume the role of a patient and external incentives, such as economic gain or avoiding legal responsibility, are absent. In malingering, the symptoms can also be physical or psychological, but the individual is consciously aware of external pragmatic incentives, such as gaining financial compensation, acquiring drugs, avoiding work or school, et cetera, and when the external incentives are removed, the symptoms resolve. Beyond a categorical diagnostic classification, it is often very intricate, especially initially, to face with a patient having PMDs and make a differential diagnosis among somatoform disorders, factious disorders, and malingering. Simplification may arise however, in the course further and exhaustive evaluation, by reinforcing the agreement between physician and patient and ensuring patient's confidence in the treatment plan (Williams et al.,2006). Moreover, most patients with PMDs have a coexisting   variety of different psychiatric disturbances such as dysthymia, major depression, anxiety, adjustment disorders, obsessive-compulsive disorder, panic attacks, bipolar disorders and others (Williams et al., 2005; Bhatia & Schneider, 2007). Yet, it is important to add that many organic movement disorders have an important incidence of the above-named psychiatric diagnoses (Reich, 2006). Finally, the common occurrence of movement disorders complicating primary mental illness and their treatment makes it important for psychiatrists to be able to recognize the various movement disorders, some of which have singular phenomenology such as tardive akathisia, tardive dystonia, tourettism and some unusual form of parkinsonism or tremor (Factor et al., 2005).

A) Historical	
1.	**Abrupt onset**
2.	**Static course**
3.	**Spontaneous remission**
4.	**Precipitated by minor trauma**
5.	**Obvious psychiatric disturbance**
6.	**Multiple somatization**
7.	**Employed in health profession**
8.	**Pending litigation or compensation**
9.	**Presence of secondary gain**
10.	**Young age (female>male) Inconsistent character of movement (amplitude, frequency, distribution, selective ability)**
B) Clinical	
1.	**Paroxysmal movement disorder**
2.	**Movements increase with attention or decrease with distrction**
3.	**Ability to trigger or relieve the abnormal movements with unusual or non physiological interventions (e.g.trigger points on the body, tuning fork)**
4.	**False weakness**
5.	**False sensory complaints**
6.	**Self-inflected injuries**
7.	**Deliberate slowness of movements**
8.	**Functional disability out of proportion to exam findings**
9.	**Movement abnormality that is bizarre, multiple or difficult to classifyUnresponsive to appropriate medications**
C) Therapeutic responses	
1.	**Response to placebos**
2.	**Unresponsive to appropriate medication**
3.	**Remission with psychotherapy**

Table 2. General clues suggesting that a movement disorder may be psychogenic (Miyasaki et al., 2003; Lang, 2006)

4.1 Types of psychogenic movement disorders
4.1.1 Psychogenic tremor

Although many patients has a mixture of different movement disorders, psychogenic tremor is the prevalent movement disorder, up to 55%, of all PMDs. Clinical sites affected include the hand (84%), the leg (28%), and generalized body tremor 20% (Thomas & Jankovic 2004). Clinically, absence of finger tremor can be a positive diagnostic sign for psychogenic tremor (Jankovic & Thomas, 2006; Bhatia & Schneider, 2007) and attempting to immobilize the affected limb often makes a functional tremor worse, as well as loading the limb with weights tends to make the tremor worse, whereas organic tremor usually improves with this operation.

The diagnosis may be supported by the "coactivation sign". As in the testing procedure for rigidity, the physician feels the increased muscle tone in the tremulous extremity in both directions and this cogwheel-like resistance is strictly related to tremor or if the patient can be made to relax completely (Deuschl et al. 1998). The technique of back-averaging electroencephalographic activity preceding the electromyographic ones, can be useful to detect premovement potential in subjects with psychogenic tremor, absent in organic involuntary movement (Brown & Thompson, 2001). Zeuner et al. using accelerometry to measure frequency changes during tapping showed that in contrast to parkinsonian and essential tremor, patients with psychogenic tremor revealed larger tremor frequency changes and marked variability in tapping (Zeuner et al., 2003). Entrainment of tremulous movements of different body parts into a single rhythm has been used clinically as a means of distinguishing these tremor forms. If functional tremor involves more than one limb, it usually has the same frequency. On the other hand, organic tremor usually has slightly different frequencies in different body parts. A quantified electrophysiological entrainment test performed on accelerometer or surface EMG tremor signals may provide supportive evidence of a functional tremor (McAuley & Rothwell 2004). Recently, Czarnecki and colleagues revealed distinct patterns of cerebral perfusion, during rest and motor task, as measured by SPECT that distinguish psychogenic tremor from essential tremor and controls (Czarnecki et al. 2011).

4.1.2 Psychogenic dystonia

Dystonia exemplifies one of the longest history of misdiagnosis: for many centuries it was considered a psychogenic condition, then, after torsion dystonia was accepted as an organic entity in the early-20th century and different aetiologies of this condition were recognized, it was thought that psychogenic dystonia rarely occurred (Fahn, 2006). In general, psychogenic dystonia represents only approximately 5% of subjects with dystonia, but in most centers, it is the second most commonly encountered among PMDs and accounts for 20% to 50% of cases (Miyasaki et al., 2003). Psychogenic dystonia, classified as a secondary dystonia, largely remains a clinical diagnosis and there are no physiologic tests available that distinguish a psychogenic aetiology from an organic form (Peckham & Hallett, 2009).

Psychogenic dystonia may not occur with the typical variability and distractibility of other PMDs and presents with fixed dystonic postures (Fig. 1) without return to the neutral position at rest from the beginning. Leg involvement is uncommon in adult-onset organic dystonia, as well as lack sensory tricks or relief by certain inexplicable trick action, and presence of severe pain suggest psychogenic dystonia, even if not in a specific way (Schrag, 2006).

Controversial patients are those with dystonia developing within ours or days after a minor injury, with a fixed distonic posture and severe pain. This kind of dystonia may be associated with features of complex regional pain syndrome type I. A study by Schrag and co-workers show that a substantial proportion of patients with fixed dystonia clearly fulfils criteria for a psychogenic dystonia (37%) or somatization disorder (29%). Although fixed dystonia sometimes developed in patients in whom a diagnosis of somatization disorder had already been made, a history of somatization was often unrecognized and, in many cases, only became evident after examination of primary care records (Schrag et al., 2004; Miyasaki et al., 2003). Various features of complex regional pain syndrome-related fixed dystonia suggest abnormal regulation of inhibitory interneuronal mechanisms at the brainstem or spinal cord level and impairment central synaptic reorganisation due to an interaction between neuroplastic activities and anomalous environmental necessities (Munts & Koehler, 2010).

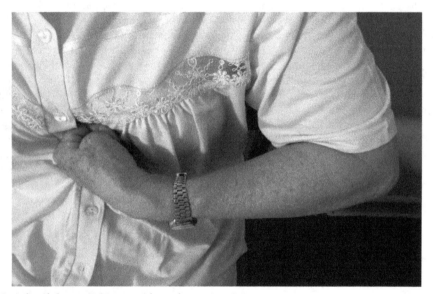

Fig. 1. A fixed dystonic posture of psychogenic origin

4.1.3 Psychogenic parkinsonism

Psychogenic parkinsonism is a rare syndrome accounting for 0.17–0.5% of all parkinsonism cases and representing nearly 10% of PMDs (Factor et al., 1995; Benaderette et al., 2006). In this disorder, atypical tremor occurs in conjunction with extremely slow movements that are often accompanied by grimacing, sighing, or whole-body movements when patients do a simple motor task. Common characteristics of organic parkinsonism, such as hypomimia, decreased blink rate, axial rigidity, and "cogwheel" phenomenon are usually absent in psychogenic parkinsonism. On postural stability testing, patients may have bizarre responses including flailing of the arms and reeling backward without falling (Thomas & Jankovic, 2004). Additionally, patients with psychogenic parkinsonism may also suffer from depression, which can cause psychomotor retardation, a clinical condition which may be difficult to distinguish from the bradyphrenia associated to Parkinson's disease (Morgan &

Sethi, 2006). It should be also remarked that parkinsonism or akinetic-rigid syndrome not uncommonly occur in the setting of major psychiatric disease and exposure to pharmacological agents.

Electrophysiology studies can be supportive in distinguishing a Parkinson's psychogenic tremor from other forms of tremor. Functional neuroimaging can be helpful in confirming a diagnosis of psychogenic parkinsonism. Loss of dopamine nerve function seen in organic parkinsonism can be measured by decreases in dopamine transporter density or presynaptic dopamine deficiency (I 123 B-CIT) on single positron emission computed tomography (SPECT) and Fluorodopa positron emission tomography (F-DOPA-PET). In psychogenic parkinsonism, these features are absent, but keeping in mind that other conditions, i.e. drug induced parkinsonism, dopa responsive dystonia-parkinsonism, have normal SPECT or F-DOPA-PET scans (Benaderette et al., 2006; Scherfler et al., 2006).

Table 3 summarizes the differences of clinical findings in Psychogenic parkinsonism, Drug-induced parkinsonism and Parkinson Disease.

	Psychogenic Parkinsonism	Drug-Induced Parkinsonism	Parkinson Disease
Onset	Abrupt, varied age of onset	Bilateral and symmetric, more common in the elderly	Gradual,unilateral or asymmetric, typically in the 6th or 7th decade
Cours	Usually static with maximum disability early, condition may abruptly or gradually remit	Acute or subacute	Insidious, slowly progressive
Tremor type	Unilateral or bilateral, rest, postural, action; usually involving the dominant hand, varying frequency and amplitude, spreads when immobilizing the affected limb	Not always present, bilateral, symmetric, postural or rest	Unilateral or asymmetric at rest, 4-6 Hz, worsens with distraction
Bradykinesia	Extremely slow movement often with fatigue, arrest or decrement; grimacing, sighing or whole body movements when performing simple task; normal speed of movements when not being examined	Often the earliest and commonest manifestation, facial hypomimia	Slowing of rapid repetitive movements without fatigue, arrest or decrement

Rigidity	Cogwheel absent, voluntary resistance which may decrease with distraction	Often uniform, inconstant cogwheel rigidity	Cogwheel rigidity
Postural instability	Impaired early, may have exaggerated or bizarre response to minimal backwards	Mild stooping, decreased arm swing	Impaired in moderate to advanced disease, retropulsion on pull test
Speech	Stuttering, bizarre dysarthria, distractible	Mild stuttering	Hypophonic, stuttering, tachyphemia
Motor fluctuation	Very rare complaint of "extra movements" on levodopa, no dyskinesias after long-term levodopa treatment	Absent	Dyskinesias in half of patients on levodopa after 5-7 years, on-off fluctuations
Psychiatric history	Previous conversion disorders, somatisation, factious disorder, anxiety, and depression	Relevant, particularly schizophrenia but also depression	Depression may precede diagnosis
Medication response	Usually unresponsive to multiple medical trials	Responds well to anticolinergic drugs, remittance within weeks or months when withdrawal of offending drug	Responds well to levodopa and dopamine agonist
Nonmotor problems	Sexual dysfunction and sleep disturbances occur	Possible swallowing less than normal, hallucination, rare costipation	Dysautonomia, constipation, sexual dysfunction, sleep problem, hallucination

Table 3. Clinical features of Psychogenic parkinsonism, Drug-induced parkinsonism and Parkinson Disease. Adapted from Morgan & Sethi, 2006.

4.1.4 Psychogenic gait

Abnormal gaits frequently occur in the setting of major psychiatric disease and represent 8% to 10% of all PMDs (Sudarsky, 2006). Psychogenic gate disorders are characterized by exaggerated effort or fatigue with grimaces, excessive slowness, convulsive shaking, often with knee buckling especially when the patient has unilateral functional weakness, astasia-abasia, arms are outstretched like a tightrope walker (Fig. 2), unusual uneconomic posture and bizarre movements (Bhatia, 2001; Baik & Lang, 2007). Patients with psychogenic require further strength and balance than an indifferent gait and they seem to be frightened of falling, and this gait allows them to be closer to the floor (Stone & Carson, 2010). The movement disorder is commonly accompanied by other psychogenic neurological symptoms, such as false weakness or sensory findings, or by excessive pain and tenderness (Thomas & Jankovic, 2004). Okun et al. described 9 consecutive patients who presented with a psychogenic gait disorder who underwent "chair testing." Each patient was asked to walk 20-30 feet forward and backward toward the examiner. Patients were then asked to sit in a swivel chair with wheels and to propel the chair forward and backward. Compared with their walking, 8 of the 9 patients in the psychogenic group performed well on the chair test, showing improved ability to propel a chair forward when seated. By contrast, all 9 control patients with nonpsychogenic gait problems, performed equally when walking or propelling utilizing the chair (Okun et al., 2007).

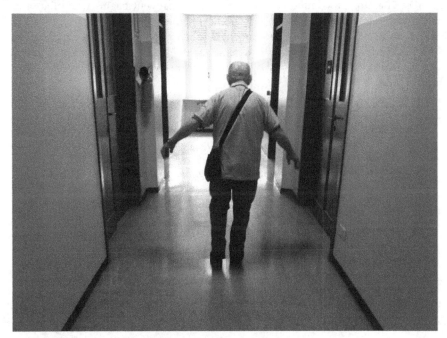

Fig. 2. Tightrope walking: the patient walks very slowly on a broad base with his arms extended.

4.1.5 Psychogenic myoclonus
Myoclonus account for 10% to 20% of PMDs. The clinical features of psychogenic myoclonus usually includes segmental or generalizes jerking, occurring at rest and during movement, commonly changing pattern, frequency, amplitude and anatomic distribution and may be stimulus sensitive (Monday & Jankovic 1993; Williams et al., 1995).

Neurophysiologic methods are particularly useful in distinguishing between voluntary jerking and cortical or brainstem myoclonus (Brown & Thomson, 2001). Organic myoclonus is characterized by burst length of less than 70 ms, and jerks lasting longer than that are suggestive of a psychogenic etiology. Functional myoclonus is often associated with a Bereitschaftpotential before the movement, which requires recording multiple events using an electroencephalogram and back averaging according to an electromyogram. In the absence of a Bereitschaftpotential, it is not possible to exclude a psychogenic etiology, as the Bereitschaftpotential can be absent in normal subjects (Brown & Thomson, 2001; Peckham & Hallett, 2009). Interestingly, in a recent case series of 35 consecutive patients with jerks of the trunk referred as possible proriospinal myoclonus, 34 patients showed features suggestive of a psychogenic origin even in the presence of a classic polymyography pattern or in the absence of a Bereitschaftpotential (van der Salm et al., 2010).

5. Treatment

There is no consensus even among the experts about the best treatment approach to patients with PMDs. Therefore, a common agreement is that treatment begins when the physician has made the diagnosis and mostly depending on the way of explaining PMDs to the patient, as well as a very close working relationship between neurologist, consulting psychiatrist, and frequently physical therapist, is crucial in obtaining symptom remission in many subjects. Table 4 emphasizes, by the acronym form THERAPIST, the essential basis for a treatment process.

Terminology must engage and not alienate the patient
Hear out the patient with interest, compassion, and empathy (and patience)
Explain the diagnosis and the mechanism of symptoms
Reassure that there is no evidence of neurologic damage
Address psychosocial and family issues
Prognosis is likely favorable, the patient has the potential to recovery fully
Individualize the therapy and customize it
Self-help is a crucial part of getting better
Treat concurrent psychiatric and medical illness (if present)

Table 4. Nine essential steps for an approach to management of patients with PMDs.

The objective of effective treatment is not only to provide symptoms remission in the short term, but to evaluate the causes that produced the heterogeneous symptomatology and to assess feasible strategies to remove them.

The issue about the terminology to use for the diagnosis is unresolved. Some authors find that "functional" disorder is an accurate term, which describe a disorder of the way the brain is working. Others find "psychogenic" an acceptable term with vagueness implication. Still others think that the latter arouses too much a "crazy" condition in the patient and family's mind and prefer the more broad word "neuropsychiatric" (Williams et al., 2005; Stone & Carson, 2010). In any case, whatever term is used it is important to find an explanatory language that engages the patient and gives a scenario within which to understand the disorder. In this regard, a self-rating approach reported that 49% of patients attributed a favorable outcome to a physician's described treatment (Jankovic & Thomas, 2006).

It is very important to reassure the patient early on, for example emphasizing that this is an "involuntary" condition and is most likely the result of an impairment of neural pathways. Another option is to explain that some of the symptoms are stress-related symptoms, pointing out that stress is a common cause of many physical afflictions. A sincere, supportive, hopeful and, professional manner of approach will allow to understand and, at the same time, have patients understand what the movement disorder means, what is its functions, why and when it evolved. Some experts and the authors also suggest an active physiotherapy program, from the beginning, in order to desensitized the stress-induced contraction that generate the anomalous muscle jerks. Overall, this aspect of the treatment may corroborate the "physical" dimension of the disorder and may allow decreasing the symptom without activating psychological defence mechanisms (Williams et al., 2006; Rosebush & Mazurek, 2006). Besides, the physiotherapist frequently recognizes the fears and unhelpful preconceptions which patients have, and can stimulate and compliment patients in their activity in a much more confidential mode than the allied psychotherapist.

Medication treatment can be initiated and the choice of a particular drug depends on the accompanying psychiatric or medical conditions. In authors experience these most frequently include anxiety, depression, insomnia and headache, and a low dose of tricyclic antidepressants or benzodiazepine can help with symptoms of pain and muscle tension.

Large randomized studies in patients with PMDs are lacking, and evidence for treatment is largely based on retrospective, case control, and case report studies. Several other clinical trials, not specifically designed for PMDs but for other forms of conversion or somatoform disorders, are treated more in detail elsewhere in this book.

In a study by Voon and co-workers, 23 patients were identified with PMDs, and 15 patients agreed to be treated with antidepressant drugs. Of the 15 patients, 10 were diagnosed with primary PMDs, and the remaining 5 were diagnosed with PMDs and another somatoform disorder. Patients were treated with either citalopram or paroxetine. Those who did not respond were switched to venlafaxine. Of the primary PMDs patients, 80% (8 patients) had marked improvement, and 7 patients had complete remission. None of the 5 patients with PMDs and other somatoform disorders improved. (Voon, & Lang, 2005).

An open-label trial of somatisation disorder studied the efficacy of nefazodone in patients with and without comorbid depression and showed improvement in clinical global impression and functioning in 73% of patients (Menza et al., 2001).

In a study by Rampello and colleagues, 18 patients were treated (6 with haloperidol and 12 with sulpiride). The latter group showed remarkable improvement in 8 patients, partial improvement in 2 patients, and no improvement in 1 patient. The haloperidol group showed 1 patient with remarkable improvement, 3 with partial improvement, and 2 with no improvement. This study showed a possible positive correlation between dopamine blockade, drug-induced plasma prolactine concentration, and improvement in a patient's conversion symptoms.

Hinson and colleagues recruited ten patients with PMDs for a single-blind clinical trial to receive 12 weeks of treatment with outpatient psychodynamic psychotherapy and use of antidepressants or anxiolytic drugs, depending on comorbid psychiatric diagnosis. The movement disorder was videotaped before and after treatment and rated in a random order by a rater unaware of treatment allocation using PMDRS. All patients were diagnosed with conversion disorder. Nine of ten recruited patients completed the study. Total mean PMDRS and total mean PMDRS function scores improved with psychotherapeutic intervention. There were significant treatment effects in Hamilton depression scores, Beck anxiety scores, and global assessment of function.

Shapiro and Teasell described a case series of 39 consecutive patients with conversion disorder who were told that they had a musculoskeletal problem that could resolve completely if they had an organic etiology. If the patients did not improve after 4 weeks, then they were told that it was a psychiatric condition, and the treatment would be modified to help them improve completely. If they did not improve, then they were given a final diagnosis of conversion disorder, and they were told that they could not improve because of an unconscious need to remain disabled. In 8 of 9 patients with acute conversion disorder (symptoms <2 months), the treatment was successful. In 1 of 28 chronic (>6 months duration) patients, behavioral treatment was successful (Shapiro & Teasell, 2004). In a randomised controlled clinical trial, Moene and colleagues assigned 48 patients to receive either hypnosis or a control intervention consisting of generic elements of psychotherapy. Outcome measures were a video rating scale for motor conversion symptoms, the symptom checklist-90, and elements of the international classification of impairments, disabilities, and handicaps. Independent of the treatment condition, 65% of patients showed substantial improvement at post-treatment assessment and 84% at 6-month follow-up, which suggests that both psychotherapy and hypnosis have a role in the treatment of conversion disorder.

A meta-analysis of studies of cognitive behavioral therapy for various somatisation syndromes showed a definite or possible treatment effect of cognitive behavioral therapy in 71 of patients (Kroenke et al., 2000). Randomized controlled studies support the efficacy of individual cognitive behavioral therapy for the treatment of hypochondriasis, body dysmorphic disorder, and undifferentiated somatoform disorders including medically unexplained symptoms, chronic fatigue syndrome, and noncardiac chest pain (Looper & Kirmayer, 2002; Allen et al., 2006).

In a single-blind study, 16 patients with PMDs completed a thrice-weekly, 12-weeks mild walking program. Assessments included DSM-IV interview, PMDRS, Beck Anxiety Inventory, Hamilton Depression Scale, V02 Max, and body mass index. A comparison of all measures taken at study onset and after completing the exercise program indicates statistically significant improvements. We observed a relevant improvement in 10 of 16 patients (62%). The mean difference for the primary outcome (PMDRS total) corresponded to about 70%. Compliance was good, and there were no adverse effects. This study provides preliminary evidence for regular low-medium intensity exercise as a safe, adequate, and pleasing intervention for PMD. (Dallocchio et al., 2010).

A retrospective study was performed in 10 patients with psychogenic gait. Patients were treated with physical therapy, occupational therapy, and recreational therapy, and psychological interventions were used in appropriate cases. All patients were able to ambulate normally before discharge (Speed, 1996).

A successful management of the three cases described in another report involved a combination of behavioral modification and physical therapy interventions Abnormal movement patterns were ignored, and correct movement patterns were reinforced using feedback and praise. All three patients showed complete resolution of their symptoms (Ness, 2007).

There is one published abstract report where EMG biofeedback as used as a treatment for psychogenic tremor; this open label study estimated the effectiveness of biofeedback therapy and found improvement in 60% of 15 subjects (Levy et al., 2006). One case report described a dramatic response to acupuncture in a patient with chronic, treatment-resistant PMD (Van Nuenen et al. 2007).

A preliminary experience with the application of transcranial magnetic stimulation to achieve symptom relief in psychogenic tremor showed its effectiveness in conversion disorder of motor subtype. In a group of 8 patients, 4 responded, 2 showed temporary improvement, and 2 did not respond. (Dafotakis et al., 2008). In a case report, a patient with psychogenic dysphonia was reported to have a dramatic improvement after 2 sessions of repetitive transcranial magnetic stimulation over the prefrontal cortex (Chastan et al., 2009).

6. Prognosis

The outcome of patients with PMDs is variable, and several elements that influence recovery have been described. These include the nature, chronicity, seriousness of the veiled psychopathology, the influence of external factors, the attitude of the patient, the capability of the patient's support system, as well as the modalities and the effectiveness of treatment. Predominantly, data are available on the outcome of conversion disorders in general.

Williams et al. found a permanent benefit in 52% of 131 patients, with complete, considerable and moderate relief in 25%, 21%, and 8% respectively, after a follow-up of an average of 1,8 years. They found that age, gender, intelligence, chronicity of illness, and types of symptoms had no influence on the outcome. In another longitudinal study of 228 patients with PMDs improvement symptoms was noticed in 56% of patients, 21% reported no change, and 22% were worse after an average duration of 3.4 years' follow-up. In this study, poor prognostic factors were inconsistent movements, dissatisfaction with the physician, long duration of illness, positive history of smoking, and suggestibility. Good prognostic factors were good physical health, positive social life, patients' perception of receiving effective treatment by the physician, elimination of a stressor, comorbid diagnosis of anxiety, and attribution of a specific medication (Thomas et al., 2006). A follow up report compared 66 patients with PMDs to 704 with Parkinson's disease and showed comparable levels of of disability and physical quality of life, increased psychiatric comorbidity and more severe mental health disorders, even if patients with PMDs were 20 years younger and had a shorter pathological condition (Anderson et al., 2007).

Feinstein et al. reported persistence of abnormal movements in 90% of 88 patients followed up for an average of 3,2 years. Poor outcome was associated with psychiatric, long duration of symptoms, and insidious onset of symptoms (Feinstein, (2001). Much higher rates of improvement was reported in another longitudinal study of 127 patients with psychogenic tremor followed for at least 3 years, 55% reported improvement in tremor. Dissatisfaction with the physician was identified as the stronger prognostic risk factor of poor long term outcome; good prognostic factors were physician's prescribed treatment, elimination of stressor, specific medication, stress management, biofeedback, and psychotherapy (Jankovic et al., (2004). Other authors described the presenting features and long-term outcomes of 33 patients with electrophysiologically-confirmed psychogenic tremor by a follow-up questionnaire. After a median follow-up of 3.2 years, 64% of patients valued their disability as moderate severe, 27% had complete resolution of symptoms, and 9% reported mild unchanged symptoms. Of the patients who had resolution of symptoms, in 15% the resolution occurred spontaneously and in 12% it occurred after an intervention (1 with an antidepressant, 1 with psychology/rehabilitation, 1 with hypnotherapy, 1 with behavioral therapy). (McKeon et al., (2008). In a follow study involving 64 patients affected by medically unexplained movement disorders, 28% showed complete resolution of symptoms, 20% improved, 14% remained unchanged, and 38% worsened after 6 years of follow-up (Crimlisk et al., 1998). Finally, other data showed that 83% of 42 patients with functional weakness or sensory symptoms, who have been investigated as inpatients, have symptoms and disability after a median of 12 years following initial assessment. In this study patients with only sensory symptoms and signs at presentation had significantly better outcome in terms of higher physical functioning, social functioning , and pain than patients with any symptoms or signs of weakness , a higher age of onset predicted lower physical functioning at follow up (Stone et al., 2003). If untreated, PMDs are inclined to become chronic, and follow-up data in several studies demonstrate 65-95% of patients are left with a high level of disability (Factor et al., 1995; Williams et al., 2005), undoubtedly asserting the necessity for un effective early intervention to convert the "sick role" of the patient and return to the suitable level of function as quickly as possible.

7. Conclusion

PMDs are important and underdiagnosed cause of major neurologic disability. Signs and symptoms must be interpreted in the overall clinical and psychological context. Neurophysiological and imaging findings may provide important understanding and confirmation of the diagnosis, but some cases pose a arduous challenge to both neurologists and psychiatrists. An adequate explanation of the symptoms to patients is a prerequisite to successful further treatment (Stone & Carson, 2010; Friedman & LaFrance, 2010). To date, the treatment for each patient with PMDs is individualized and may include psychotherapeutic interventions, behavioral therapy, pharmachotherapy, physical therapy, hypnosis and others. Recovery is sometimes delayed and can take place over the course of months and several patients are left with a high level of disability, but a supportive, nonjudgmental, and persistent multidisciplinary approach can divert the illness course to an excellent clinical outcome (Rosebush & Mazurek, 2006). Further researches are required, not only to improve the understanding and management of these heterogeneous diseases, but also for reconsidering conversion disorder terminology and positive rather than negative diagnostic criteria.

8. References

Allen, L.A., Woolfolk, R.L., Escobar JI, et al. (2006). Cognitive-behavioral therapy for somatization disorder: a randomized controlled trial. Arch Intern Med. 166(14):1512–8.

Anderson, K.E., GruberBaldini, A.L., Vaughan, C.G. et al. (2007). Impact of psychogenic movement disorders versus Parkinson's on disability, qualiy of life, and psychopathology. Movement Disord. 22:2204-2209.

Baik, J.S., Lang, A.E. (2007). Gait abnormalities in psychogenic movement disorders. Mov Disord. 22(3):395–9.

Barsky, A.J., Orav E.J., Bates D.W. (2005) Somatization increases medical utilization and costs independent of psychiatric and medical comorbidity. Arch Gen Psychiatry. 62(8):903-10.

Benaderette, S., Zanotti, F.P., Apartis, E. et al. (2006). Psychogenic parkinsonism: a combination of clinical, electrophysiological, and [(123)I]-FP-CIT SPECTscan explorations improves diagnostic accuracy. Mov Disord. 21(3):310–7.

Bhatia, K.P., (2001). Psychogenic gait disorders. Adv Neurol. 87: 251–54.

Bhatia, K.P., Schneider, S.A. (2007) Psychogenic tremor and related disorders. J Neurol. 254(5):569-74.

Breuer, J., Freud S., Studies on hysteria (1893-1895). In: Strachey J, Strachey A, eds. The standard edition of the complete psychological works of Sigmund Freud, (Vol. 2). London: Hogart Press & Institute of Psycho-Analysis, 1955.

Brown, P., Thomson, P.D. (2001). Electrophysiological aids to jerks, spasms and tremor. Mov Disord. 16:595.99.

Brown, R.J. Dissociation and conversion in psychogenic illness. In: Hallet M, Yudofsky SC, Lang AE, et al., editors. To psychogenic movement disorders. Philadelphia, USA: Lippincott Williams & Wilkins; 2006, pp. 131-143.

Carson, A., Stone, J., Hibberd C. et al. (2011). Disability, distress and unemployment in neurology outpatients with symptoms 'unexplained by disease'. J Neurol Neurosurg Psychiatry, in press.

Charcot, J.M. (1889). Clinical Lectures on Diseases of the Nervous System. In New Sydenham Society, London, pp. 220–259.

Chastan, N., Parain, D, Verin, E. et al. (2009). Psychogenic aphonia: spectacular recovery after motor cortex transcranial magnetic stimulation. J Neurol Neurosurg Psychiatr. 80(1):94.

Cojan, Y., Waber L., Carruzzo, A., Vuilleumier, P. (2009). Motor inhibition in histerical conversion paralisis; 47(3):1026-37.

Crimlisk, H.L., Bhatia, K., Cope, H., David, A., Marsden, C.D., Ron, M.A. (1998). Slater revisited: 6 year follow up study of patients with medically unexplained motor symptoms. Br. Med. J. 316, 582–586.

Criswell, S., Sterling, C., Swisher, L. et al. (2010). Sensitivity and specificity of the finger tapping task for the detection of psychogenic movement disorders. Parkinsonism Relat Disord. 16(3):197-201.

Cubo, E., Hinson, V.K., Goetz, C.G. et al. (2005). Transcultural comparison of psychogenic movement disorders. Mov Disord;20:1343-45.

Czarnecki, K., Jones, D.T., Burnett, M.S. et al. (2011). SPECT perfusion patterns distinguish psychogenic from essential tremor. Parkinsonism and related disorders (in press).

Deuschl, G., Koster, B., Lucking, C., Scheidt, C. (1998). Diagnostic and pathophysiological aspects of psychogenic tremors. Mov. Disord. 13, 294–302.

Espay, A.J., Goldenhar, L.M, Voon, V., et al. (2009). Opinion and clinical practices related to diagnosing and managing patients with psychogenic movement disorders: an international survey of Movement Disorder Society Members. Mov Disord. 24(9):1366-74.

Fahn, S. (1994). Psychogenic movement disorders. In: Marsden CD, Fahn S (eds) Movement Disorders 3. Buttenw Heinem, Oxford, pp. 359-72.

Fahn, S. The history of psychogenic movement disorders. In: Hallet M, Yudofsky SC, Lang AE, et al., editors. To psychogenic movement disorders. Philadelphia, USA: Lippincott Williams & Wilkins; 2006, pp. 24–31.

Factor, S.A., Podskalny,G.D., Molho, E.S. (1995). Psychogenicmovement disorders. Frequency, clinical profile and characteristics. J. Neurol. Neurosurg. Psychiatry 59, 406–412.

Factor, S, Lang, A.E, Weiner WJ. Drug Induced Movement Disorders. Mount Kisko, NY: Futura; 2005.

Feinstein A, Stergiopoulus V, Fine J, Lang AE. (2001). Psychiatric outcome in patients with a psychogenic movement disorder: a prospective study. Neuropsychiatry Neuropsychol Behav Neurol. 14:169-76.

Fink, G.R., Halligan, P.W., Marshall J.C. Neuroimaging og hysteria. In: Hallet M, Yudofsky SC, Lang AE, et al., editors. To psychogenic movement disorders. Philadelphia, USA: Lippincott Williams & Wilkins; 2006, pp. 230-237.

Friedman, J.H., LaFrance. W.C. Jr. (2010). Psychogenic disorders: the need to speak plainly. Arch Neurol. 67(6):753-5.

Freud, S., (1910). Psycho-analytic view of psychogenic disturbance of vision. The Standard Edition of the Complete Psychological Works of Sigmund Freud, 11. The Hogarth Press, London, pp. 209-218.

Gupta, A. Lang A.E. (2009). Psychogenic movement disorders. Current Opin Neurol. 22:430-436.

Hallet, M. (2010). Physiology of psychogenic movement disorders. J Clin Neuroscience. 17:959-65.

Hinson, V.K., Cubo, E., Comella, C., Leurgans, S., Goetz, C.G., (2005). Rating scale for psychogenic movement disorders: scale development and clinimetric testing. Mov Disord; 20: 1592-97.

Hinson, V.K., Cubo, E., Comella, C.L, Goetz, C.G., Leurgans, S. (2005) Rating scale for psychogenic movement disorders: scale development and clinimetric testing. Mov Disord;20:1592-1597.

Hinson, V.K., Weinstein, S., Bernard B., Leurgans, S.E, Goetz C.G., (2006) Single-blind clinical trial of pychotherapy for treatment of psychogenic movement disorders. Parkinsonism Relat Disord;12:177-180.

Hinson, V.K, Blacke Haren, W. (2006). Psychogenic movement disorders. Lancet Neurol;5:695-700.

Janet P., (1889). L'automatisme psychologique. Paris, NE: Felix Alcan.

Janet P., (1907) The major symptoms of hysteria. New York; Macmillan.

Jankovic, J., Thomas, M., Vuong, K.D. (2004). Long term outcome of psychogenic tremor. Neurology. 62(Suppl.5):A501.

Jankovic, J., Thomas, M., 2006. Psychogenic tremor and shaking. In: Hallett, M., Fahn, S., Jankovic, J., Lang, A.E., Cloninger, C.R., Yudofsky, C. (Eds.), Psychogenic Movement Disorders. InLippincott Williams and Wilkins, Philadelphia, pp. 42–47.

Jankovic, J., Cloninger, C.R., Fahn, S., Hallet, M., Lang, A.E,, Williams, D.T. Therapeutic approaches to psychogenic movement disorders. In: Hallet M, Yudofsky SC, Lang AE, et al., editors. To psychogenic movement disorders. Philadelphia, USA: Lippincott Williams & Wilkins; 2006, pp. 323-328.

Kagi, G., Bathia, K.P, Tolosa, E. (2010). The role of DAT-SPECT in movement disorders. J Neurol Neurosur Psychiatry. 81:5-12.

Kroenke, K., Swindle, R. (2000).Cognitive behavioral therapy for somatization and symptom syndromes: a critical review of controlled clinical trials. Psychother Psychosom. 69: 205-15.

Lang, A.E. General overview of psychogenic movement disorders: epidemiology, diagnosis, and prognosis. In: Hallet M, Yudofsky SC, Lang AE, et al., editors. To psychogenic movement disorders. Philadelphia, USA: Lippincott Williams & Wilkins; 2006, pp. 35-41

Lempert, T., Dieterich, M., Huppert, D., Brandt, T., (1990). Psychogenic disorders in neurology. Frequency and clinical spectrum. Acta Neurol. Scand. 82, 335–340.

Levy J.K., Thomas, M. Biofeedback therapy for psychogenic movement disorders. In: Hallet M, Yudofsky SC, Lang AE, et al., editors. To psychogenic movement disorders. Philadelphia, USA: Lippincott Williams & Wilkins; 2006. p 343–344.

Looper, K. J., Kirmayer, L. J. (2002). Behavioral medicine approaches to somatoform disorders. *J Consult Clin Psychol.* 70(3), pp. 810-827.

Mace, C.J., Trimble, M.,R. (1996). Ten year prognosis of conversion disorder. Br. J. Psychiatry 169, 282-288.

McAuley, J., Rothwell, J. (2004). Identification of psychogenic, distonic, and other organic tremors by a coherence entraiment test. Mov Disord. 19:253-67.

McKeon, A., Ahlskog, J.E., Bower, J.H. et al. (2008). Psychogenic tremor: long term prognosis in patients with electrophysiologically-confirmed disease.MovDisord. 24(1):72-6.

Menza, M., Lauritano, M., Allen, L. et al. (2001). Treatment of somatization disorder with nefazodone: a prospective, open-label study. Ann Clin Psychiatry. 13: 153–58.

Miyasaki, J.M., Sa, D.S., Galvez-Jmenez N. et al. (2003). Psychogenic movement disorders. Can J Neurol Sci; (30 Suppl 1):S94-100.

Moene, F.C., Landberg, E.H., Hoogduin, K.A. et al. (2000). Organic syndromes diagnosed as conversion disorder: identification and frequency in a study of 85 patients. J Psychosom Res. 49(1):7-12.

Monday, K., Jankovic, J. (1993). Psychogenic myoclonus. Neurology. 43(2):349–52.

Morgan. J.C., Sethi, K.D. (2006). Psychogenic parkinsonism. In: Hallet M, Yudofsky SC, Lang AE, et al., editors. To psychogenic movement disorders. Philadelphia, USA: Lippincott Williams & Wilkins. pp. 62–68.

Munhoz, R.P., Zavala, J.A., Becker. N., Teive H.A. (2010). Cross-cultural influences on psychogenic movement disorders - a comparative review with a Brazilian series of 83 cases. Clin Neurol Neurosurg. 113(2):115-8.

Munts, A.G., Koehler, P.J. (2010). How psychogenic is dystonia? Views from past to present. Brain. 133; pp. 1552-1564.

Ness, D. (2007). Physical therapy management for conversion disorder: case series. J Neurol Phys Ther. 31(1):30–9.

Ng, B.Y. (1999). Hysteria: a cross-cultural comparison of its origins and history. Hist Psychiatry. 10(39, pt 3):287-301.

Nowak, D., A., Fink, G.R. (2009). Psychogenic movement disorders: aetiology, phenomenology, neuroanatomical correlates and therapeutic approach. Neuroimage. 47:1015-25.

Okun, M.S., Rodriguez, R.L., Foote, K.D., et al. (2007). The "chair test" to aid in the diagnosis of psychogenic gait disorders. Neurologist. 13(2):87–91.

Ovsiew, F. An overview of the psychiatric approach to conversion disorder. In: Hallet M, Yudofsky SC, Lang AE, et al., editors. To psychogenic movement disorders. Philadelphia, USA: Lippincott Williams & Wilkins; 2006; pp. 115–121.

Peckham, E.L., Hallett, M. (2009). Psychogenic movement disorders. Neurol Clin. 27:801-819.

Rampello, L., Raffaele, R., Nicoletti. G. et al. (1996) Hysterical neurosis of the conversion type: therapeutic activity of neuroleptics with different hyperprolactinemic potency. Neuropsychobiology 1996; 33: 186–88.

Reich, S.G., (2006) Psychogenic movement disorders. Semin Neurol;26:289-206.

Rosebush, P., Mazurek, M.F. (2006). Treatment of conversion disorder. . In: Hallet M, Yudofsky SC, Lang AE, et al., editors. To psychogenic movement disorders. Philadelphia, USA: Lippincott Williams & Wilkins; 2006; pp. 289–301.

Scherfler, C., Schwarz, J., Antonini, A., et al. (2007). Role of DAT-SPECT in the diagnostic work up of parkinsonism. Mov Disord;22(9):1229–38.

Schrag, A., Trimble, M., Quinn, N., et al. (2004). The syndrome of fixed dystonia: an evaluation of 103 patients. Brain. 127:2360-72.

Schrag, A. Psychogenic dystonia and reflex sympathetic dystrophy. In: Hallett M, Yudofsky SC, Lang AE, et al, eds. Psychogenic movement disorders. Philadelphia, USA: Lippincott Williams & Wilkins, 2006: 53–61.

Shapiro, A.P., Teasell, R.W. (2004). Behavioural interventions in the rehabilitation of acute v. chronic non-organic (conversion/factitious) motor disorders. Br J Psychiatry. 185:140–6.

Shibasaky, H., Hallett, M. What is the Bereitschaftspotential? Clin Neurophysiol. 117:2341-56.

Shill, H., Gerber, P. (2006). Evaluation of clinical diagnostic criteria for psychogenic movement disorders. Mov Disord;21(8):1163–8.

Smith, G.R. Jr, Monson, R.A., Ray, D.C. (1986) Patients with multiple unexplained symptoms. Their characteristic, functonal health, and health care utilization. Arch Intern Med. 146(1):69-72.

Speed, J. (1996). Behavioral management of conversion disorder: retrospective study. Arch Phys Med Rehabil. 77(2):147–54.

Stone, J., Sharpe, M., Rothwell, P.M., et al. (2004). The 12 year prognosis of unilateral functional weakness and sensory disturbance. J Neurol Neurosurg Psychiatry. 74:591–6.

Stone, J., Carson, A. (2010). Functional neurologic symptoms: assessment and management. Neurol Clin. 29:1-18.

Stone, J., Vuilleumier, P., Friedman, J.H. (2010). Conversion disorders. Separating "how" from "why". Neurology; 74:190-91.

Sudarsky, L. Psychogenic gait disorders. (2006). Semin Neurol;26(3):351–6.

Thomas, M., Jankovic, J. (2004). Psychogenic movement disorders: diagnosis and management. CNS Drugs. 18(7):437–52.

Thomas, M., Vuong, K.D., Jankovic. J. (2006). Long-term prognosis of patients with psychogenic movement disorders. Parkinsonism Relat Disord. 12(6):382–7.

Van Nuenen, B.F., Wohlgemuth, M., Wong Chung, R.E. et al. (2007). Acupuncture for psychogenicmovement disorders: treatment or diagnostic tool? Mov Disord. 22(9):1353–5.

Voon, V., Lang, A.E. (2005) Antidepressant treatment outcomes of psychogenic movement disorder. J Clin Psychiatry;66:1529–1534.

Voon, V., Gallea, C., Hattori. et al. (2010). The involuntary nature of conversion disorder. Neurology. 19;74(3):223-8.

Vuilleumier, P., 2005. Hysterical conversion and brain function. Prog. Brain Res.150, 309–329.

Williams, D.T., Ford B, Fahn S. (1995). Phenomenology and psychopathology related to psychogenic movement disorders. Adv Neurol;65:233-57.

Williams D.T., Ford B., Fahn, S. (2005). Treatment issues in psychogenic-neuropsychiatric movement disorders. Adv Neurol. 96:350-63.

Williams, D.T., et al. Natural history of psychogenic movement disorder. In: Hallet M, Yudofsky SC, Lang AE, et al., editors. To psychogenic movement disorders. Philadelphia, USA: Lippincott Williams & Wilkins; 2006; pp. 274-286.

Zeuner K.E.,, Shoge, R.O., Goldstein, S.R. et al. (2003). Accelerometry to distinguish psychogenic from essential or parkinsonian tremor. Neurology. 61:548-550.

Permissions

The contributors of this book come from diverse backgrounds, making this book a truly international effort. This book will bring forth new frontiers with its revolutionizing research information and detailed analysis of the nascent developments around the world.

We would like to thank Assoc. Prof. Dr. Toru Uehara, for lending his expertise to make the book truly unique. He has played a crucial role in the development of this book. Without his invaluable contribution this book wouldn't have been possible. He has made vital efforts to compile up to date information on the varied aspects of this subject to make this book a valuable addition to the collection of many professionals and students.

This book was conceptualized with the vision of imparting up-to-date information and advanced data in this field. To ensure the same, a matchless editorial board was set up. Every individual on the board went through rigorous rounds of assessment to prove their worth. After which they invested a large part of their time researching and compiling the most relevant data for our readers. Conferences and sessions were held from time to time between the editorial board and the contributing authors to present the data in the most comprehensible form. The editorial team has worked tirelessly to provide valuable and valid information to help people across the globe.

Every chapter published in this book has been scrutinized by our experts. Their significance has been extensively debated. The topics covered herein carry significant findings which will fuel the growth of the discipline. They may even be implemented as practical applications or may be referred to as a beginning point for another development. Chapters in this book were first published by InTech; hereby published with permission under the Creative Commons Attribution License or equivalent.

The editorial board has been involved in producing this book since its inception. They have spent rigorous hours researching and exploring the diverse topics which have resulted in the successful publishing of this book. They have passed on their knowledge of decades through this book. To expedite this challenging task, the publisher supported the team at every step. A small team of assistant editors was also appointed to further simplify the editing procedure and attain best results for the readers.

Our editorial team has been hand-picked from every corner of the world. Their multi-ethnicity adds dynamic inputs to the discussions which result in innovative outcomes. These outcomes are then further discussed with the researchers and contributors who give their valuable feedback and opinion regarding the same. The feedback is then collaborated with the researches and they are edited in a comprehensive manner to aid the understanding of the subject.

Apart from the editorial board, the designing team has also invested a significant amount of their time in understanding the subject and creating the most relevant covers. They scrutinized every image to scout for the most suitable representation of the subject and create an appropriate cover for the book.

The publishing team has been involved in this book since its early stages. They were actively engaged in every process, be it collecting the data, connecting with the contributors or procuring relevant information. The team has been an ardent support to the editorial, designing and production team. Their endless efforts to recruit the best for this project, has resulted in the accomplishment of this book. They are a veteran in the field of academics and their pool of knowledge is as vast as their experience in printing. Their expertise and guidance has proved useful at every step. Their uncompromising quality standards have made this book an exceptional effort. Their encouragement from time to time has been an inspiration for everyone.

The publisher and the editorial board hope that this book will prove to be a valuable piece of knowledge for researchers, students, practitioners and scholars across the globe.

List of Contributors

Arthur J. Lurigio
Department of Psychology, Department of Criminal Justice, Loyola University Chicago, USA

Scott P. Novak, Sara L. Calvin and Cristie Glasheen
RTI International, Department of Behavioral Epidemiology, USA

Mark J. Edlund
University of Arkansas School of Medicine, Department of Psychiatry, USA

Stephan Muehlig
Chemnitz University of Technology, Germany

Marja Aartsen
VU-University Amsterdam, The Netherlands

Rafael S. Maior, Marilia Barros and Carlos Tomaz
University of Brasilia, Brazil

Krzysztof Krysta, Irena Krupka-Matuszczyk, Małgorzata Janas-Kozik and Małgorzata Stachowicz
Medical University of Silesia, Katowice, Poland

André Rex
Department of Neurology, Center for Stroke Research, Charité University Medicine, Berlin, Germany

Heidrun Fink
Institute of Pharmacology and Toxicology, School of Veterinary Medicine, Freie Universität Berlin, Berlin, Germany

Taiichi Katayama
United Graduate School of Child Development, Osaka University, Kanazawa University and Hamamatsu University School of Medicine, Japan

Shinsuke Matsuzaki and Masaya Tohyama
United Graduate School of Child Development, Osaka University, Kanazawa University and Hamamatsu University School of Medicine, Japan Department of Anatomy and Neuroscience, Graduate school of Medicine, Osaka University, Japan

Tsuyosi Hattori
Department of Molecular Neuropharmacology, Graduate School of Medicine, Osaka University, Japan

Carlo Dallocchio
Department of Medical Specialities, Division of Neurology, Ospedale Civile, Voghera (Pavia), Italy